WHEN IT COMES TO PRESCRIPTION DRUGS, WHAT A WOMAN DOESN'T KNOW CAN HURT HER. GET THE FACTS.

* Breathing difficulties, skin rash, and/or hives indicate a potentially serious drug reaction; learn how to spot these deadly warning signs early.

* Some antibiotics can interfere with the effectiveness of oral contraceptives—know which ones before you call the doctor.

* A plant-derived synthetic estrogen drug is a popular alternative to Premarin in the relief of hot flashes, mood changes, night sweats, and other menopausal symptoms. Is it right for you?

* One common over-the-counter drug can play a lifesaving role in reducing the risk of death or complications from heart attack if taken at the first sign of an attack.

* Potentially life-threatening drug interactions can occur with analgesics containing codeine. Know the facts.

* Heart disease is the leading cause of death in American women over 35. Find out more about the new drugs available.

* Once thought to be a "man's" disease, ulcers now affect women equally—half of the 500,000 new cases each year—but remarkable new combination drug therapies are proving highly successful.

* Certain drugs, including Prozac, remain in the body for a long period of time, and drug interactions can occur even after you stopped taking it. Find out if you're at risk.

The Women's Pharmacy

THE WOMEN'S PHARMACY

An Essential Guide to What
Women Should Know about
Prescription Drugs

Introduction by Robert L. Rowan, M.D.

**Julie Catalano
with Robert L. Rowan, M.D.**

A DELL BOOK

Published by
Dell Publishing
a division of
Random House, Inc.
1540 Broadway
New York, New York 10036

Dell books may be purchased for business or promotional use or for special sales. For information please write to: Special Markets Department, Random House, Inc., 1540 Broadway, New York; NY 10036.

Dell® is a registered trademark of Random House, Inc., and the colophon is a trademark of Random House, Inc.

ISBN: 0-440-23537-5

Printed in the United States of America

Published simultaneously in Canada

September 2000

10 9 8 7 6 5 4 3 2 1

OPM

Acknowledgments

Many thanks to Agnes Birnbaum, the most patient, understanding, and persevering literary agent in the world. Without her, this book would not exist.

Thank you to senior editor Danielle Perez for her patience and expert editing, and to the entire production and design team at Random House/Dell. A special thanks to Christine Zika for getting the book off to such a good start.

For their generous professional help: thanks to *American Druggist, Drug Store News, Pharmacy Times,* and *FDA Consumer,* along with the FDA offices in San Antonio and Dallas for their assistance; *Women's Health Research Issues* from the American Pharmaceutical Association; Rose Valdez Jackson of the Women's Health Initiative at the University of Texas Health Science Center at San Antonio; Kim Roberson of the Texas Pharmacy Association; The Council of Family Health and The National Women's Health Network, Washington, DC; The National Library of Medicine, Bethesda, MD; Mary Ann Maryn of Rubenstein Associates, New York; Angela O'Meara and Eric Morgan of The Professional Image, Newport Beach; Reeta Owczarek; and many others whom I am probably forgetting but also have my gratitude and thanks.

Thanks to my mother and father, family, and friends, especially the following. All have provided either moral support, gainful employment, or inspiration, but most of all, the invaluable gifts of fun, friendship, and growth: Ricardo Cedillo, Doris Taggart, Jim Harford, Susan Blumert, Dora Fitzgerald, Bill and Diana Lamm, Rick Kroninger, Angela Zarnoti, Ruth Papazian, Mona Lane, Helen Lozano, John and Mary Martinez, Kristin Athas, Ann Schlosser, Pat Barnes, John Hardiman, Jesse Cardona, Sister Rose Marie Gallatin, Mel and Nancy Wheeler, Arline Zatz, Dorothy Beach, Gene Scheer, Michele Krier, Doug Smart, Thomas Sergiovanni, Michael Smith, Angela Youngheim, Renato Perez; Buddy and Susan Treviño of The University of the Incarnate Word; the gang at EHR Design; Larry Felder and PCI Publishing; and Kristina Paledes of the *San Antonio Express-News.* A special thanks to Daniel Presswood, who is always there in good times, bad times, and worse times, all of which occurred during the writing of this book.

Thanks to Suki, my four-footed Siamese writing partner of almost 20 years, for being the best furry feline friend, companion, and sounding board anyone could ask for.

A huge thank-you to Cynthia Dueñes Villafranco, my wonderful assistant whom I'm happy to also call a friend. Her positive energy, unflappable good mood, and cheery notes (with helpful reminders to *breathe*) kept me going during frantic times when it appeared that there was no end in sight. Thanks, Cynthia. Your skills and talent will no doubt serve you well in your own writing career.

Finally, thanks to Dr. Bob Rowan, a veteran author who undertook the ultimate act of bravery by getting his first computer—and learning how to use it—during the process of writing this book. His boundless energy and kindness were welcome bonuses to the knowledge and experience that helped to shape this book. It is my hope that his medical expertise of more than four decades will help every woman who reads these pages.

Julie Catalano

Contents

Introduction

In my forty years as a practicing physician, I have seen few fields explode in the vast amount and diversity of information as the subject of women's health. And where women's health goes, so go the pharmaceutical companies, searching for new treatments for one of their largest group of consumers—women. Hardly a day goes by that we don't hear about the latest developments in promising new drugs for breast cancer, menopause, cardiovascular disease, rheumatoid arthritis, reproductive health, and dozens of other topics that affect women either exclusively or in greater numbers than men. The sheer number and variety of prescription drugs—5,200 at last count—make them a complex and powerful force, and one that is virtually unavoidable for most women during almost every stage of their lives.

Fortunately for women, this explosion of information coincides with unprecedented access to that information. From her morning newspaper to the evening news to the hundreds of thousands of women's health links on the Internet, a woman no longer has to rely only on her doctor to find out almost everything she wants to know about the medicines she's taking.

But with all that information comes responsibility—and often confusion. There is no doubt that prescription drugs are a mixed blessing. They save lives, and they can also threaten them. Along with the good news about prescription drugs comes the cold, hard fact that prescription and nonprescription drugs kill more than 100,000 Americans every year, and another 2.1 million are hospitalized for adverse drug reactions. This year's miracle drug becomes next year's horror story with the ultimate unhappy ending—a prescription drug recall due to associated deaths and disabilities—leaving a bewildered public wondering which drug will be next, and if it is already in their medicine cabinets.

Women have a huge stake in this scenario. The proliferation of specialists means that more women are seeing more doctors more often. In the past, a woman might have had one general practitioner and an ob/gyn. These days, women are streaming into the offices of oncologists, neurologists, rheumatologists, urologists, psychiatrists, allergists, and cardiologists in unprecedented numbers. Chances are they're walking out with one or more prescriptions in hand, along with the very real possibility that none of their doctors knows about the others—and the corresponding prescriptions—unless their patients tell them. The changing environment of managed care also plays a part in this scenario. At the very time when doctors should be spending more time with their patients—especially female patients—HMOs are limiting that time, resulting in increasingly shorter office visits.

Add to that the women-only health care issues—pregnancy, breast-feeding, hormone fluctuations, menopause, vaginal infections, a host of minor and major ailments, along with constant reminders to do breast self-exams, get annual Pap smears and pelvic exams, use effective birth control, practice safe sex, and take enough calcium. It's no wonder that women can easily become overwhelmed at the prospect of being told repeatedly to take a more active role in their own health care. And so every day, millions of women take millions of pills based on nothing more than blind faith and implicit trust in the doctors who prescribed them.

It is good to trust your doctor. Working with your doctor in a relationship of mutual respect and honesty is even better. No woman should have to be alone in the management of her drug therapy, but she may have to become more informed and assertive to ensure that she is getting the maximum benefits with the minimum adverse reactions. Weighing the benefits against the risks is an indispensable aspect of drug management.

What do I suggest to women with regard to working with their physicians, nurses, physician's assistants, nurse practitioners, and pharmacists in order to use prescription drugs safely and wisely?

It's very simple. Despite major technological advances, computerized diagnostics, and state-of-the-art products and services, what high-quality health care comes down to remains constant: one-on-one communication; the open and honest exchange of information with all of your health care providers, and never settling for less. Most doctors are doing their best in an assembly-line environment where they, too, are overwhelmed by information and time constraints. But an intelligent doctor welcomes an intelligent patient—one who is actively involved in her health care and who works with her doctors to make every office visit an informative and productive one:

- The average office visit is eight to ten minutes, so you need to stay organized and on the subject. Write down your questions and/or list of symptoms. Give your doctor an overview so you both will know exactly what you want to accomplish in that visit. "I have three things I need to discuss with you."
- Take notes or use a tape recorder, or take along a friend who will help you remember what was said.

- Always tell your doctor if you are pregnant or trying to become pregnant. This is essential when prescription drugs are involved, as little is known about the effects of most drugs on a woman's reproductive system.
- Inform your doctor of any drug allergies you have, or if you've experienced severe side effects from any drug. Drugs in the same category can cause similar reactions. When you're having a prescription filled or refilled, also tell your pharmacist about any drug allergies or serious side effects.
- Take a complete list of every prescription and nonprescription drug you are taking, along with vitamins, herbal remedies, and dietary supplements. Never assume that any doctor knows all of the medications you are taking.
- Provide a complete medical history, even if some of it is painful or embarrassing. This information may prove crucial in deciding which drug to prescribe.

When a doctor prescribes a drug, ask the following questions:

- How long will I need to take it?
- What common side effects can I expect, and when should they be considered severe?
- What are the consequences of long-term use?
- What is the exact brand name and generic name, and is it safe to take the generic equivalent?
- Are there any specific medicines, food, or drinks (especially alcohol) that may interact with this drug or interfere with its effectiveness?

If you have a doctor who won't listen to you, who looks at your desire for accurate information as a personal threat to his or her expertise, who treats your very real symptoms as purely emotionally based or hypochondriacal without taking the appropriate tests, and most important, won't give you satisfactory answers about any drug you are taking—then it's time to find another doctor. Nothing is more important than your health, and for women that means being armed with as much information as possible and working with doctors and all other health care providers to make sure that any drug therapy—whether it's one pill or ten—is exactly the right one for you.

In my job as clinical professor, teaching at New York University School of Medicine, I am pleased and delighted to see that half of my class is female—a far cry from the days when a single woman in an otherwise all-male class was the norm. This increase in the number of women doctors will undoubtedly influence the future of women's health care for the better.

But in the end it will all come down to you, the patient. The best patients are active, not passive. The best questions are informed, not random. The massive amount of information on women's health will continue to proliferate at breakneck speed. Although no book should ever be used as a substitute for the advice of a medical professional, women will continue to need every resource they can find to make sure they are getting the best medical care possible. *The Women's Pharmacy* is just a part of that, and one that we hope will be a useful addition to your health care library.

Robert L. Rowan, M.D.
Clinical Professor, New York University Medical School

Taking Charge: What Women Need to Know about Prescription Drugs

From the moment a young girl is given her first over-the-counter pain reliever for menstrual cramps to the time when she has to weigh the pros and cons of hormone-replacement therapy after menopause, women carry on a lifelong relationship with a vast and often confusing array of medicines, having to make decisions regarding drugs in ways that men never have to make.

Women are by far the largest consumers of medications—both prescription and nonprescription—just as they are by far the largest consumers of medical care. According to the National Council on Patient Information and Education, two-thirds of the approximately 137 million physician and pharmacist visits each year are by women. Correspondingly, an estimated two-thirds of the more than 2.4 billion prescriptions a year are written to women. Women over age 45 use more medication than any other group. Not surprisingly, women have a powerful presence as majority purchasers of more than 600,000 over-the-counter treatments available. As managers of medications for their families, more women than men buy more of these products for themselves and their children.

The list of the top 200 prescription drugs (see appendix 2) shows the drugs most often prescribed in the United States, but there is no comprehensive list of what prescriptions are most often filled for women. Obviously, drugs for premenstrual syndrome, menstrual pain, endometriosis, menopause, vaginitis, oral contraception, and fertility are used exclusively by women. But women also use a higher percentage of drugs for anxiety and depression, not necessarily because they have a predisposition toward these disorders, but because 1) women routinely seek appropriate treatment more often than do men, and 2) traditionally, doctors are more likely to prescribe these types of medications for women than for men, even outside a psychiatric or psychological setting. It's not unusual for a woman to be prescribed numerous drugs to treat an array of *symptoms* as opposed to addressing the underlying *disorder*—being given a sedative to treat insomnia, for example, instead of investigating the possibility of a physical or psychological cause and the appropriate treatment for it. Or being prescribed an antidepressant or antianxiety drug in lieu of having a complete medical workup to determine the overall health picture.

Women also suffer from urinary tract infections, osteoporosis, lupus, multiple sclerosis, and rheumatoid arthritis in greater numbers than men do. Even disorders that would appear to have no specific gender disposition can strike disproportionately: Of the 23 million migraine sufferers in this country, for example, 18 million are women. More than 14,000 women die from Alzheimer's disease each year. It can be difficult to diagnose, but a woman's longer life span may predispose her to developing it. More than half of people over 85 have probable Alzheimer's. In addition, women represent 80 percent of caregivers. And while heart disease was once considered the exclusive domain of men, it is now the leading killer of women in the United States, accounting for 500,000 fatalities each year. Nearly twice as many women die from heart disease and stroke as from all forms of cancer combined.

Although we know statistically that women take more drugs than do men, there is still a need for more information about what drugs they are taking, their ingredients, their effects during pregnancy and breast-feeding, their interactions with other drugs, food, and alcohol, and their side effects and complications. At the very least, women are at a much higher risk for an assortment of drug-related problems: overmedication, adverse side effects, addiction, withdrawal, and drug interactions.

Add to this a tendency to self-diagnose and self-medicate, and the potential for serious problems multiplies as over-the-counter treatments proliferate. Women are much more likely to self-medicate—if they take proper care of their health at all. Women often move themselves and their medical needs to the back of the line—after home, children, parents, work, school—as they routinely juggle commodities that are frequently in short supply: time and money. So instead of discussing thorough treatments and making informed choices with family practitioners, gynecologists, or pharmacists, women often head for the drug aisles, buying over-the-counter diuretics, appetite suppressants, laxatives, sleep aids, and a host of other readily available medications.

Donna Shalala, Secretary of Health and Human Services, has advised: "It is far less costly, and less painful, to prevent disease than to treat it. Prevention for women means, among other things, an annual Pap smear, clinical and self-breast exams and mammography, prenatal care, regular exercise, and good nutrition."

While prevention—and the sound advice given above—is naturally the ideal way to avert disease, the fact is that sooner or later women are going to be ingesting, applying, or inhaling some form of medication in much greater numbers than are men. When she does, she might ask herself the following:

- Why am I taking this drug?
- What was this medication designed to do?
- How does it work in my body?
- How long does it take to begin working?
- What are the side effects, and when should I notify my doctor about them?
- What about the other drugs I'm taking with this? Are there any food or alcohol interactions?
- What if I'm pregnant, or trying to become pregnant, or nursing?

These questions and more are just some of the issues that are addressed in drug trials, the procedure by which a drug is tested before it is made available to consumers. Drug development is enormously expensive and time-consuming. It takes an average of twelve years and approximately $500 million to complete successfully the FDA's approval process, and only one in five drugs tested in people is approved.

Women and Drug Studies: Where Have We Been?

Ironically, the population that uses the greater proportion of medications is the very population that has been largely neglected in the trials that determine a drug's efficacy and safety. Women have been seriously underrepresented in medical research and, until recently, drug trials have been performed exclusively on men. There has been long-standing frustration by both the medical community and women over the exclusion of women from several landmark medical studies, most notably cardiovascular disease and aging. For example, an exhaustive study in the late 1970s helped to define the risk factors for coronary disease as blood pressure, dietary fat, and cholesterol levels. It involved 13,000 men and not one woman. In fact, three out of four major clinical trials on cholesterol-lowering drugs were conducted using only middle-aged men, yet half the prescriptions for those drugs subsequently were written for women over age 60. In the early 1980s, when estrogen was first studied for its protective properties against heart disease, it was tested only in men.

Several explanations stand out for why women have been excluded from drug trials. First, in our increasingly litigious society, researchers and drug companies fear liability if drug treatments affect conception, reproduction, or fetal development in women of childbearing age; second, some believe that a woman's fluctuating hormone levels during menstruation, ovulation, pregnancy, and lactation would complicate the study or possibly render the information useless.

Low disease prevalence is another factor cited in the past. In the cardiovascular study mentioned above, the reason for limiting the research to men was justified by the belief that the disease was seen more often in middle-aged men than in women. But because heart disease usually occurs at a later life stage in women than in men, due to menopause and the loss of potentially protective estrogen, and because women tend to live longer than men, we now know that many older women develop cardiovascular disease. According to the American Heart Association, one in nine women age 45 to 64 has some form of heart or blood vessel disease—a ratio that climbs to one in three at age 65 and over.

Women and Drug Studies: Where Are We Now?

So, what are the consequences of excluding women from drug research? According to a report on women's health research issues published by the American Pharmaceutical Association (APhA), women may receive improper medication doses and have unfavorable side effects when information obtained exclusively from men's drug trials is applied to women. Elderly women especially have a higher incidence of adverse side effects than do men, for example.

There are other gender-related differences as well, such as how a drug is absorbed, metabolized, and eliminated, all of which may be affected by hormonal changes during premenstruation, menstruation, pregnancy, and menopause. Further, higher body-fat content and smaller body size are factors in how women and men respond differently to drugs. In some instances, dosages have to be adjusted for women on birth control pills; oral contraceptives can decrease the body's clearance of certain drugs such as some asthma medications, some antidepressants, and corticosteroids. Few drugs have been adequately studied to determine the extent of these differences, but preliminary findings show that gender is an essential element in any discussion of women and prescription drugs:

- Some antidepressants can take a long time to clear a woman's body, increasing the risk for potentially dangerous side effects.
- Other drugs clear out faster with equally adverse results. Heart transplants are rejected by women more often than by men. Some researchers believe this may be because antirejection drugs like cyclosporine are cleared faster in women.

• Women wake up from anesthesia almost twice as fast as men do, according to a study reported by the American Society of Anesthesiologists.

Even at this early stage of discovery, gender-related differences in drug use represent important knowledge for women. Fortunately, the picture for women in drug trials is improving, albeit slowly. As far back as the mid-1980s, the APhA was the first pharmacy organization to advocate the inclusion of women in clinical research. It took almost ten years, in 1993, for the U.S. Congress to require the National Institutes of Health, the nation's largest research funder, to include women in all applicable clinical trials of medical treatments. That same year the Food and Drug Administration also issued guidelines that encouraged researchers to use women in tests of new drugs. Before that, women had been virtually banned from participating in Phase I and early Phase II studies—the stages at which doses are determined—because of fears of effects on reproduction. At an FDA meeting in 1995, researchers were urged to include women in Phase I trials in order to discover the potential for gender-related variables before drugs are approved for widespread use.

Finally, research on women and heart disease is getting the attention it deserves from a federal health standpoint: In 1998, the women's Health Research and Prevention Amendments were signed into law to designate funds for research on women and cardiovascular disease at the National Heart, Lung, and Blood Institute.

New Drugs for Women

When Dr. Rowan said in his introduction, "Where women's health goes, so go the pharmaceutical companies," he was referring to an unprecedented revolution in women's health that has motivated drug manufacturers to address women's special needs. A 1999 survey by the Pharmaceutical Research and Manufacturers of America (PhRMA) found a 75% increase in drug research on women's health since their 1991 survey. This increase represents 348 medicines in development for diseases that disproportionately affect women, including

- 24 medicines for rheumatoid arthritis, which causes pain and disability in 1.5 million women
- 60 medicines for breast cancer, which kills 43,000 women each year in the U.S.
- 38 medicines for ovarian cancer, which claims 14,500 lives each year
- 23 new treatments for Alzheimer's disease
- 24 medicines for osteoporosis, which causes two fractures in American women every minute.
- 80 new medicines under study to combat heart disease, with special attention to how the drugs work in women

Other new medicines on the horizon target osteoarthritis, multiple sclerosis, psoriasis, cervical cancer, endometrial cancer, migraine headache, anxiety, and depression. Also in the pipeline are 102 medicines for AIDS and AIDS-related conditions, including 11 preventive vaccines and a new class of drugs called anti-HIV fusion inhibitors that block the virus before it enters and infects blood cells.

Along with encouraging development news, however, comes a growing concern over rising drug prices. People over age 65 will double to about 70 million by 2030. Women live longer than men, earn less than men, and are generally lower on the socioeconomic ladder. Barring a major overhaul of the health care system, it's difficult to imagine a scenario where all women will benefit equally from new-generation drugs that can cost up to $15 per pill.

Gaining Ground: The Women's Health Initiative

Until recently there was little research on menopause, osteoporosis, ovarian cancer, or breast cancer. In 1987, a report by the General Accounting Office stated that only 13 percent of the National Institutes of Health $14.7 billion in research funds were being spent on diseases that affect women disproportionately (e.g., rheumatoid arthritis, systemic lupus, mental affective disorders such as depression, and autoimmune thyroid disease).

The GAO report helped to pave the way for the increased focus on women's health. Thanks to activists and advocates of women's equality in health care, Bernadine P. Healy was appointed the first female director of the NIH in 1991; shortly thereafter, she launched the fourteen-year, $625 million Women's Health Initiative. The WHI is a study of some 160,000 women between the ages of 50 and 79 at forty centers nationwide that will examine primarily diseases of utmost importance to women—specifically heart disease, breast cancer, and osteoporosis, as well as stroke and depression. The study will determine how hormones affect women with such diseases; whether hormones affect memory loss; and how calcium and vitamin D affect women's diets. It is the first and largest study of its kind dedicated exclusively to women's health issues. (For information on the study or to inquire about participating, see the Women's Resource Directory at the back of this book.)

Your doctor and your pharmacist will most likely be your main sources of information about prescription and nonprescription drugs. (*Remember, this book is not a substitute for expert professional advice or treatment.*) There is little question that women are at a turning point in the management of their health care and drug therapy. As more women realize the importance of taking charge of their health care, awareness and education will be their best weapons against an increasingly overwhelming onslaught of information about the safety and effectiveness of prescription drugs. As the population ages, the cost of medical care and drugs skyrockets, HMOs chip away at the traditional doctor-patient relationship, and we are inundated with more health care information than at any other time in history. Books like this one are part of what is undeniably a constructive trend toward women assuming a greater responsibility for their health and well-being.

How to Use This Book

The Women's Pharmacy is a convenient, easy-to-use pill guide covering the most often prescribed drugs plus selected over-the-counter medications that may be of primary interest to women based on their special needs. Because of the sheer number of prescription drugs on the market, it was not designed to be a definitive, all-inclusive reference, but one that would highlight information of most interest to you.

We hope that we have compiled a useful selection of the prescription drugs that are commonly used in the treatment of diseases, disorders, or conditions that either primarily or disproportionately affect women. This includes drugs used exclusively by women—contraceptives, fertility drugs, and estrogens, for example—as well as antihypertensives, nonsteroidal antiinflammatory drugs (NSAIDs), antidepressants, antimigraines, cholesterol-lowering drugs, anticancer drugs, and many more.

What you will *not* find is specific information on over-the-counter medications, including products such as home pregnancy kits, douches, feminine hygiene products, birth control methods other than oral contraceptives, or similar items; herbal products, vitamins, or dietary supplements (unless they have potential interactions with prescription drugs); cosmetic products; or any nonprescription treatments or products that have not been subjected to the usual process of drug testing as conducted by the Food and Drug Administration (FDA).

The book is divided into the following sections:

Part 1: Prescription Drug Profiles

This section contains more than two hundred prescription-drug profiles covering more than three hundred drugs, listed alphabetically by brand name and cross-referenced by generic name. If you do not see a drug's brand name, look it up under its generic name. Each drug profile contains the following information:

Brand name:

This is the patented name of the drug (always capitalized) as given by the pharmaceutical company that researched and developed it, followed by selected additional brand names, if any. For example, the listing for Fastin reads: "Fastin (also Adipex-P, Ionamin)." (Note: Not every brand name for every drug is listed.) Competition among drug companies to come up with memorable brand names for new drugs has resulted in some drugs starting to look and sound eerily similar—Elavil and Eldepryl, Monopril and Monurol, Symmetrel and

Synarel, to name just a few. With the proliferation of new drugs every year, it is extremely important to know both the brand names and the generic names of the drugs you take. However, keep in mind that because of drug patents, not every brand name prescription drug has a generic counterpart available for sale. In fact, newer drugs are almost exclusively brand name. An asterisk next to a brand name indicates that the drug appeared on the list of the Top 200 Prescriptions in 1998, based on more than 2.4 billion prescriptions. (Source: *American Druggist*, February 1999.)

Generic name:

If you can remember only one name of the drug you are taking, choose its generic name (always lower case here). The reason for this is that the same drug can have many brand names but only one generic name. As drug costs rise, so does the popularity of less expensive and—with few exceptions—equally effective generic drugs. The generic name of a drug is based on its active ingredient. If you are taking a generic drug but would like to know its brand name, look through the alphabetical drug profiles to find the generic name (example: lovastatin, see Mevacor), which will refer you to one of the more popular brand names. An asterisk next to a generic name indicates that the drug appeared on the list of the Top 200 Prescriptions in 1998, based on more than 2.4 billion prescriptions. (Source: *American Druggist*, February 1999.)

Availability and dosage:

This refers to selected forms—or availability—of a drug (tablet, capsule, oral syrup, topical cream, etc.) in varying strengths (2 mg, 5 mg, 10 mg). Oral solutions are usually measured by the amount of active ingredient in a liquid base: 5 mg per 5 ml (milliliter). Topical drugs are usually measured by the percentage of active ingredient in a cream or ointment (2 percent, 4 percent). Occasionally, standard dosages are indicated. For example: "Claritin is usually taken once a day." Otherwise, specific dosage information is not provided here, as that is something your physician or nurse practitioner should determine. *Do not use this or any other book to attempt to estimate the proper dosage of any medication.* Always follow your doctor's directions, and never reduce, increase, or stop a medication without first discussing it with him or her. If a drug has special instructions on how to take it (e.g., with or without food, or at certain times of the day) it will be noted here.

Side effects:

Any drug carries the risk of side effects, and sometimes side effects are a sign that the drug is working, although that may not be much consolation when they affect your ability to function, or worse. Every year, approximately 100,000 Americans die of adverse drug reactions and 1.5 million are hospitalized. Generally speaking, side effects fall into four categories: annoying but tolerable, tolerable but disruptive to your normal routine, potentially serious, and life-threatening. The side effects in this listing are divided into "more common" and "other." A long list of side effects is not necessarily indicative of a high level of risk; they may have been reported by only one or two people during the clinical trial phase. Occasionally, interactions can be minimized by changing the dosage or the dosage schedule, and some initial side effects diminish over time. Life-threatening side effects usually manifest as severe allergic reactions: difficulty breathing, rash, and hives, but you might also experience heart arrhythmia, extreme dizziness, and any number of other reactions depending on the drug. If you experience any particularly uncomfortable or persistent side effects, consult your pharmacist or your physician, and always ask if there are any consequences to long-term use of a drug. If you suspect that a drug caused potentially serious side effects, you or your doctor can report them to the FDA's MedWatch Program, which tracks adverse drug reactions (see the listing under "Medications" in the Women's Resource Directory at the back of this book for more information).

Drug interactions:

This section contains selected drug interactions between two or more drugs or classes of drugs. Although much publicity has been generated concerning dangerous drug interactions, the fact is that many drugs—even when they have the potential to interact—can be managed through careful monitoring by your doctor along with your cooperation in taking the drug exactly as prescribed. There are varying degrees of drug interactions, ranging from whether the drug's effectiveness is altered in any way to serious adverse reactions—including disability and death—that have resulted from dangerous drug combinations. With newer drugs, there may be little evidence of dangerous interactions until the drug has been used by the public for some time. The interactions listed here do not necessarily reflect every potential drug interaction possible, but there are certain classes of drugs that warrant special cautions when used concurrently: central nervous system depressants, drugs for heart conditions and hypertension, antihistamines, anticoagulants (blood thinners), diuretics, monoamine oxidase (MAO) inhibitors (for depression), and others. Always provide all of your doctors with a complete and current list of all prescription and nonprescription drugs you take, as well as vitamins, herbal remedies, and dietary supplements.

Food/alcohol interactions:

Alcohol warnings will be listed here. Alcohol interacts with many drugs and therefore should be avoided while taking particular medications. Drug/food interactions are less common, except in the case of monoamine oxidase (MAO) inhibitors used to treat depression, anxiety, and phobias. If you are on any MAO inhibitors you will be given a list of foods to avoid. If you are unsure about a potential drug/alcohol interaction, it's best to avoid alcohol until your doctor or pharmacist verifies that it's safe. Grapefruit juice may intensify the effects of some medications. Always ask your doctor or pharmacist if there is a potential grapefruit juice/drug interaction.

Pregnancy/nursing:

In an ideal world, pregnancy would be a drug-free state, as very little is known about the effects of most drugs on a developing fetus and few expectant mothers are willing to take even the slightest risk. However, there are times when a pregnant woman must take prescription drugs for chronic conditions. Health providers may disagree about what is and isn't safe during which trimesters of pregnancy, so you and your ob/gyn will need to discuss whether the benefits of prescription drug use outweigh the risks. This also applies to breast-feeding. *Note: There are drugs that should never under any circumstances be taken by a pregnant woman (or, in some cases a woman planning to become pregnant).*

Seniors:

In general, drugs are often metabolized and eliminated more slowly in older people. Special information for this group is noted here. A lower dose may be initially prescribed, but you should never adjust your dosage without consulting your doctor. If there are no known cautions for seniors, it will indicate "no special warnings," but this does not mean that a drug could not affect an older individual adversely. Take your medicine as prescribed and notify your doctor of any persistent or troublesome side effects.

Warnings:

This category is reserved for especially serious or potentially life-threatening side effects as well as to reiterate pregnancy warnings. Severe side effects may warrant immediate medical treatment. Any breathing difficulties, skin rash, and/or hives indicate a potentially serious drug reaction. If you are experiencing any intense or unusual side effects, call your doctor immediately.

Comments:

Other important or interesting facts about the drug are mentioned here.

Part 2: You and Your Pharmacist

This section discusses how women can work with their pharmacists to derive the most benefit from their medications. Guidelines for safe drug use, questions for your pharmacist, information about generic drugs, tips for keeping home medication records, and information on selected categories of nonprescription, over-the-counter medications are also included.

Appendix 1: Medical Conditions

This appendix alphabetically lists diseases and disorders along with the prescription drugs—both brand name and generic—that may be used in the course of treatment. If you have been diagnosed with a particular disorder, check this appendix first for an overview of drugs that you might encounter in treatment, and then refer to the individual drug profiles in part 1 for details. (Note: Only the drugs mentioned in this book are listed here. There may be many more drugs available under a variety of brand names.)

Women's Resource Directory

This section contains names, addresses, and phone numbers (in most cases, toll-free) for national health organizations and support groups that are either exclusively for women or have departments devoted to women's health. Where applicable, Web site addresses are also provided.

Disclaimer: Now that you know how to use this book, it's important that you also know how not to use this book. *Do not use this book to self-diagnose, self-medicate, or make any changes in how you take your prescribed medications.* This book should never replace the advice of your doctor or other health care provider, including your pharmacist. No book of this type should be interpreted as all-inclusive or used as a substitute for expert medical care. This book offers no endorsement of products, recommendations for dosages or administration, or any implied promise of relief. The inclusion or exclusion of a brand name does not imply endorsement or otherwise. Every attempt was made to present correct information at the time of publication, but the subject of prescription drugs, interactions, warnings, and drug recalls is a highly volatile one. Always discuss any questions or concerns you have about any prescription or nonprescription drugs with your doctors and your pharmacist.

Part 1. Prescription Drug Profiles

Points to remember:

- An asterisk (*) following a brand name or a generic name indicates that that drug is one of the Top 200 Prescriptions, based on more than 2.4 billion prescriptions in the United States in 1998. (Source: *American Druggist*, February 1999.)
- Do not attempt to self-diagnose or self-medicate using the information or dosage forms listed in this book. Only your doctor can determine the proper dosage depending on your particular condition. Do not change your dosage in any way or stop taking a prescribed medication without consulting your doctor.
- We have attempted to list the most common side effects here, along with the ones most pertinent to women. They do not include every side effect ever reported in clinical trials or actual use. If you experience any side effect that you suspect may be caused by any drugs you are taking, notify your doctor or your pharmacist.
- Potentially hazardous drug/drug, drug/food, and drug/alcohol interactions are being discovered all the time. We have attempted to include the most common ones here. Never assume that because a specific interaction is not listed in this or any other book that it does not exist. Your pharmacy should provide an instruction sheet with every prescription. Always confirm with your doctor whether the medications you are taking have the potential to interact.
- If you are pregnant, you are probably seeing your doctor, nurse practitioner, or other health care provider on a regular basis anyway. If you plan to become pregnant, your gynecologist and any other specialists you are seeing should be made aware of this. As a general rule, drugs should not be taken during pregnancy, but depending on your overall health they may be required. You and your doctors should discuss the benefits versus the risks when managing drug therapy during pregnancy and breast-feeding. If you are pregnant, never take any prescription or nonprescription drug, herbal remedy, or dietary supplement without consulting your health care provider.
- Make sure that your doctors have a complete, up-to-date medical history. People with a history of asthma, anemia, glaucoma, diabetes, kidney or liver failure, heart disease, or

thyroid disorders, among other ailments, may be at a higher risk of potentially serious side effects from certain drugs. Also, make a note of any drug allergies or adverse effects to any prescription or nonprescription drugs you have taken in the past.

- *Always provide all of your doctors with a complete and current list of all prescription and over-the-counter drugs you are taking, including vitamins, herbal remedies, and dietary supplements.*

A/T/S

See Ery-Tab

abacavir sulfate

See Ziagen

Brand Name
Accolate*

Generic Name
zafirlukast

Type of Drug
Antileukotriene. This drug is not a steroid or a theophylline. In people with asthma, the body produces natural chemicals known as leukotrienes. These cause the muscles in the airways to contract and lung tissue to swell, resulting in difficulty in breathing. Taken regularly, zafirlukast can block the effects of these chemicals.

For
Prevention and treatment of chronic asthma. Not to be used for acute asthma.

Availability and Dosage
Tablets: 20 mg. Usual dosage is twice daily. This drug should be taken as prescribed, even during symptom-free periods. Food may interfere with the absorption of zafirlukast, so it is best taken 1 hour before or 2 hours after a meal.

Side Effects

More common include headache, nausea, diarrhea, and mild to moderate upper respiratory tract infections. Others include generalized pain, abdominal pain, dizziness, fever, back pain, and vomiting.

Drug Interactions

This drug may interact with anticoagulants (blood thinners), erythromycin, theophylline, aspirin, some calcium channel blockers, phenytoin, and carbamazepine. Always inform your doctors of every medication you are taking, including nonprescription medicines, vitamins, herbal remedies, and dietary supplements. *Do not take any over-the-counter medications unless approved by your doctor.*

Food/Alcohol Interactions

No special warnings.

Pregnancy/Nursing

No special warnings, although any drug during pregnancy and breast-feeding should be avoided if possible. Before taking this drug, discuss with your doctor the benefits versus the potential risks. Zafirlukast passes into breast milk. Bottle-feed your baby while on this drug.

Seniors

In clinical trials, patients age 55 and older reported mild to moderate infections, predominantly of the upper respiratory tract. Take as prescribed and immediately inform your doctor of any persistent or troublesome side effects.

Warning

A rare side effect of zafirlukast is elevation of liver enzymes. If you experience abdominal pain, nausea, fatigue, lethargy, jaundice, or any flu-like symptoms, contact your physician immediately.

Comments

Zafirlukast is not a bronchodilator and should not be used to treat acute episodes of asthma. Improvement in symptoms usually occurs within 1 week of starting treatment.

Brand Name
Accupril*

Generic Name

quinapril

Type of Drug

ACE (angiotensin-converting enzyme) inhibitor. ACE inhibitors are antihypertensives used to treat high blood pressure (hypertension). They work by blocking an enzyme in the body that is required to produce a substance that causes blood vessels to tighten. When this enzyme is blocked, blood vessels are relaxed, blood pressure is lowered, the workload of the heart and arteries is reduced, and blood and oxygen supplies are increased. ACE inhibitors do not cure hypertension; they control it for as long as the medication is used. Controlling high blood pressure may reduce the risk of heart attack, stroke, or kidney failure.

For

High blood pressure; congestive heart failure.

Availability and Dosage

Tablets: 5 mg, 10 mg, 20 mg, 40 mg. Should be taken on an empty stomach, either 1 hour before or 2 hours after meals. It should be taken at the same time every day.

Side Effects

A side effect that appears to occur more frequently in women than in men is a dry, hacking cough. More common side effects include dizziness, fatigue, and headache. Others include abdominal pain, nausea, vomiting, changes in heart rhythm, fainting, nervousness, insomnia, constipation, dry mouth, skin rash, itching, sore throat, and depression.

Drug Interactions

This type of drug has the potential to interact with diuretics, digoxin, indomethacin, allopurinol, potassium supplements, beta blockers, tetracycline drugs, and lithium. Antacids may interfere with absorption of quinapril. Do not take within 2 hours of each other. Always inform your doctors of every medication you are taking, including nonprescription medicines, vitamins, herbal remedies, and dietary supplements. *Do not take any over-the-counter medications unless approved by your doctor.*

Food/Alcohol Interactions

Taking quinapril with food that has a high fat content may interfere with the absorption of this drug. Do not use any salt substitute.

Pregnancy/Nursing

Not recommended, especially during the second and third trimesters. Birth defects or fetal death may result. This drug passes into breast milk. Bottle-feed your baby while on this drug.

Seniors

Due to loss of kidney function associated with aging, dosage may have to be adjusted accordingly. Your doctor may prescribe a low dose.

Warning

Call your doctor if you experience swelling of the face, hands, or feet, difficulty in breathing, chest pains, fever, palpitations, sore throat, rash, or loss of taste. Make sure your doctor has your complete medical history, including a history of kidney disease, diabetes, or systemic lupus.

Comments

Use caution when taking any over-the-counter medicine while on this drug. Nonprescription diet pills and decongestants contain ingredients that may raise blood pressure when taken with quinapril. Check with your pharmacist or your physician if you have questions. It may take several weeks before the full effects of this drug are noticed.

Brand Name
Accutane

Generic Name

isotretinoin

Type of Drug

Antiacne.

For

Acne, particularly severe cystic acne.

Availability and Dosage

Capsules: 10 mg, 20 mg, 40 mg. Should be taken with food. Your doctor will prescribe it for use every day for several months, then instruct you to stop for a rest period of at least two months. A second course of treatment may be prescribed if the acne does not improve.

Side Effects

More common include dry skin, cracked or inflamed lips, dry nose, dry mucous membranes, thinning of hair, drowsiness, conjunctivitis (pinkeye), and headache. Others include loss of appetite, stomach or intestinal discomfort, intolerance to contact lenses, diminished night vision, peeling palms or soles of the feet, and urinary discomfort.

Drug Interactions

Do not take supplements that contain vitamin A. Isotretinoin is chemically related to vitamin A, and taking them together could cause toxic levels. Tetracycline antibiotics should also be avoided while taking this medication.

Food/Alcohol Interactions

Avoid alcohol. It can cause increased elevations of blood triglyceride levels. Also avoid excess consumption of apricots, beef liver or chicken liver, carrots, pumpkin, and other foods high in vitamin A. Your doctor or your pharmacist may provide you with a list of foods to avoid or restrict.

Pregnancy/Nursing

A woman must never take this drug during pregnancy, or if she is trying to become pregnant. Isotretinoin has been shown to cause severe birth defects. If you are a woman of childbearing age, you will be given verbal and written warnings about avoiding pregnancy during the course of treatment, and you will be required to sign an informed-consent sheet saying that you have been told of the drug's side effects. Not recommended for nursing mothers.

Seniors

No special warnings. Take as prescribed and immediately inform your doctor of any persistent or troublesome side effects.

Warning

Call your doctor if you experience severe headaches, nausea, vomiting, or vision changes while taking this drug. These may be symptoms of increased fluid pressure inside the head.

Comments

Isotretinoin is being prescribed in record numbers as an acne preventive, so the pregnancy warnings are especially important. In the last three years, the number of users has doubled, especially among women in their twenties and thirties with mild acne who are not responding to traditional treatment. Your skin may become especially sun-sensitive while taking this drug.

acetaminophen and codeine phosphate*

See Tylenol with codeine

acetaminophen and hydrocodone bitartrate

See Vicodin

acetaminophen and oxycodone hydrochloride

See Percocet

acetaminophen and propoxyphene hydrochloride

See Daypro

Brand Name
Actigall

Generic Name

ursodiol

Type of Drug

Bile acid. This medication works by suppressing the secretion of cholesterol and inhibiting the intestinal absorption of cholesterol, both factors in gallstone formation.

For

Prevention of gallstone formation in obese patients experiencing rapid weight loss.

Availability and Dosage

Capsules: 300 mg. Should be taken with food.

Side Effects

More common include constipation, diarrhea, and headache. Others include abdominal pain, nausea, fatigue, and muscle aches and pains.

Drug Interactions

Estrogens and oral contraceptives increase cholesterol secretion and encourage gallstone formation and thus may counteract the effectiveness of this medication. Cholesterol-lowering drugs may also reduce the effectiveness of ursodial. Do not take antacids within 2 hours of taking this drug. Always inform your doctors of every medication you are taking, including nonprescription medicines, vitamins, herbal remedies, and dietary supplements.

Food/Alcohol Interactions

No special warnings. However, you may be placed on a special diet by your doctor while taking this drug.

Pregnancy/Nursing

No special warnings, although all drugs during pregnancy and breast-feeding should be avoided if possible. Before taking this drug, discuss with your doctor the benefits versus the potential risks.

Seniors

No special warnings. Take as prescribed, and immediately inform your doctor of any persistent or troublesome side effects.

Warning

This drug will not have any effect on a severe gallstone attack. If you experience severe pain traveling from your abdomen to your right shoulder, seek emergency medical treatment immediately. Your doctor may suggest surgery to remove gallstones that are too large to respond to drug therapy.

Comments

Rapid weight loss sometimes results in the formation of gallstones, which are clusters of solid materials comprised mostly of cholesterol that form in the gallbladder. Complete dissolution does not occur in all cases. Recurrence of stones within 5 years has been observed in up to 50 percent of patients whose stones are dissolved by bile-acid therapy.

Brand Name
Actos

Generic Name

pioglitazone

Type of Drug

Antidiabetic. When combined with dietary changes and exercise habits, antidiabetic drugs provide relief of symptoms and enable most diabetics to lead healthy and productive lives.

For

Type II non-insulin–dependent diabetes mellitus (NIDDM).

Availability and Dosage

Tablets: 15 mg, 30, mg, 45 mg. May be taken with or without food. Any drug therapy for diabetes is highly individualized. Always follow your doctor's directions.

Side Effects

More common include upper respiratory-tract infection, headache, and sinusitis. Others include a worsening of diabetes.

Drug Interactions

If you are using an oral contraceptive (particularly the combination of norethindrone and ethinyl estradiol), this drug may reduce the effectiveness of your birth control pill by 30 percent. Patients receiving pioglitazone in combination with insulin or oral hypoglycemic drugs may be at risk for hypoglycemia. Always inform your doctor of every medication you are taking, including nonprescription medicines, vitamins, herbal remedies, and dietary supplements. *Do not take any over-the-counter medications unless approved by your doctor.*

Food/Alcohol Interactions

No special warnings. Your doctor or other health care provider should provide you with guidelines for a healthy diet.

Pregnancy/Nursing

Not recommended. Your doctor may prescribe insulin during your pregnancy. Bottle-feed your baby while on this drug.

Seniors

No special warnings. Take as prescribed and immediately inform your doctor of any persistent or troublesome side effects.

Warning

If you are premenopausal and no longer ovulating, this drug may result in resumption of ovulation. Be sure to use additional birth control methods if you do not wish to become pregnant. Seek immediate medical treatment for unexplained nausea, vomiting, abdominal pain, fatigue, anorexia, or dark urine.

Comments

Type II diabetes affects women and men equally, but a disproportionate number of minorities: More than 33 percent of Hispanics and nearly 25 percent of African Americans develop this disease by ages 65 to 74. Gestational diabetes occurs only during pregnancy. Women over 35 who have a family history of diabetes, are overweight, or have had gestational diabetes during a previous pregnancy are at greatest risk. *Regular monitoring by your doctor is essential if you have diabetes and are taking any antidiabetic drugs.* Another drug in the thiazolidinedione class, Rezulin (troglitazone) has been associated with liver failure and death, and was recalled in 2000. Although Actos (pioglitazone) has shown no evidence of liver failure in studies, patients on this drug should be checked for liver function at the start of therapy and every two months during the first year.

acyclovir

See Zovirax

Adalat

See Procardia XL*

Brand Name

Adderall*

Generic Name

amphetamine mixed salts

Type of Drug

Amphetamine.

For

Attention deficit hyperactivity disorder (ADHD), a chronic behavior disorder characterized by disruptive behavior, hyperactivity, impulsiveness, and difficulty sustaining concentration or focus. Although ADHD is usually associated with children, adults of any age can exhibit symptoms. There are no biological tests for ADHD. Diagnoses are based on guidelines set by the American Psychiatric Association. Behavior management is usually a major part of the treatment.

Availability and Dosage

Tablets: 5 mg, 10 mg, 20 mg, 30 mg.

Side Effects

More common include heart palpitations, a rise in blood pressure, restlessness, dizziness, and insomnia. Others include tremor, headache, dry mouth, diarrhea, constipation, anorexia, and changes in sex drive.

Drug Interactions

This drug has the potential to interact with tricyclic antidepressants, monoamine oxidase (MAO) inhibitor antidepressants, antihypertensives or other heart drugs, and some anticonvulsants. Always inform your doctors of every medication you are taking, including nonprescription medicines, vitamins, herbal remedies, and dietary supplements. *Do not take any over-the-counter medications unless approved by your doctor.*

Food/Alcohol Interactions

Avoid alcohol. Acidic fruit juices lower the absorption of amphetamines. Some sources advise avoiding sugar and limiting the intake of additives and preservatives.

Pregnancy/Nursing

No special warnings, although all drugs during pregnancy and breast-feeding should be avoided if possible. Before taking this drug, discuss with your doctor the benefits versus the potential risks. Bottle-feed your baby while on this drug.

Seniors

No special warnings. Take as prescribed and immediately inform your doctor of any persistent or troublesome side effects.

Warning

Amphetamines should not be used by people who have glaucoma, hypertension, tics (twitching), or Tourette's syndrome. This type of drug has a high potential for abuse and dependence. Your doctor will probably prescribe this type of drug sparingly.

Comments

Preliminary studies show that once-a-day dosage of Adderall may be able to replace multiple doses of Ritalin (methylphenidate) for some patients with ADHD. The gender gap in this disorder is narrowing. Men taking medication for ADHD outnumbered women 10 to 1 in 1985 but only 5 to 1 in 1995.

Adipex-P

See Fastin

Alatone

See Aldactone

albuterol

See Proventil*

Brand Name
Aldactone (also Alatone)

Generic Name

spironolactone

Type of Drug

Diuretic; antihypertensive. Diuretics promote the loss of water and salt from the body, which results in the lowering of blood pressure. Antihypertensives work to reduce abnormally high pressure of the blood against the walls of the blood vessels. Hypertension can cause strokes and heart attacks, as well as damage to the eyes and kidneys. Antihypertensives do not cure high blood pressure; they control it for as long as the medication is taken.

For

High blood pressure; edema.

Availability and Dosage

Tablets: 25 mg, 50 mg, 100 mg. Usual dosage is once daily. May be taken with food or milk (not low-sodium milk) if stomach upset occurs, unless your doctor instructs otherwise.

Side Effects

More common include nausea, vomiting, dry mouth, increased urination, dizziness, and headache. These side effects may subside as your body adjusts to the medication. Other side effects include irregular menstruation, diarrhea, lethargy, and rash.

Drug Interactions

This drug has the potential to interact with many other drugs, including lithium, digoxin, anticoagulants (blood thinners), other blood-pressure–lowering drugs, and laxatives. Always inform your doctors of every medication you are taking, including nonprescription medicines, vitamins, herbal remedies, and dietary supplements. *Do not take any over-the-counter medications unless approved by your doctor.*

Food/Alcohol Interactions

Avoid or limit alcohol. Do not use salt substitutes. Avoid foods high in potassium (e.g., salt substitutes, dried fruit, low-sodium milk) to reduce the risk of hyperkalemia, an excess of potassium in the blood.

Pregnancy/Nursing

Not recommended. Spironolactone passes into breast milk. Bottle-feed your baby while on this drug.

Seniors

Your doctor may prescribe a low dose. Older adults may be more susceptible to hyperkalemia (excess potassium) due to decreased kidney function.

Warning

Report to your doctor immediately any of the following: muscle weakness, numbness or tingling in the hands and feet, clumsiness, anxiety, rapid weight gain, deepening of the voice, increased hair growth, menstrual disturbances, or postmenopausal bleeding.

Comments

For women, diuretics are occasionally recommended for fibro-cystic breast changes (fluid-filled cysts) to relieve discomfort associated with fluid retention. Hypertension is often referred to as "the silent killer" because it has no symptoms, yet it forces the heart to work harder. Heart disease is the leading cause of death among women in the United States. People with hypertension should be monitored regularly to keep track of their blood pressure.

Brand Name
Aldara

Generic Name

imiquimod

Type of Drug

Antimitotic; chemical remover.

For

External genital and perianal warts.

Availability and Dosage

Topical cream: Each gram of the 5 percent cream contains 50 mg of imiquimod in an off-white, oil-in-water vanishing cream base. Usual dosage is 3 times a week, prior to bedtime, and is left on the skin for 6 to 10 hours.

Side Effects

More common are mild local skin reactions such as redness, peeling, itching, burning, pain, erosion, rash, and edema at the site of application or surrounding areas. In trials, side effects were more common and more intense with daily application rather than 3 times a week. Other side effects may include headache, flu-like symptoms, and muscle pain.

Drug Interactions

No known interactions with other topically applied drugs. However, imiquimod is not recommended until genital/perianal tissue is healed from any previous drug or surgical treatment.

Food/Alcohol Interactions

No special warnings.

Pregnancy/Nursing

No special warnings, although all drugs during pregnancy and breast-feeding should be avoided if possible. Before taking this drug, discuss with your doctor the benefits versus the potential risks.

Seniors

No special warnings. Take as prescribed and immediately inform your doctor of any persistent or troublesome side effects.

Warning

If you experience a severe skin reaction to this cream, wash off immediately and notify your doctor.

Comments

Imiquimod is not a cure for external genital and perianal warts. New warts may develop during therapy. Sexual contact should be avoided while the cream is on the skin; sexual precautions are necessary.

alendorate sodium

See Fosamax*

Alesse 28*

See Oral Contraceptives

Brand Name
Allegra*

Generic Name

fexofenadine hydrochloride

Type of Drug

Antihistamine. These drugs counteract the effect of histamine, a chemical released in the body that can cause itching and swelling.

For

Relief of symptoms associated with seasonal allergic rhinitis, including sneezing, itchy nose/palate/throat, and itchy or watery eyes.

Availability and Dosage

Tablets or capsules: 60 mg.

Side Effects

More common include nausea, drowsiness, fatigue, and dysmenorrhea (painful menstrual periods).

Drug Interactions

No special warnings, although any drug has the ability to interact with any other drug. Report any problems to your doctor or your pharmacist. Always inform your doctors of every medication you are taking, including nonprescription medicines, vitamins, herbal remedies, and dietary supplements.

Food/Alcohol Interactions

No special warnings.

Pregnancy/Nursing

No special warnings, although all drugs during pregnancy and breast-feeding should be avoided if possible. Before taking this drug, discuss with your doctor the benefits versus the potential risks.

Seniors

Your doctor may initially prescribe a low dose, especially for patients with decreased kidney function.

Comments

In addition to prescription antihistamines, there are dozens of over-the-counter antihistamines available. Many people self-medicate with antihistamines for everything from hay fever to hives to insomnia. Both prescription and nonprescription antihistamines have the potential to interact with many different drugs, including those taken for heart disease, diabetes, and other conditions. Always check with your doctor or your pharmacist before combining over-the-counter antihistamines with any prescription drug. Follow package directions carefully and notify your doctor if you have any problems.

allopurinol*

See Zyloprim

alprazolam*

*See Xanax**

Brand Name
Altace*

Generic Name

ramipril

Type of Drug

Angiotensin-converting enzyme (ACE) inhibitor. ACE inhibitors are antihypertensives used to treat high blood pressure (hypertension). They work by blocking an enzyme in the body that is required to produce a substance that causes blood vessels to tighten. When this enzyme is blocked, blood vessels are relaxed, blood pressure is lowered, the workload of the heart and arteries is reduced, and blood and oxygen supplies are increased. ACE inhibitors do not cure hypertension; they control it for as long as the medication is used. Controlling high blood pressure may reduce the risk of heart attack, stroke, or kidney failure.

For

High blood pressure; congestive heart failure.

Availability and Dosage

Capsules 1.25 mg, 2.5 mg, 5 mg, 10 mg. Should be taken on an empty stomach, either 1 hour before or 2 hours after a meal, as food can affect the absorption of this drug.

Side Effects

More common in women may be a chronic cough that usually disappears within a few days of stopping the medication. Other side effects include fatigue, nausea, headache, dizziness when rising from a sitting or lying position, abnormal heart rhythms, tingling in the hands or feet, hair loss, rash, increased sensitivity to sunlight, nervousness, and difficulty in sleeping.

Drug Interactions

ACE inhibitors have the potential to interact with a wide variety of drugs, including diuretics, potassium supplements, tetracycline antibiotics, lithium, other blood-pressure–lowering drugs including beta blockers, allopurinol, and digoxin. Always inform your doctors of every medication you are taking, including nonprescription medicines, vitamins, herbal remedies, and dietary supplements. Nonprescription diet pills and decongestants may raise blood pressure when taken with ramipril. Do not take antacids within 2 hours after taking this drug. *Do not take any over-the-counter medications unless approved by your doctor.*

Food/Alcohol Interactions

Taking ramipril with food may affect the absorption of this drug. Do not use salt substitutes.

Pregnancy/Nursing

Not recommended. Ramipril taken during the second and third trimesters is known to cause birth defects and even death to the newborn. Bottle-feed your baby if you must take this drug.

Seniors

Your doctor may prescribe a low dose, especially for patients with decreased kidney function.

Warning

If you experience swelling of the face or throat, difficulty in breathing, chest pain, mouth sores, abnormal heartbeat, or loss of taste, seek emergency medical treatment.

Comments

Regular and careful monitoring by your doctor is recommended while you are on this drug. Make sure that your doctor knows your complete medical history, especially a history of diabetes, kidney or liver disease, or systemic lupus.

alzapam

See Ativan

amantadine

See Symmetrel

Brand Name
Amaryl*

Generic Name

glimepiride

Type of Drug

Antidiabetic. When combined with dietary changes and exercise habits, antidiabetic drugs provide relief of symptoms and enable most diabetics to lead healthy and productive lives. You should wear a medical identification tag at all times and carry an ID card that lists your medications.

For

Type II non-insulin–dependent diabetes mellitus (NIDDM).

Availability and Dosage

Tablets: 1 mg, 2 mg, 4 mg. Usually taken 30 minutes before a meal.

Side Effects

More common include nausea, headache, upset stomach, loss of appetite, diarrhea, and tingling in the hands or feet. Others include jaundice, itching, rash, tremors, dizziness, and drowsiness.

Drug Interactions

This drug has the potential to interact with a wide variety of drugs, including any medication that can decrease blood sugar: nonsteroidal antiinflammatory drugs (NSAIDs), aspirin, enalapril, cimetidine, and fluconazole; medications that can increase blood sugar; oral contraceptives, estrogens, phenytoin, steroids, amphetamines, and thyroid drugs; ranitidine, famotidine, nizatidine, and anticoagulants (blood thinners). Always inform your doctors of every medication you are taking, including nonprescription medicines, vitamins, herbal remedies, and dietary supplements. *Do not take any over-the-counter medications unless approved by your doctor.*

Food/Alcohol Interactions

Avoid alcohol. Any use of alcohol can increase the possibility of adverse side effects, including skin flushing, difficulty in breathing, chest pains, low blood pressure, dizziness, and palpitations. You will probably be on a special diet to help control your diabetes.

Pregnancy/Nursing

Not recommended. Pregnant diabetic women are usually treated with insulin. Glimepiride passes into breast milk. Bottle-feed your baby if you must take this drug.

Seniors

Because of the usual decline in kidney function that occurs with age, you may be started on a lower dose. The potential for side effects is greater because of the slower elimination of this drug. If you are going to have surgery, this drug will have to be stopped temporarily.

Warning

People with chronic kidney or liver problems should not take this drug. Symptoms of low blood sugar (hypoglycemia) may be alleviated by drinking fruit juice or other foods containing sugar. However, if severe symptoms occur (seizures, convulsions, faintness, chest pains, low blood pressure, sweating) do not eat or drink anything, as choking could result. *Seek emergency medical attention.*

Comments

Type II diabetes affects women and men equally, but a disproportionate number of minorities: More than 33 percent of Hispanics and nearly 25 percent of African Americans develop this disease between age 65 and 74. Gestational diabetes occurs only during pregnancy. Women over 35 who have a family history of diabetes, are overweight, or have had gestational diabetes during a previous pregnancy are at greatest risk. *Regular monitoring by your doctor is essential if you have diabetes and are taking any antidiabetic drugs.*

Brand Name
Ambien*

Generic Name

zolpidem

Type of Drug

Sedative (nonbenzodiazepine); central nervous system (CNS) depressant.

For

Short-term treatment of insomnia, including difficulty in staying asleep or awakening too early.

Availability and Dosage

Tablets: 10 mg. Usual dose is 10 mg at bedtime, taken on an empty stomach. Follow your doctor's instructions when taking this drug. Do not take more of this medicine than is prescribed. Do not abruptly stop taking this drug without consulting your doctor.

Side Effects

More common include dizziness, nausea, diarrhea, and drowsiness. Long-term use (1 month or more) may cause headaches, back pain, constipation, memory loss, lethargy, vomiting, loss of appetite, flu-like symptoms, anxiety, and vivid dreams.

Drug Interactions

Zolpidem has the potential to interact with a variety of medications, including other CNS depressants, tricyclic antidepressants, benzodiazepines, tranquilizers, narcotic pain relievers, monoamine oxidase (MAO) inhibitor antidepressants, and antihistamines. The combination of zolpidem with any of these drugs may increase the sedative effect. Always inform your doctors of every medication you are taking, including nonprescription medicines, vitamins, herbal remedies, and dietary supplements. *Do not take any over-the-counter medications unless approved by your doctor.*

Food/Alcohol Interactions

Avoid alcohol. The combination of zolpidem and alcohol could be potentially life-threatening.

Pregnancy/Nursing

No special warnings, although all drugs during pregnancy and breast-feeding should be avoided if possible. Before taking this drug, discuss with your doctor the benefits versus the potential risks. Bottle-feed your baby if you must take this drug.

Seniors

Older adults can be more sensitive to zolpidem. Your doctor may prescribe a low dose. Falling and confusion are more common side effects in the elderly, especially with doses of 20 mg or more.

Warning

Some prescription sleep medications may cause amnesia, especially in doses larger than 10 mg per night. This drug should be taken only at bedtime, but there may be some residual effects the day after. Use caution when driving, operating machinery, or performing tasks that require mental alertness until you know how this drug will affect you the following day.

Comments

Drugs for insomnia affect only the symptoms of a possible physical or psychological disorder and not the underlying cause. Zolpidem is usually prescribed for short-term treatment of insomnia—7 to 10 days—and its effectiveness may be decreased if used for longer than 2 weeks.

Brand Name
Amerge

Generic Name

naratriptan hydrochloride

Type of Drug

Antimigraine. Naratriptan hydrochloride is used for the short-term treatment of most migraine attacks in adults. It is not used to prevent migraines, or to decrease the number of migraine attacks. There is no cure for migraine, although the condition can spontaneously disappear. Migraine headaches are more common in women, especially those of childbearing age, and they tend to run in families.

For

Short-term relief from acute migraine, characterized by severe pain and often accompanied by one or more of the following symptoms: nausea, vomiting, and sensitivity to light, sound, and smell. Attacks can last from 4 to 72 hours. This drug is not used to prevent migraines, or to treat basilar or hemiplegic migraines.

Availability and Dosage

Tablets: 1 mg, 2.5 mg. May be taken at the first sign of symptoms. Dosage should not exceed 5 mg within any 24-hour period.

Side Effects

More common include dizziness, drowsiness, fatigue, and general malaise. Others include pain or tightness in chest or throat, and feelings of tingling, heat, or skin flushing.

Drug Interactions

Do not take this drug within 24 hours of taking Imitrex (sumatriptan), other antimigraines, or medications containing ergotamine, dihydroergotamine, or methysergide. Other interactions have been reported with fluoxetene, fluvoxamine, paroxetine, and sertraline.

Food/Alcohol Interactions

Avoid alcohol and caffeine. Do not skip meals or fast. Your doctor should provide you with a list of foods, drinks, and additives that may trigger a migraine. Smoking increases the likelihood of heart-related side effects.

Pregnancy/Nursing

No special warnings, although all drugs during pregnancy and breast-feeding should be avoided if possible. Before taking this drug, discuss with your doctor the benefits versus the potential risks. Naratriptan may pass into breast milk. Bottle-feed your baby if you must take this drug.

Seniors

Not recommended. No studies of naratriptan were conducted in patients age 65 and older.

Warning

Make sure your physician has your complete medical history, especially a history of heart disease, angina, stroke, hypertension, high cholesterol, obesity, diabetes, hemiplegic or basilar migraine, smoking, and kidney or liver disease.

Comments

Migraines are the most common neurological disease, with an estimated 28 million sufferers (migraineurs) in the United States, 18 million of them women. About half of all women's migraine headaches are believed to be linked to estrogen; in these cases, migraines can disappear entirely after menopause. Migraine "triggers" include certain foods, bright lights, glare, changes in temperature, cigarette smoke, emotional factors, movement from riding in cars, planes, trains, etc., hormonal changes and medications. Migraineurs may experience an "aura"—flashing lights, zigzag lines, blind spots, loss of vision, and numbness. Medications prescribed to treat or prevent frequent migraines include calcium channel blockers, beta-blockers, and some tricyclic antidepressants. Over-the-counter medications specifically formulated for migraine are now available, but always check with your doctor or your pharmacist before self-medicating. There is no cure for migraine, but many people are finding nondrug therapeutic relief in biofeedback, massage, and acupuncture.

amitriptyline*

See Elavil

amlodipine

See Norvasc*

amlodipine/benazepril

See Lotrel*

amoxicillin*

See Amoxil*

amoxicillin and potassium clavulanate

See Augmentin*

Brand Name

Amoxil* (also Biomox, Polymox, Trimox*, Wymox)

Generic Name

amoxicillin*

Type of Drug

Antibiotic. This large class of drugs is among the most commonly prescribed, resulting in such widespread use that the bacteria they were developed to kill have become resistant to them. These "resistant" forms are then passed from person to person, further causing the spread of infections that become even more difficult to treat. Some antibiotics work against a limited number of microorganisms. Broad-spectrum antibiotics are effective against a variety of bacteria. Your doctor will prescribe the correct antibiotic depending on the type of infection. Antibiotics are useless against viral infections such as colds and flu. It is essential to take the complete course of antibiotics prescribed. If you fail to do so, increased drug resistance by any leftover bacteria is likely to occur.

For

Various infections, including urinary-tract infections (UTIs), and respiratory-tract infections; skin infections; gonorrhea.

Availability and Dosage

Tablets: 500 mg, 875 mg. Capsules: 250 mg, 500 mg. Oral suspension: 125 mg, 250 mg per 5 ml. Chewable tablets: 125 mg, 200 mg, 250 mg, 400 mg. May be taken with or without food, but should be taken with a full glass of water (not juice or soda). Take this drug at evenly spaced intervals; amoxicillin works best when the level is kept constant in the bloodstream. Always take the full course of treatment prescribed.

Side Effects

More common include nausea, vomiting, upset stomach, diarrhea, colitis, abdominal pain, and coated tongue. Other side effects include loss of appetite, itchy rash, vaginal irritation, and fungal infections.

Drug Interactions

Amoxicillin may decrease the effectiveness of oral contraceptives containing estrogen. Unplanned pregnancies have resulted from this combination. You should use additional birth control while taking this medication. This drug may also interact with a wide variety of medications, including beta-blockers, atenolol, anticoagulants (blood thinners), and other antibiotics including erythromycin. Always inform your doctors of every medication you are taking, including nonprescription medicines, vitamins, herbal remedies, and dietary supplements.

Food/Alcohol Interactions

Avoid or limit alcohol. Do not take this drug with juices or carbonated beverages.

Pregnancy/Nursing

No special warnings, although all drugs during pregnancy and breast-feeding should be avoided if possible. Before taking this drug, discuss with your doctor the benefits versus the potential risks. Bottle-feed your baby if you must take this drug.

Seniors

No special warnings. Take as directed and immediately notify your doctor of any persistent or troublesome side effects.

Warning

Before taking amoxicillin, be sure to tell your doctor if there have been any previous allergic reactions to penicillin. Serious and fatal reactions have occurred in patients if there is a history of allergy to penicillin. If you experience difficulty in breathing, skin rash, hives, wheezing, vomiting, fever, or swelling, seek emergency medical treatment.

Comments

As with any antibiotic, you should take all of the medication prescribed unless instructed otherwise. Do not stop taking this drug even if you feel that your condition is improved. Bacteria may continue growing even if symptoms are no longer present, and the infection could recur. Long-term or repeated use of antibiotics may result in secondary infections of the vagina.

anastrozole

See Arimidex

Brand Name
Ansaid

Generic Name

flurbiprofen

Type of Drug

Nonsteroidal antiinflammatory drug (NSAID). Drugs in this group reduce pain, inflammation, and stiffness associated with a wide range of conditions affecting the bones, joints, and muscles.

For

Relief of symptoms of rheumatoid arthritis and osteoarthritis, including joint pain, inflammation, stiffness, and swelling; menstrual pain; migraine.

Availability and Dosage

Tablets: 50 mg, 100 mg. May be taken with or without food, but will get into the bloodstream quicker if you take it 1 hour before or 2 hours after meals. If there is stomach irritation, however, your doctor may direct you to take it with food. Ocufen Eyedrops is the brand name of the eyedrop form of this drug, prescribed prior to eye surgery.

Side Effects

Most common include diarrhea, constipation, nausea, and drowsiness. Other side effects include stomach ulcers, fluid retention, kidney damage, jaundice, dizziness, nervousness, heart palpitations, and ringing or buzzing in the ears.

Drug Interactions

Do not combine NSAIDs with prescription or over-the-counter acetaminophen or aspirin products; they can increase stomach irritation. Flurbiprofen can also interact with anticoagulants (blood thinners), furosemide, spironolactone, beta-blockers, lithium, cimetidine, and some diuretics. Always inform your doctors of every medication you are taking, including nonprescription medicines, vitamins, herbal remedies, and dietary supplements.

Food/Alcohol Interactions

Avoid alcohol, as it may increase the possibility of stomach ulceration.

Pregnancy/Nursing

This drug is not recommended during pregnancy, especially during the last trimester. NSAIDs, including flurbiprofen, may pass into breast milk. Bottle-feed your baby if you must take this drug.

Seniors

Older people may be at increased risk for side effects, especially gastrointestinal problems.

Warning

There have been rare severe allergic reactions to flurbiprofen, including anaphylactic shock and severe skin rash. NSAIDs can cause several potentially serious side effects, including gastrointestinal disorders, dizziness, and gastric bleeding. Seek immediate medical treatment if you experience vomiting, diarrhea, rapid heartbeat, confusion, or abdominal pain. Make sure that your physician has your complete medical history, especially a history of ulcers, anemia, asthma, kidney or liver disease, or lupus.

Comments

Your physician may routinely prescribe a series of different NSAIDs in order to find the one best suited for you. Many NSAIDs can be obtained over-the-counter and are routinely used in self-medication. Side effects and interactions remain the same with nonprescription NSAIDs. When using any nonprescription NSAID, follow package directions carefully and consult your doctor if problems arise. If you are going to have surgery, you may need to discontinue this drug temporarily. Women may have a higher risk of developing ulcers while taking NSAID, particularly if you smoke or drink alcohol, are over age 60, or use corticosteroid drugs.

Brand Name
Antivert

Generic Name

meclizine

Type of Drug

Antihistamine; antiemetic. This drug affects the part of the brain that controls nausea, vomiting, and episodes of extreme dizziness (vertigo).

For

Prevention of vomiting and nausea from motion sickness; vertigo or dizziness from inner-ear disorders or other medical conditions.

Availability and Dosage

Tablets: 12.5 mg, 25 mg, 50 mg. Capsules: 50 mg. Chewable tablets: 25 mg. May be taken with or without food. When using meclizine to prevent motion sickness, the usual administration is 30 minutes to 1 hour before travel. Do not take more of this medicine than is prescribed.

Side Effects

More common include drowsiness. Others include dizziness, dry mouth, blurred vision, headache, constipation, diarrhea, upset stomach, rapid heartbeat, restlessness, and difficulty in urinating.

Drug Interactions

Meclizine interacts with central nervous system (CNS) depressants including drugs used to treat anxiety or insomnia, including diazepam; narcotic pain relievers, other antihistamines, some anticonvulsants, digoxin, some antidepressants, and some muscle relaxants. Always inform your doctors of every medication you are taking, including nonprescription medicines, vitamins, herbal remedies, and dietary supplements. *Do not take any over-the-counter medications unless approved by your doctor.*

Food/Alcohol Interactions

Avoid alcohol, as it increases the sedative effect of meclizine and may cause dizziness.

Pregnancy/Nursing

Not recommended. This drug may pass into breast milk. Bottle-feed your baby if you must take this drug.

Seniors

Meclizine has the potential to cause more adverse side effects in older adults because of its sedative qualities. Your doctor may prescribe a low dose.

Warning

Meclizine can cause drowsiness and dizziness. Do not drive, operate machinery, or perform any tasks requiring mental alertness and coordination until you know how this drug will affect you. If you are taking this medication on a regular basis for dizziness caused by inner-ear disorders, it is important to be regularly monitored by your physician.

Comments

Taking this drug with over-the-counter antihistamines, sleep aids, or cough, cold, sinus, or allergy medications may intensify drowsiness and can also cause severe dizziness. Check with your pharmacist or doctor before taking any nonprescription medication while on meclizine.

Brand Name
Arava

Generic Name

leflunomide

Type of Drug

Antirheumatic. These drugs are frequently used when aspirin and other nonsteroidal antiinflammatory drugs (NSAIDs) are not sufficient to relieve the symptoms of rheumatoid arthritis. This drug works by blocking the overproduction of immune cells that cause most arthritic inflammation.

For

Slowing of damage to joints and reduction of symptoms of rheumatoid arthritis, including joint stiffness and inflammation, during all stages of the disease.

Availability and Dosage

Tablets: 10 mg, 20 mg, 100 mg. May be taken with or without food, at the same time every day.

Side Effects

More common include hair loss, diarrhea, and skin rash. Others include elevated liver enzymes, headache, loss of appetite, changes in taste, nausea, back pain, bronchitis, and nasal congestion.

Drug Interactions

This drug has the potential to interact with methotrexate, ketoconazole, phenytoin, anticoagulants (blood thinners), and some oral antidiabetics. Do not take charcoal tablets while on this drug. Always inform your doctors of every medication you are taking, including nonprescription medicines, vitamins, herbal remedies, and dietary supplements. *Do not take any over-the-counter medications unless approved by your doctor.*

Food/Alcohol Interactions

Avoid alcohol. It can increase dizziness and the possibility of liver damage.

Pregnancy/Nursing

A woman must never become pregnant while taking this drug. You will have to take a pregnancy test before beginning treatment. Leflunomide causes birth defects or fetal death. Use reliable birth control while on this drug or if your male partner is on this drug. If you suspect you may be pregnant during your course of treatment, notify your doctor at once. Do not breast-feed while taking this drug.

Seniors

No special warnings. Take as prescribed and immediately inform your doctor of any persistent or troublesome side effects.

Warning

You must continue to use reliable birth control even after stopping use of this drug. Leflunomide remains in the body for up to 6 months and can affect a developing fetus. Discuss with your doctor the procedure necessary to completely eliminate this drug from your body before you safely become pregnant. Make sure that your doctor has your complete medical history, including a history of liver disease, hepatitis B or C, kidney disease, or other immune system disorders. You will need to be regularly monitored while on this drug to check for liver damage.

Comments

Rheumatoid arthritis—which affects three times more women than men—is a disabling form of arthritis. The cause of rheumatoid arthritis is unknown but is believed to begin with a breakdown in the immune system. It can appear at any age, although it commonly begins between ages 25 and 50. Symptoms include swelling of the hands and wrists, inflammation in three or more joints, and, in its most severe form, can become crippling and disfiguring. There are more than 100 forms of arthritis, and the total number of arthritis patients is expected to reach 60 million by 2020.

Brand Name
Aricept

Generic Name

donepezil

Type of Drug

Acetylcholinesterase inhibitor (chemical nerve-muscle coordinator). Acetylcholinesterase breaks down the neurotransmitter acetylcholine, thought to be associated with memory and learning. Acetylcholine is in short supply in patients with Alzheimer's disease. This drug is not a cure for Alzheimer's, but it produces improvement in mild to moderate symptoms, including loss of memory, language skills, alertness, and the ability to perform simple activities. Clinical trials in more than 900 patients indicated that more than 80 percent of patients taking donepezil either experienced improvement or showed no further deterioration in cognitive skills.

For

Alzheimer's disease.

Availability and Dosage

Tablets: 5 mg, 10 mg. Usual dosage is once daily at bedtime. May be taken with or without food. If the patient does not respond to the lower dose, it may be increased to 10 mg.

Side Effects

More common include nausea, vomiting, diarrhea, insomnia, fatigue, loss of appetite, and muscle cramps. Others include fainting, headache, dizziness, and depression. Side effects appear more frequently with 10 mg dosage.

Drug Interactions

This drug may interact with carbamazepine, phenytoin, dexamethasone, rifampin, some surgical muscle relaxants, dicyclomine, and phenobarbital. Always inform your doctors of every medication you are taking, including nonprescription medicines, vitamins, herbal remedies, and dietary supplements. *Do not take any over-the-counter medications unless approved by your doctor.*

Food/Alcohol Interactions

Avoid alcohol. Patients should not smoke while taking this drug.

Pregnancy/Nursing

Not recommended.

Seniors

No special warnings. Caregivers should immediately inform the doctor of any persistent or troublesome side effects.

Warning

Those patients at increased risk for developing ulcers should be closely monitored while on donepezil, especially those who also take nonsteroidal antiinflammatory drugs (NSAIDs). Make sure that the doctor has a complete medical history of the patient, including a history of heart disease, asthma, or seizures. Regular medical examinations are imperative for suspected Alzheimer's patients to evaluate the progression of the disease.

Comments

Although there are more than twenty-two new drugs in the research and development stage for this devastating and incurable disease, Aricept (donepezil) and Cognex (tacrine hydrochloride) are the only medications currently prescribed for Alzheimer's. Neither drug slows the progression or delays the onset of the disease. Recent studies on vitamin E and the antiparkinsonian drug Eldepryl (selegiline) suggest that using them may postpone the need for nursing-home care; some doctors are currently recommending vitamin E. Findings from other studies suggest that estrogen replacement therapy may slow the onset or even help to prevent Alzheimer's in postmenopausal women. Additional research indicates that antiinflammatory medications such as ibuprofen and naproxen may also help to postpone symptoms. Preliminary studies also point to the possibility of a vaccine that may prevent or even reverse brain lesions. More than 4 million Americans are affected by Alzheimer's—1 in 10 of those age 65 and older, nearly half of those age 85 and older—a figure that is expected to rise to 14 million by 2050. One of the most significant discoveries about this disease is that we now know that changes in the brain can take place from 20 to 40 years before any symptoms are seen. With the boomer generation aging and life spans increasing, the number of people with Alzheimer's could be as high as 14 million by mid-century.

Brand Name
Arimidex

Generic Name
anastrozole

Type of Drug
Anticancer (antineoplastic). This drug is a member of a new class of medications available to treat advanced breast cancer in postmenopausal women whose disease has progressed following therapy with Nolvadex (tamoxifen citrate).

For
Breast cancer.

Availability and Dosage

Tablets: 1 mg. Usual dosage is once daily. May be taken with or without food, at the same time every day. Do not stop taking this drug without consulting with your doctor.

Side Effects

More common include fatigue, nausea, headache, hot flashes, pain, and back pain. Others include dizziness, weight gain, weakness, loss of appetite, cough, and vaginal bleeding.

Drug Interactions

No special warnings, although all drugs have the ability to interact with other drugs. Report any problems to your doctor. Always inform your doctors of every medication you are taking, including nonprescription medicines, vitamins, herbal remedies, and dietary supplements. *Do not take any over-the-counter medications unless approved by your doctor.*

Food/Alcohol Interactions

Avoid alcohol. Follow a healthy diet and drink plenty of fluids while on any form of chemotherapy.

Pregnancy/Nursing

A woman must never become pregnant while taking this drug. Anastrozole is not prescribed for premenopausal women. Make sure you are not pregnant before beginning treatment. Bottle-feed your baby if you must take this drug.

Seniors

Older adults may be more susceptible to adverse reactions.

Warning

You will need to be regularly monitored while on this drug. Report any vaginal bleeding to your doctor at once.

Comments

Approximately two-thirds of breast cancers are hormone dependent, meaning that tumor growth is promoted by estrogen or progesterone. Anastrozole selectively suppresses aromatase—an enzyme that converts male hormones (androgens) to female hormones (estrogens)—leading to reduction of estrogens. The drug trials included patients whose cancer had progressed after they had received Nolvadex (tamoxifen citrate) as part of their initial breast-cancer therapy or as therapy for advanced cancer. Breast cancer is the second-leading cause of cancer death in women in the United States.

atenolol

See Tenormin

Brand Name
Ativan (also Alzapam)

Generic Name
lorazepam*

Type of Drug
Benzodiazepine tranquilizer. These drugs are central nervous system (CNS) depressants, and work on the part of the brain that controls emotion by slowing nervous system transmissions. They are often used to relieve the symptoms of anxiety but do not address the underlying cause.

For
Anxiety; agitation; panic attacks; irritable bowel syndrome (IBS); insomnia.

Availability and Dosage
Tablets: 0.5 mg, 1 mg, 2 mg. Oral solution: 2 mg per ml. Should be taken without food but may be taken with food if stomach upset occurs. Do not take more of this medicine than is prescribed. Do not abruptly stop taking this medication; doing so may cause adverse reactions including seizures, abdominal cramps, and confusion.

Side Effects
More common include drowsiness, unsteadiness, dizziness, weakness, and light-headedness. Others include confusion, headache, nausea, rash, change in sex drive, constipation, fatigue, and weight loss or weight gain.

Drug Interactions
This drug has the potential to interact with other central nervous system (CNS) depressants, resulting in increased sedation. These interactions can occur with antianxiety drugs, antihistamines, some antidepressants, narcotic pain relievers, antipsychotics, and drugs used for insomnia. Other interactions may occur with digoxin, erythromycin, oral contraceptives, levodopa, and cimetidine. Always inform your doctors of every medication you are taking, including nonprescription medicines, vitamins,

herbal remedies, and dietary supplements. *Do not take any over-the-counter medications unless approved by your doctor.*

Food/Alcohol Interactions

Avoid alcohol, as it will increase the sedative effects of lorazepam.

Pregnancy/Nursing

Not recommended at any time, but especially during the first trimester. Bottle-feed your baby if you must take this drug.

Seniors

Older adults may experience an increase in side effects, especially oversedation. Your doctor may prescribe a low dose.

Warning

Lorazepam has a high risk of physical and psychological dependency. Make sure your doctor has your complete medical history, including a history of alcohol or drug abuse, depression or other mental disorder, suicidal tendencies, sleep apnea, hyperactivity, or kidney or liver disease. Do not drive, operate machinery, or perform tasks requiring concentration or mental alertness until you know how this drug will affect you.

Comments

This drug is usually prescribed for short-term treatment of the above conditions, for anywhere from 2 to 4 months. This drug may lose its effectiveness over time. If you must take this drug for a longer period of time, regular and careful monitoring by your doctor is essential. When it is time to stop taking this drug, your dose will have to be reduced gradually to avoid symptoms of withdrawal.

Brand Name
Atrovent*

Generic Name

ipratropium

Type of Drug

Anticholinergic; bronchodilator.

For

Bronchial spasms associated with bronchitis and emphysema.

Availability and Dosage

Inhalation aerosol, 14 gram metered-dose inhaler: 18 mcg per inhalation. This medication comes with directions for use. Follow instructions carefully for using and cleaning the aerosol spray device. If you have questions, your pharmacist or doctor will demonstrate proper use of the inhaler. Do not abruptly stop taking this medication without consulting your doctor even if you begin to feel better; doing so may cause your symptoms to worsen.

Side Effects

More common include dizziness, headache, dry mouth, and nasal irritation. Side effects may diminish as your body adjusts to this medication.

Drug Interactions

No special warnings, although all drugs have the ability to interact with other drugs. If you are using other types of inhalation drugs while taking ipratropium, ask your doctor about properly spacing the dosages of each. Report any problems to your doctor or your pharmacist.

Food/Alcohol Interactions

No special warnings.

Pregnancy/Nursing

No special warnings, although all drugs during pregnancy and breast-feeding should be avoided if possible. Before taking this drug, discuss with your doctor the benefits versus the potential risks.

Seniors

No special warnings. Take as prescribed and immediately inform your doctor of any persistent or troublesome side effects.

Warning

Adverse reactions are rare, but if you experience difficulty in swallowing, hives, sores in mouth or on lips, or eye pain, notify your doctor immediately.

Comments

If you have glaucoma, use extra caution to avoid spraying this medication into your eyes. It may cause blurred vision and irritation. Rinse with cool water immediately and call your doctor or your pharmacist if irritation persists.

Brand Name
Augmentin*

Generic Name
amoxicillin and clavulanic acid

Type of Drug
Antibiotic. This large class of drugs is among the most commonly prescribed, resulting in such widespread use that the bacteria they were developed to kill have become resistant to them. These "resistant" forms are then passed from person to person, further causing the spread of infections that become even more difficult to treat. Your doctor will prescribe the correct antibiotic depending on the type of infection. Antibiotics are useless against viral infections such as colds and flu.

For
Bacterial infections.

Availability and Dosage
Tablets: 250 mg amoxicillin and 125 mg clavulanic acid, 500 mg amoxicillin and 125 mg clavulanic acid. Chewable tablets: 125 mg amoxicillin and 31.25 mg clavulanic acid; 250 mg amoxicillin and 62.5 mg clavulanic acid. Oral suspension: 125 mg amoxicillin and 31.25 mg clavulanic acid per 5 ml; 250 mg amoxicillin and 62.5 mg clavulanic acid per 5 ml. May be taken with or without food, but should be taken with a full glass of water (not juice or soda). It is essential to take the complete course of antibiotics prescribed. If you fail to do so, increased drug resistance by any leftover bacteria is likely to occur.

Side Effects
More common are nausea, diarrhea, rash, stomach pain, headache, mouth pain, white patches in mouth or on tongue, and vaginal discharge. Others include loss of appetite, weakness, and anemia.

Drug Interactions
This antibiotic may decrease the effectiveness of oral contraceptives containing estrogen. Unplanned pregnancies have resulted from this combination. You should use additional birth control while taking this medication. This drug should not be used in combination with other antibiotics, including erythromycin, tetracycline, and neomycin. Other interactions may occur with methotrexate, allopurinol, some beta blockers, and atenolol.

Food/Alcohol Interactions

Avoid or limit alcohol. Drink plenty of water while on this medication.

Pregnancy/Nursing

No special warnings, although all drugs during pregnancy and breast-feeding should be avoided if possible. Before taking this drug, discuss with your doctor the benefits versus the potential risks.

Seniors

No special warnings. Take as prescribed and immediately inform your doctor of any persistent or troublesome side effects.

Warning

Before taking amoxicillin, be sure to tell your doctor if you have had any previous allergic reaction to penicillin. Serious and fatal reactions have occurred in patients if there is a history of allergy to penicillins. People who have hay fever, asthma, or allergies may be more susceptible to penicillin reactions. If you experience difficulty in breathing, skin rash, hives, wheezing, vomiting, fever, or swelling, seek emergency medical treatment.

Comments

As with any other antibiotic, you should take all of the medication prescribed unless instructed otherwise. Do not stop taking this drug even if you feel that your condition has improved. Bacteria may continue growing even if symptoms are no longer present, and the infection could recur. Long-term or repeated use of antibiotics may result in secondary infections of the vagina.

auranofin

See Ridaura

Brand Name
Avandia

Generic Name

rosiglitazone

Type of Drug

Antidiabetic. When combined with dietary changes and exercise habits, antidiabetic drugs provide relief of symptoms and enable most diabetics to lead healthy and productive lives. You should wear a medical identification tag at all times and carry an ID card that lists your medications.

For

Type II non-insulin–dependent diabetes mellitus (NIDDM).

Availability and Dosage

Tablets: 2 mg, 4 mg.

Side Effects

More common include pain, headache, weight gain, edema, and infection.

Drug Interactions

No special warnings, although all drugs have the ability to interact with other drugs. Report any problems to your doctor or your pharmacist. Always inform your doctors of every medication you are taking, including nonprescription medicines, vitamins, herbal remedies, and dietary supplements. *Do not take any over-the-counter medications unless approved by your doctor.*

Food/Alcohol Interactions

Avoid or limit alcohol. You will probably be on a special diet to help control your diabetes.

Pregnancy/Nursing

Not recommended: Pregnant diabetic women are usually treated with insulin. Rosiglitazone may pass into breast milk. Bottle-feed your baby if you must take this drug.

Seniors

No special warnings. Take as prescribed and immediately inform your doctor of any persistent or troublesome side effects.

Warning

Rosiglitazone has not been linked with the increased risk of liver damage associated with Rezulin (troglitazone). Studies of more than 4,000 patients showed no evidence of liver damage. However, liver-function tests are recommended before beginning treatment with rosiglitazone and should be continued periodically as long as you are on this drug. If you experience nausea, vomiting, jaundice, abdominal pain, dark urine, or fatigue, notify your doctor immediately.

Comments

This drug may cause ovulation to resume in premenopausal women who have stopped ovulating. Use a reliable form of birth control while on this medication.

Brand Name
Avonex

Generic Name

interferon beta 1-a

Type of Drug

Interferon. This drug is not a cure for multiple sclerosis, but its antiviral effect does slow the progression of the disease in patients with relapsing forms of the disease. It also reduces the annual relapse rate of multiple sclerosis. This drug has not been evaluated in patients who have chronic progressive multiple sclerosis.

For

Multiple sclerosis.

Availability and Dosage

Intramuscular injection: 30 mcg once a week. This drug is intended for use under the guidance and supervision of a physician. Patients may self-inject interferon beta 1-a with proper training in intramuscular injection technique and medical follow-up as necessary. A four-week supply contains four administration dose packs, each of which includes: a single-use vial of interferon beta 1-a 30 mcg, a 10 cc vial, a 3 cc syringe, a Micro Pin® vial access pin, a needle, two alcohol swabs, and an adhesive bandage.

Side Effects

More common include flu-like symptoms, muscle aches, fever, chills, weakness, and reactions at the injection site. Some side effects may diminish as your body adjusts to the medication.

Drug Interactions

This drug may interact with zidovudine (AZT), used to treat HIV infection.

Food/Alcohol Interactions

No special warnings.

Pregnancy/Nursing

Not recommended. Use reliable birth control while on this drug. Bottle-feed your baby if you must take this drug.

Seniors

No special warnings. Take as prescribed and immediately inform your doctor of any persistent or troublesome side effects.

Warning

Interferon beta 1-a should be used with caution in patients who have depression. Depression and suicide have occurred in patients receiving other interferon compounds. Make sure your doctor knows your complete medical history, including a history of heart disease, angina, arrhythmia, or seizures. You must be regularly monitored by your doctor while on this drug.

Comments

Approximately 250,000 people in the United States have multiple sclerosis, two-thirds of them women. This inflammatory disease of the central nervous system—in which scarring of nerve fibers in the brain and spinal cord occurs—typically starts in young adults age 20 to 40. Symptoms vary, but include weakness, fatigue, vision problems, impaired coordination, slurred speech, short-term memory loss, depression, partial or complete paralysis, and bladder or bowel dysfunction. In the relapsing forms of the disease, symptoms may appear and disappear; the progressive form is marked by steady worsening of symptoms. Another interferon drug, Betaseron (interferon 1-b), is also used to treat the relapsing form of MS; it is self-injected every other day.

Brand Name
Axid*

Generic Name

nizatidine

Type of Drug

Histamine H_2 blocker; antiulcer. Histamine is a chemical that produces a variety of effects, including increased secretion of stomach acid. Antihistamines traditionally used for allergies do not block the effect of histamine on stomach acid.

For

Stomach and duodenal ulcers; heartburn; gastroesophageal reflux disease (GERD).

Availability and Dosage

Capsules: 150 mg, 300 mg. May be taken with or without food. Take with water (not juice or soda). Dosages vary depending on the condition being treated. Do not take more of this medicine than is prescribed. Do not stop taking this drug even if you feel better before the prescribed course of treatment is finished.

Side Effects

More common include headache, diarrhea, nausea, fatigue, and drowsiness.

Drug Interactions

Nizatidine has been shown to increase blood levels of aspirin in patients who take high doses (3,900 mg per day) of aspirin. Always inform your doctors of every medication you are taking, including nonprescription medicines, vitamins, herbal remedies, and dietary supplements.

Food/Alcohol Interactions

Avoid alcohol. Avoid or limit foods and beverages high in acid content, including citrus and tomatoes. Avoid or limit caffeine in foods and beverages.

Pregnancy/Nursing

Not recommended.

Seniors

Older patients who have impaired kidney function may experience increased side effects. Your doctor may prescribe a low dose.

Warning

Make sure your doctor has your complete medical history, including a history of liver or kidney disease. Patients who have impaired kidney function will need to be regularly monitored while on this drug. If you have an ulcer, notify your doctor immediately if any of the following occurs: diarrhea, black or tarry stools, vomiting, fever, chills, or worsening stomach pain. These may be signs of a bleeding ulcer.

Comments

Gastroesophageal reflux disease (GERD) occurs when stomach contents flow back into the esophagus, irritating the sensitive lining and causing heartburn. A severe form of GERD (erosive esophagitis) can result in sores or erosions in the esophagus. Histamine H_2 blockers (which include cimetidine, famotidine, nizatidine, and ranitidine) are among the most prescribed drugs in the United States. Axid AR is the nonprescription form of nizatadine. Follow package directions, do not take more often than needed, and consult your doctor if symptoms worsen. Smoking is known to aggravate stomach ulcers by increasing stomach acid secretion and may interfere with the effectiveness of this medication.

azithromycin

See Zithromax*

Brand Name
Azmacort Aerosol* (also Nasacort Aerosol)

Generic Name
triamcinolone acetonide

Type of Drug
Corticosteroid inhaler.

For
Chronic asthma. (Nasacort Aerosol is prescribed only to relieve symptoms of hay fever and allergic rhinitis: runny nose, postnasal drip, sneezing, and nasal congestion.)

Availability and Dosage
Inhalation aerosol, 0.1 mg per metered spray. Dosage for each patient must be determined individually. Triamcinolone is also available in tablets, topical cream, topical ointment, topical lotion, injectable, and dental paste. The tablet form can be used as an antiinflammatory. Do not increase frequency or dosage of this medication.

Side Effects

More common include cough and dry mouth. Others include headache, nausea, bad taste in mouth, nosebleed, loss of taste, and throat irritation.

Drug Interactions

Triamcinolone has the potential to interact with nonsteroidal antiinflammatory drugs (NSAIDs), anticoagulants (blood thinners), phenytoin, oral contraceptives, antidiabetics, diuretics, other corticosteroids, and digoxin. Serious interactions have occurred with certain vaccinations. Always inform your doctors of every medication you are taking, including nonprescription medicines, vitamins, herbal remedies, and dietary supplements.

Food/Alcohol Interactions

No special warnings.

Pregnancy/Nursing

Not recommended.

Seniors

No special warnings. Take as prescribed and immediately inform your doctor of any persistent or troublesome side effects.

Warning

Do not use this drug to treat an acute asthma attack in progress. This drug is used to prevent asthma attacks. Long-term use requires supervision by a physician. If triamcinolone is used in high doses or for an extended period of time, there is an increased possibility of adverse reactions. If you develop white patches or sores in your mouth, have difficulty in breathing, or notice increased wheezing, notify your doctor immediately.

Comments

The inhalation forms of triamcinolone for asthma come with detailed instructions for use of the inhaler. Consult your doctor or your pharmacist if you need a demonstration of how to use and clean the inhaler properly. Nasacort nasal spray should be used regularly to be effective against allergic rhinitis; it may take several days before you notice improvement in symptoms.

Brand Name
Bactrim (also Septra, Septra DS, Cotrim, Cotrim DS)

Generic Name

trimethoprim and sulfamethoxazole

Type of Drug

Antiinfective. Combination of two antibiotics.

For

Urinary-tract infections (UTIs); bronchitis.

Availability and Dosage

Tablets: 100 mg (80 mg trimethoprim and 400 mg sulfamethoxazole); 200 mg (160 mg trimethoprim and 800 mg sulfamethoxazole). Oral suspension: 40 mg trimethoprim and 200 mg sulfamethoxazole per 5 ml. Take this medicine with a full glass of water, and be sure to finish the complete course of treatment.

Side Effects

More common include skin rash, itching, and increased sensitivity to sunlight. Others are aches and pains in joints, allergic reactions, diarrhea, dizziness, headache, and nausea.

Drug Interactions

This drug may enhance the effect of some oral antidiabetic drugs, which can cause low levels of blood sugar. Other potential interactions can take place with blood thinners, anticonvulsants, methotrexate (Rheumatrex), and thiazide diuretics (water pills). Always inform your doctors of every medication you are taking, including nonprescription medicines, vitamins, herbal remedies, and dietary supplements.

Food/Alcohol Interactions

No special warnings. Drink plenty of water while on this medication to reduce the possibility of kidney problems.

Pregnancy/Nursing

Not recommended. You and your doctor will need to discuss whether the potential benefits outweigh the risks.

Seniors

The potential for side effects is increased in older people. Contact your doctor immediately if you have any type of allergic reaction: difficulty breathing, increased thirst, lower back pain, or pain or difficulty in urinating.

Warning

This drug should be used cautiously by people who have kidney or liver disease or any kind of blood disorder (including AIDS patients). It can result in anemia or other serious blood disorders. If you experience unusual bleeding or bruising, bluish nails or lips, fever, chills, jaundice, or sore throat, seek immediate medical help.

Comments

If you must take this drug for a long time, it is important that your doctor do periodic blood tests to check for folic acid deficiency, among other problems. Wear protective clothing when outdoors, and apply sunscreen with an SPF factor of at least 15 to exposed areas, including your lips. Do not use tanning beds or tanning lamps.

Brand Name
Bactroban*

Generic Name

mupirocin

Type of Drug

Topical antibiotic.

For

Impetigo and minor bacterial skin infections.

Availability and Dosage

Topical ointment: 2%. Dosage is to be determined individually. If the infection is still present after the initial course of treatment, consult your doctor about other treatments.

Side Effects

Itching, redness, rash, swelling, pain. Report these to your doctor if they become persistent or severe.

Drug Interactions

No special warnings. However, all drugs, have the potential to interact with other drugs. Always inform your doctors of every medication you are taking, including nonprescription medicines, vitamins, herbal remedies, and dietary supplements.

Food/Alcohol Interactions

No special warnings.

Pregnancy/Nursing

No special warnings, although the use of all drugs during pregnancy and breast-feeding should be kept to a minimum.

Seniors

No special warnings. Take as prescribed and immediately inform your doctor of any side effects.

Warning

Notify your doctor if you have ever had an allergic reaction to other topical antibiotics. In order to minimize problems, do not use any cosmetic skin products such as creams, lotions, or perfumes on the affected area.

Comments

A newer form of mupirocin, called Bactroban Nasal, is formulated to kill staphylococcus (staph) bacteria found in the nasal passages.

beclomethasone

See Vancenase AQ

Beconase AQ

See Vancenase AQ

benazepril

See Lotensin*

Brand Name
Bentyl

Generic Name
dicyclomine hydrochloride

Type of Drug
Antispasmodic.

For
Irritable bowel syndrome (IBS); spastic colon.

Availability and Dosage
Tablets: 20 mg. Capsules: 10 mg. Oral syrup: 10 mg per 5 ml. Should be taken with water on an empty stomach, 30 minutes to 1 hour before meals, or 2 hours after a meal.

Side Effects
More common include dry mouth, constipation, headache, and sensitivity to light (eyes). Others are drowsiness, blurred vision, and reduction in breast milk. Because this medication causes reduced perspiration, you may be at risk for heatstroke. Avoid excessive activity in hot weather.

Drug Interactions
Antacids, antiulcers, and antifungals (ketoconazole) can interfere with absorption. Drugs that have a sedative effect such as antihistamines and benzodiazepines can enhance the sedative effect of this drug. This drug should not be taken with other drugs of its type (anticholinergic). Always inform your doctors of every medication you are taking, including nonprescription medicines, vitamins, herbal remedies, and dietary supplements.

Food/Alcohol Interactions
Avoid alcohol, as it may increase the sedative effects of this drug.

Pregnancy/Nursing
No special warnings, although the use of all drugs during pregnancy should be kept to a minimum. Not recommended for nursing mothers as it has been shown to reduce the amount of breast milk.

Seniors

Your doctor may prescribe a lower dose, as older people may experience increased side effects, especially agitation, confusion, memory loss, and dizziness.

Warning

Do not drive or operate machinery until you have determined how this medication affects you. Drowsiness, dizziness, and blurred vision are possible side effects that could interfere with your ability to perform tasks requiring mental alertness and concentration. Notify your doctor if you have heart disease, hiatal hernia, high blood pressure, or glaucoma, as this drug should be used with caution in these instances.

Comments

Dicyclomine works by relieving cramping caused by spasms in the gastrointestinal tract. It slows the movement of the GI tract and decreases the production of digestive secretions.

betamethasone and clotrimazole

See Lotrisone*

Brand Name
Betapace

Generic Name

sotalol HCL

Type of Drug

Beta-blocker. These drugs block the response of the heart and blood vessels, lower the pulse rate, and reduce the force of the heartbeat, thereby reducing the workload of the heart. They are sometimes prescribed after a heart attack to help prevent future attacks.

For

High blood pressure; heart arrhythmia; migraines.

Availability and Dosage

Tablets: 80 mg, 120 mg, 160 mg, 240 mg. Should be taken on an empty stomach, 1 hour before meals or 2 hours after.

Side Effects

More common include fatigue, bradycardia (pulse rate under 50 beats per minute), and shortness of breath. Others include increased arrhythmia, weakness, and dizziness. If you are planning to have surgery, make sure the anesthesiologist knows you are on this medication.

Drug Interactions

Drugs given for heart disease have the most potential for interaction with sotalol, including calcium channel blockers and digitalis drugs. Other interactions may occur with migraine medications in the ergot-alkaloid drug class, thyroid hormone replacements, and anticonvulsants. Notify your doctor if you are taking an MAO inhibitor such as Nardil or Parnate. Always inform your doctors of every medication you are taking, including nonprescription medicines, vitamins, herbal remedies, and dietary supplements.

Food/Alcohol Interactions

No special warnings.

Pregnancy/Nursing

Not recommended. Sotalol should not be taken by women who might become pregnant while on this drug. The drug also passes into breast milk. You should bottle-feed your baby while on this drug.

Seniors

Your doctor may start with a lower dose to minimize the possibility of side effects.

Warning

This drug should be used with caution in patients who have bronchial asthma, congestive heart failure, heart block, or liver or kidney disease. Make sure your doctor has your entire medical history if you are prescribed this drug.

Comments

Do not abruptly stop taking this drug without consulting your doctor. Sudden withdrawal may result in irregular heartbeat, difficulty in breathing, or chest pain.

Betaseron

See **Avonex**

Brand Name
Biaxin*

Generic Name

clarithromycin

Type of Drug

Antibiotic. Drugs in this class are among the most commonly prescribed, resulting in such widespread use that there now exists the danger of "resistant" bacteria that have become even more difficult to treat. Your doctor will prescribe the correct antibiotic depending on the type of infection. Antibiotics are useless against viral infections such as colds and flu.

For

Sinus and respiratory-tract infections; "strep" throat; pneumonia.

Availability and Dosage

Tablets: 250 mg, 500 mg. Also available in oral suspension in varying dosages. Should be taken with a full glass of water, with or without food. Food may alleviate possible nausea or stomach upset. Be sure to finish the entire course of treatment while on this or any other antibiotic. Antibiotics are most effective when taken at evenly spaced intervals on a daily basis.

Side Effects

More common are stomach upset, diarrhea, nausea, and stomach cramps.

Drug Interactions

Some antibiotics have been known to interfere with the effectiveness of oral contraceptives. Potential drug interactions can also occur with blood thinners (anticoagulants), anticonvulsants, and digitalis drugs. Always inform your doctors of every medication you are taking, including nonprescription medicines, vitamins, herbal remedies, and dietary supplements.

Food/Alcohol Interactions

No special warnings.

Pregnancy/Nursing

Not recommended.

Seniors

Your doctor may initially prescribe a lower dose to minimize the possibility of adverse effects. Notify your doctor if you have kidney disease.

Warning

If you have any allergic reaction to this medication, such as skin rash, vomiting, difficulty in breathing, swelling, or severe diarrhea, notify your doctor immediately.

Comments

Long-term or repeated use of antibiotics can result in secondary infections of the vagina.

Biomox

See Amoxil*

bisoprolol HCTZ

See Ziac*

Brevicon

See Oral Contraceptives

budesonide

See Rhinocort*

bupropion

See Wellbutrin

bupropion HCL

See Zyban*

Brand Name
BuSpar*

Generic Name

buspirone

Type of Drug

Antianxiety; tranquilizer

For

Anxiety; symptoms of premenstrual tension (PMS), including aches, cramps, and fatigue.

Availability and Dosage

Tablets: 5 mg, 10 mg. Can be taken with or without food. Take with water at regular intervals, and do not take more of this medicine than is prescribed.

Side Effects

More common include dizziness, drowsiness, nausea, headache, nervousness, light-headedness, and excitement. Others include nightmares, ringing in the ears, and weakness.

Drug Interactions

A potentially dangerous interaction exists between buspirone and any monoamine oxidase (MAO) inhibitors such as Nardil and Parnate. Interactions may also occur with any drugs that affect the central nervous system, such as benzodiazepines and other antianxiety drugs. Always inform your doctors of every medication you are taking, including nonprescription medicines, vitamins, herbal remedies, and dietary supplements.

Food/Alcohol Interactions

Avoid alcohol as it may increase drowsiness and dizziness.

Pregnancy/Nursing

If possible, the use of all drugs during pregnancy should be avoided. This drug should be used during pregnancy only if clearly needed as determined by your doctor.

Seniors

No special warnings. Take as prescribed and notify your doctor of any troublesome side effects.

Warning

Make sure that the doctor prescribing this or any other antidepressant knows your entire medical history. Avoid driving or operating machinery until you know the effects of this drug on your mental alertness and concentration.

Comments

This drug is usually prescribed for persistent anxiety that has lasted six months or more, along with other physical and mental symptoms such as irritability, muscle tension, difficulty in concentrating, and sleep disturbances.

buspirone

*See BuSpar**

Brand Name
Calan SR (also Calan, Isoptin, Isoptin SR, Verelan)

Generic Name

verapamil SR*

Type of Drug

Calcium channel blocker; antianginal; antihypertensive. Calcium channel blockers are used for the prevention of chest pain, or angina. They are also used to correct certain heart arrhythmias (irregular heartbeats) and to lower blood pressure by blocking or slowing the flow of blood into the two chambers of the heart.

For

Angina pectoris; irregular heartbeat; high blood pressure. Calan SR (sustained-release formula) is used only to treat high blood pressure.

Availability and Dosage

Tablets: 40 mg, 80 mg, and 120 mg. Sustained-release tablets: 120 mg, 180 mg, and 240 mg. Sustained-release capsules: 120 mg, 180 mg, and 240 mg. Regular form of verapamil should be taken on an empty stomach, 1 hour before or 2 hours after meals. Sustained-release forms can be taken with or without food.

Side Effects

More common include headache, constipation, and palpitations. Others include low blood pressure, weakness, nausea, diarrhea, ringing in the ears, and rash.

Drug Interactions

Verapamil may interact with beta-blockers, other antihypertensives, cimetidine, ranitidine, carbamazepine, aspirin, digoxin, lithium, and some anticonvulsants. Always inform your doctors of every medication you are taking, including nonprescription medicines, vitamins, herbal remedies, and dietary supplements. *Do not take any over-the-counter medications unless approved by your doctor.*

Food/Alcohol Interactions

Avoid alcohol. Do not take with grapefruit juice.

Pregnancy/Nursing

Not recommended. This drug passes into breast milk but its effects are unknown. Discuss with your doctor the benefits versus the potential risks.

Seniors

Side effects may be more frequent and severe, including low blood pressure. Your doctor may prescribe a low dose.

Warning

If you experience dizziness, swelling of the lower legs or ankles, fainting, chest pain, or a pulse rate lower than 50 beats per minute, contact your doctor immediately.

Comments

Verapamil is also sometimes prescribed for mitral valve prolapse (MVP) syndrome, an inherited condition in which a "floppy" mitral valve of the heart is linked to an underlying disorder of the autonomic nervous system. Diagnosis is usually made by echocardiogram (heart sonogram). Symptoms include debilitating fatigue, "pounding" heartbeat, palpitations, dizziness, vertigo, balance disorders, chest pain, esophageal spasm, irritable bowel syndrome (IBS), panic disorder, depression, premenstrual syndrome (PMS), headache, migraine, and sleep disorders. Treatment includes dietary changes, adequate hydration, exercise, medication, and herbal or dietary supplements. Proper education and ongoing management of MVP is essential to living with this disorder, which affects primarily women. If a doctor tells you that MVP syndrome is "all in your head," find a doctor who is educated and aware of this syndrome.

calcitonin salmon

See Miacalcin Nasal*

capecitabine

See Xeloda

Brand Name
Capoten

Generic Name
captopril

Type of Drug
Angiotensin-converting enzyme (ACE) inhibitor. These drugs are used to treat high blood pressure (hypertension). They work by blocking an enzyme in the body required to produce a substance that causes blood vessels to tighten. When this enzyme is blocked, blood vessels are relaxed, blood pressure is lowered, the workload of the heart and arteries is reduced, and blood and oxygen supplies are increased.

For
High blood pressure and congestive heart failure.

Availability and Dosage
Tablets: 12.5 mg, 25 mg, 50 mg, 100 mg. Captopril is best taken on an empty stomach, 1 hour before or 2 hours after a meal.

Side Effects
Most common in women include a dry, hacking cough. Others include dizziness, fatigue, weakness, nausea, drowsiness, diarrhea, constipation, loss of appetite, dry mouth, and chest pain. Always inform your doctors of every medication you are taking, including nonprescription medicines, vitamins, herbal remedies, and dietary supplements. *Do not take any over-the-counter medications unless approved by your doctor.*

Drug Interactions

Captopril may interact with a wide variety of medications including some diuretics, potassium supplements, beta-blockers, arthritis drugs, antidiabetics, antihypertensives, lithium, capsaicin, anticoagulants (blood thinners), and nonsteroidal antiinflammatory drugs (NSAIDs). Do not take antacids within 2 hours of taking captopril. Always inform your doctors of every medication you are taking, including nonprescription medicines, vitamins, herbal remedies, and dietary supplements. *Do not take any over-the-counter medications unless approved by your doctor.*

Food/Alcohol Interactions

Avoid or limit alcohol. Do not use salt substitutes, low-sodium milk, or other foods or beverages high in potassium, but discuss any dietary changes with your doctor first.

Pregnancy/Nursing

Not recommended, especially during the second and third trimesters. This drug passes into breast milk. Bottle-feed your baby while on this drug.

Seniors

Side effects may be more severe and frequent if you have impaired kidney function. Your doctor may prescribe a low dose.

Warning

Do not self-medicate with any over-the-counter remedies for coughs, colds, allergies, stimulants, or appetite suppressants.

Comments

Congestive heart failure—when the heart cannot keep blood circulating adequately—compromises kidney function, resulting in a buildup of sodium. ACE inhibitors are among the most commonly prescribed drugs for hypertension, which is referred to as the "silent killer" because there are often no symptoms. Untreated hypertension can lead to stroke, which affects women more often than men—and the risk increases with each decade after age 35. Statistics indicate that African American women are at higher risk than are white women. A woman can decrease her risk of stroke and heart attack by making lifestyle changes—quit smoking, begin an aerobic exercise program, eat a low-fat diet, and take medications if necessary, including hormone replacement therapy that may possibly protect the heart after menopause.

capsaicin

See Zostrix

captopril

See Capoten

carbamazepine

See Tegretol

carbidopa and levodopa

See Sinemet

Brand Name

Cardizem CD* (also Cardizem, Cardizem SR, Dilacor SR)

Generic Name

diltiazem hydrochloride

Type of Drug

Calcium channel blocker. These drugs are used for the prevention of chest pain, or angina. They are also used to correct certain heart arrhythmias (irregular heartbeats) and to lower blood pressure by blocking or slowing the flow of blood into the two chambers of the heart.

For

Angina pectoris.

Availability and Dosage

Tablets: 30 mg, 60 mg, 90 mg, 120 mg. Extended-release capsules: 180 mg, 240 mg, 300 mg. Sustained-release capsules: 60 mg, 90 mg, 120 mg. Should be taken on an empty stomach, 1 hour before or 2 hours after meals.

Side Effects

More common include headache, slow pulse, palpitations. dizziness, and fluid retention. Others include diarrhea, constipation, weakness, nervousness, and insomnia.

Drug Interactions

Diltiazem may interact with beta-blockers, cimetidine, digoxin, antihypertensives, carbamazepine, lithium, and calcium supplements. Always inform your doctors of every medication you are taking, including nonprescription medicines, vitamins, herbal remedies, and dietary supplements. *Do not take any over-the-counter medications unless approved by your doctor.*

Food/Alcohol Interactions

Avoid alcohol.

Pregnancy/Nursing

Not recommended, especially during the first trimester. Bottle-feed your baby if you must take this drug.

Seniors

Side effects, including fainting and dizziness, may be more frequent or severe in older adults. Your doctor may prescribe a low dose.

Warning

If you experience shortness of breath, severe dizziness, fainting, slow or irregular heartbeat, or confusion, these may be signs of heart blockage. *Seek emergency medical treatment.*

Comments

The pain of angina comes from partial blockage in one or more of the coronary arteries in which blood flows to the heart. In addition to medication, lifestyle changes can go a long way in treating angina—stop smoking, reduce high blood pressure, lower high cholesterol, and lose weight.

Brand Name
Cardura*

Generic Name

doxazosin

Type of Drug

Antihypertensive. These drugs work to reduce abnormally high pressure of the blood against the walls of the blood vessels. They do not cure high blood pressure; they control the condition for as long as the medication is taken.

For

High blood pressure.

Availability and Dosage

Tablets: 1 mg, 2 mg, 4 mg, 8 mg. May be taken with or without food. (See Warning.)

Side Effects

More common include drowsiness, dizziness, and headache. Others include weakness, arrhythmia, constipation, diarrhea, nausea, and fatigue.

Drug Interactions

Doxazosin can interact with other antihypertensives, beta-blockers, estrogen, nonsteroidal antiinflammatory drugs (NSAIDs), and diuretics. Do not take any over-the-counter medications for coughs, colds, allergies, or appetite suppression. Always inform your doctors of every medication you are taking, including nonprescription medicines, vitamins, herbal remedies, and dietary supplements. *Do not take any over-the-counter medications unless approved by your doctor.*

Food/Alcohol Interactions

Avoid alcohol. Your doctor may recommend dietary changes to help treat hypertension.

Pregnancy/Nursing

No special warnings, although all drugs during pregnancy should be avoided if possible. Before taking this drug, discuss with your doctor the benefits versus the potential risks. Doxazosin passes into breast milk. Bottle-feed your baby if you must take this drug.

Seniors

Dizziness, drowsiness, and other side effects may be more frequent or severe in older patients. Your doctor may prescribe a low dose.

Warning

Your are likely to feel dizzy or drowsy after the first dose or the first few doses. Some doctors recommend taking this drug at bedtime, starting with 1 mg and gradually increasing it to the dose that you need. Do not rise quickly from a sitting or reclining position.

Comments

Hypertension has no symptoms. It forces the heart to work harder, which can bring about heart attacks and strokes as well as cause damage to the eyes and kidneys. Women with hypertension should be regularly monitored by health care practitioners to keep track of their blood pressure. Heart attacks kill six times more women each year than does breast cancer. Know the warning signs of a heart attack: Chest pain or pressure lasting more than a few minutes; pain radiating from your chest to shoulders, neck, arms, or jaw; fainting, nausea, shortness of breath.

carisoprodol*

See Soma

cefprozil

*See Cefzil**

Brand Name
Ceftin*

Generic Name

cefuroxime axetil

Type of Drug

Antibiotic. The drugs in this class are among the most commonly prescribed, resulting in such widespread use that the bacteria they were developed to kill have become resistant to them. These "resistant" forms are then passed from person to person, further causing the spread of infections that become even more difficult to treat. Your doctor will prescribe the correct antibiotic depending on the type of infection. Antibiotics are useless against viral infections such as colds and flu.

For

Bacterial infections, including those of the respiratory tract, urinary tract, sinuses, and ear.

Availability and Dosage

Capsules: 250 mg, 500 mg. Oral suspension: 125 mg, 187 mg, 250 mg, 375 mg per 5 ml. Should be taken with food. It is essential to take the complete course of antibiotics prescribed. If you fail to do so, increased drug resistance by any leftover bacteria is likely to occur.

Side Effects

More common include diarrhea, abdominal pain, and nausea. Others include dizziness, fatigue, muscle aches, vaginal itching, fever, rash, and joint pain.

Drug Interactions

Cefuroxime can interact with other antibiotics, including erythromycin and tetracycline, diuretics, and anticoagulants (blood thinners). Some antibiotics reduce the effectiveness of oral contraceptives. Always inform your doctors of every medication you are taking, including nonprescription medicines, vitamins, herbal remedies, and dietary supplements.

Food/Alcohol Interactions

Avoid or limit alcohol. Drink plenty of water while on this medication.

Pregnancy/Nursing

No special warnings, although all drugs during pregnancy should be avoided if possible. Before taking this drug, discuss with your doctor the benefits versus the potential risks. Cefuroxime passes into breast milk. Bottle-feed your baby if you must take this drug.

Seniors

Side effects may be more frequent or severe in older adults if there is impaired kidney function. Your doctor may prescribe a low dose.

Warning

Inform your doctor if you have ever had an allergic reaction to penicillin. If you experience difficulty in breathing, itching, swelling, rash, severe vomiting, or diarrhea, call your doctor at once.

Comments

Prolonged or repeated use of antibiotics can result in secondary infections of the vagina. This occurs when the balance of vaginal bacteria is disturbed by antibiotics that kill both "good" and "bad" bacteria, thus promoting yeast infections. Consult your doctor if you have vaginal itching or discharge, inflammation, or irritation of the vulva.

cefuroximeaxetil

*See **Ceftin****

Brand Name
Cefzil*

Generic Name

cefprozil

Type of Drug

Antibiotic. The drugs in this class are among the most commonly prescribed, resulting in such widespread use that the bacteria they were developed to kill have become resistant to them. These "resistant" forms are then passed from person to person, further causing the spread of infections that become even more difficult to treat. Your doctor will prescribe the correct antibiotic depending on the type of infection. Antibiotics are useless against viral infections such as colds and flu.

For

Bacterial infections, including those of the middle ear, skin, and upper and lower respiratory tract.

Availability and Dosage

Tablets: 250 mg, 500 mg. Oral suspension: 125 mg, 250 mg per 5 ml. It is essential to take the complete course of antibiotics prescribed. If you fail to do so, increased drug resistance by any leftover bacteria is likely to occur.

Side Effects

More common include diarrhea, abdominal pain and nausea. Others include dizziness, fatigue, muscle aches, vaginal itching, fever, rash and joint pain.

Drug Interactions

Cefprozil can interact with other antibiotics, including erythromycin and tetracycline, diuretics, and anticoagulants (blood thinners). Some antibiotics reduce the effectiveness of oral contraceptives. Always inform your doctors of every medication you are taking, including nonprescription medicines, vitamins, herbal remedies, and dietary supplements.

Food/Alcohol Interactions

Avoid or limit alcohol. Drink plenty of water while on this medication.

Pregnancy/Nursing

No special warnings, although all drugs during pregnancy should be avoided if possible. Before taking this drug, discuss with your doctor the benefits versus the potential risks. Cefprozil passes into breast milk. Bottle-feed your baby if you must take this drug.

Seniors

Side effects may be more frequent or severe in older adults if there is impaired kidney function. Your doctor may prescribe a low dose.

Warning

Tell your doctor if you have a history of allergies to any antibiotics, including penicillin. If you experience severe diarrhea, do not self-medicate with over-the-counter remedies. If you experience difficulty in breathing, itching, swelling, rash, severe vomiting, or diarrhea, call your doctor at once.

Comments

Cefprozil is one of more than twenty cephalosporin antibiotics, used to treat infections of the ear, nose, throat, skin and soft tissue, gastrointestinal tract, and kidney and urinary tract. (See Ceftin, above.)

Brand Name
Celebrex

Generic Name

celecoxib

Type of Drug

Nonsteroidal antiinflammatory drug (NSAID). This drug differs from other NSAIDs in that scientists believe that it inhibits an enzyme called COX-2, which plays a role in pain and inflammation, while not inhibiting the COX-1 enzyme, which helps maintain normal stomach lining. This means that celecoxib has been associated with fewer upper gastrointestinal ulcers than have both naproxen and ibuprofen. This drug does not slow or halt the progress of arthritis.

For

Relief of symptoms of osteoarthritis and rheumatoid arthritis.

Availability and Dosage

Capsules: 100 mg, 200 mg. Usual dose for osteoarthritis is 200 mg a day; for rheumatoid arthritis, 100 to 200 mg twice a day. Take this medicine exactly as prescribed. May be taken with or without food.

Side Effects

More common include indigestion, diarrhea, and abdominal pain. Others include headache, sinus inflammation, nausea, and fluid retention.

Drug Interactions

Celecoxib can interact with angiotensin-converting enzyme (ACE) inhibitors, furosemide, fluconazole, lithium, and anticoagulants (blood thinners). Always inform your doctors of every medication you are taking, including nonprescription medicines, vitamins, herbal remedies, and dietary supplements. *Do not take any over-the-counter medications unless approved by your doctor.*

Food/Alcohol Interactions

Avoid or limit alcohol, as it may aggravate stomach irritation.

Pregnancy/Nursing

Not recommended. It is not known whether celecoxib passes into breast milk. Discuss with your doctor the benefits versus the potential risks.

Seniors

Side effects may be more frequent and severe in older patients. Your doctor may prescribe a low dose.

Warning

Do not use this drug if you have had an allergic reaction to cele-coxib, sulfonamides, or aspirin or other NSAIDs. Although this drug has a low potential for stomach ulcers, serious gastrointestinal ulcerations can occur without warning symptoms. Notify your doctor of any burning stomach pain, black or tarry stools, or vomiting.

Comments

Celebrex was the first in a new class of "super-aspirins," designed to reduce arthritic inflammation while averting the usual side effects of aspirin and other NSAIDs. Selective COX-2 inhibitors may be the drug of choice in the future of arthritis treatment, and research continues aggressively to find new alternatives for these disabling and debilitating diseases. Almost 40 million Americans have some form of arthritis, 23 million of them women. Osteoarthritis is the breakdown of joint cartilage leading to pain and loss of movement in the affected joints. Rheumatoid arthritis is an autoimmune disease in which the joint lining becomes inflamed as part of excessive immune system activity.

Brand Name
Celexa

Generic Name

citalopram hydrobromide

Type of Drug

Selective serotonin reuptake inhibitor (SSRI) antidepressant. These drugs comprise a newer class of antidepressants that work by raising the brain's level of serotonin, a chemical associated with mood and mental alertness.

For

Depression.

Availability and Dosage

Tablets: 20 mg, 40 mg. May be taken with or without food. Do not take more of this medicine than is prescribed (see Warning).

Side Effects

More common include dry mouth, nausea, diarrhea, migraine headache, increased sweating, weight loss or gain, drowsiness, tremor, and cough. Others include abdominal pain, vomiting, anxiety, menstrual changes, and decreased sex drive.

Drug Interactions

Citalopram has the potential to interact with a wide variety of medications. The most dangerous interactions occur with monoamine oxidase (MAO) inhibitor antidepressants; do not take citalopram within 14 days of taking an MAO inhibitor. Other interactions can occur with central nervous system (CNS) depressants, sibutramine, some heart medications, antibiotics, antifungals, antimigraines, corticosteroids, narcotic painkillers, cyproheptadine, fluvastatin, and drugs for mental disorders. Do not take St. John's wort, tryptophan, kava kava, or other over-the-counter remedies for colds, coughs, or allergies. Always inform your doctors of every medication you are taking, including nonprescription medicines, vitamins, herbal remedies, and dietary supplements. *Do not take any over-the-counter medications unless approved by your doctor.*

Food/Alcohol Interactions

Avoid alcohol. Avoid grapefruit juice.

Pregnancy/Nursing

Not recommended. Bottle-feed your baby if you must take this drug.

Seniors

Side effects may be more frequent or severe. Your doctor may prescribe a low dose.

Warning

Do not abruptly stop taking this drug without your doctor's approval. Withdrawal symptoms may include dizziness, anxiety, numbness, fatigue, and flu-like symptoms. Your dose will have to be gradually decreased.

Comments

Low levels of serotonin figure prominently in many of the symptoms of depression. By increasing these levels, citalopram relieves symptoms and contributes to mood elevation. A major depressive episode is characterized by the presence of symptoms for at least 2 weeks that are interfering with normal functions. Symptoms include feelings of worthlessness or guilt, sleeping too much or not enough, loss of interest in usual activities, isolation, difficulty in concentrating, and changes in appetite. Women reportedly outnumber men 2 to 1 in treatment for major depression. For nonmajor depression (including dysthymia, a chronic, low-grade form of the disorder), the ratio jumps to 10 to 1. There is some controversy over whether women actually experience depression more often than men do, or whether they are more likely to seek treatment and therefore are more statistically visible.

celecoxib

See Celebrex

Brand Name
Cenestin

Generic Name
synthetic conjugated estrogens, A

Type of Drug
Estrogen. This is a 100% plant-derived synethetic estrogen derived from soy and yam.

For
Relief of menopausal symptoms including hot flashes, mood changes, night sweats, and vaginal dryness.

Availability and Dosage
Tablets: 0.625 mg, 0.9 mg. Should be taken with food.

Side Effects
More common include headache, insomnia, abdominal pain, palpitations, and depression. Others include joint pain, nausea, nervousness, and breast pain.

Drug Interactions
Although patient information for this drug indicates no known drug interactions, estrogens have the potential to interact with a variety of medications, including carbamazepine, cimetidine, antidiabetics, methotrexate, phenytoin, thyroid drugs, tricyclic antidepressants, and anticoagulants (blood thinners). Always inform your doctors of every medication you are taking, including nonprescription medicines, vitamins, herbal remedies, and dietary supplements.

Food/Alcohol Interactions
No special warnings. Avoid grapefruit juice.

Pregnancy/Nursing
A woman must never become pregnant while taking this drug. If you think you are pregnant, stop taking this drug immediately and consult your gynecologist. Bottle-feed your baby if you must take this drug.

Seniors

Side effects may be more frequent and severe in older women. Your doctor may prescribe a low dose.

Warning

Make sure that the doctor prescribing estrogen has your complete medical history, especially a history of breast cancer promoted by estrogen, a family history of breast cancer, fibrocystic breast disease, or a blood-clotting disorder. If you experience persistent vaginal bleeding, notify your doctor at once.

Comments

For some women, this plant-based drug may provide a more acceptable and humane alternative to Premarin, which is made from pregnant horses' urine. In recent years, the estrogenic properties in plants have been found to be beneficial in alleviating the symptoms of menopause. The decision to take or not to take estrogen is by no means a simple one. Women have to carefully weigh the pros and cons of estrogen replacement therapy (ERT). Studies indicate that estrogen protects the heart and the bones, but may increase the risk of breast, endometrial, and other cancers. The subject of hormone replacement therapy (HRT) is controversial, with no one solution that is right for every woman. The best course for a woman entering menopause (between ages 45 and 55) is to gain as much knowledge about the subject, formulate with her gynecologist a personal health profile (and get second and third opinions if necessary), and decide if the benefits of ERT or HRT outweigh the risks. Regular monitoring by your gynecologist is essential.

Brand Name
Centrax

Generic Name

prazepam

Type of Drug

Benzodiazepine. These drugs are central nervous system (CNS) depressants and work on the part of the brain that controls emotion by slowing nervous-system transmissions. They are often the drug of choice to relieve the symptoms of anxiety but do not address the underlying cause.

For

Anxiety; agitation; irritable bowel syndrome (IBS); tension, panic attacks; fatigue.

Availability and Dosage

Tablets: 10 mg. Capsules: 5 mg, 10 mg, 20 mg. May be taken with or without food. Do not take more of this medicine than is prescribed. Do not abruptly stop taking this drug without consulting your doctor.

Side Effects

More common include drowsiness, dizziness, and unsteadiness. Other include headache, nausea, vomiting, depression, mood changes, and tremors.

Drug Interactions

Prazepam has the potential to interact with a wide variety of medications, including antihistamines, anticonvulsants, cimetidine, erythromycin, levodopa, digoxin, oral contaceptives or other hormone drugs, and other CNS depressants. Take antacids at least 1 hour before or after taking this drug. Always inform your doctors of every medication you are taking, including non-prescription medicines, vitamins, herbal remedies, and dietary supplements. *Do not take any over-the-counter medications unless approved by your doctor.*

Food/Alcohol Interactions

Avoid alcohol.

Pregnancy/Nursing

Not recommended, especially during the first trimester. Bottle-feed your baby if you must take this drug.

Seniors

Side effects may be more frequent or severe if there is impaired kidney or liver function. Your doctor may prescribe a low dose.

Warning

Tell your doctor if you have a history of drug or alcohol dependence, depression, psychoses or suicidal thoughts, sleep apnea, or kidney or liver disease. Use caution when driving, operating machinery, or performing tasks that require mental alertness until you know how this drug will affect you. Combining this drug and supplements containing kava kava may result in intensified CNS-depressant effect.

Comments

You will need to be regularly monitored by your physician while on this medication. Women are often prescribed antianxiety or tranquilizing agents while the underlying cause remains untreated. If you suspect that your symptoms are being prematurely ascribed to anxiety without a complete medical checkup, get a second opinion.

cephalexin*

See Keflex

cetirizine HCl

*See Zyrtec**

chlordiazepoxide

See Librium

cimetidine*

See Tagamet

Brand Name

Cipro*

Generic Name

ciprofloxacin

Type of Drug

Antibiotic. The drugs in this class are among the most commonly prescribed, resulting in such widespread use that the bacteria they were developed to kill have become resistant to them. These "resistant" forms are then passed from person to person, further causing the spread of infections that become even more difficult to treat. Antibiotics are useless against viral infections such as colds and flu.

For

Urinary tract infections (UTIs), skin and bone infections; bronchitis; pneumonia; sinusitis.

Availability and Dosage

Tablets: 250 mg, 500 mg, 750 mg. Should be taken on an empty stomach, 1 hour before or 2 hours after meals. Take at evenly spaced intervals to keep the level of drug constant. It is essential to take the complete course of antibiotics prescribed. If you fail to do so, increased drug resistance by any leftover bacteria is likely to occur.

Side Effects

Most common include nausea, diarrhea, and increased sun sensitivity. Others include abdominal pain, yeast infections, dizziness, constipation, headache, restlessness, vomiting, gas, insomnia, drowsiness, and dry mouth.

Drug Interactions

Ciprofloxacin can interact with some antiasthmatics, phenytoin, some oral contraceptives, anticoagulants (blood thinners), and nitrofurantoin. Do not take this drug with multivitamins or multiminerals containing iron, calcium, magnesium, manganese, or zinc. Do not take antacids within 2 hours of taking this drug. Always inform your doctors of every medication you are taking, including nonprescription medicines, vitamins, herbal remedies, and dietary supplements. *Do not take any over-the-counter medications unless approved by your doctor.*

Food/Alcohol Interactions

Avoid or limit alcohol. Avoid caffeine in foods and beverages, as ciprofloxacin substantially raises caffeine levels in the blood. Avoid milk and dairy products, as they can affect absorption. Drink plenty of water while on this drug.

Pregnancy/Nursing

Not recommended. Ciprofloxacin passes into breast milk and can cause serious side effects in a nursing infant. Bottle-feed your baby if you must take this drug.

Seniors

Side effects may be more frequent and severe in older patients due to slower elimination from the body. Your doctor may prescribe a low dose.

Warnings

Notify your doctor if you have any major side effects such as blurred vision, chest pain, chills, fever, hives, nightmares, seizures, skin rash, or tremors.

Comments

Ciprofloxacin is an antibiotic that so far has not encountered significant resistance from respiratory illnesses. A recent study showed that the drug is highly effective against three microbes that are the most common causes of respiratory illnesses. Drug-resistant bacteria represents a growing health hazard, contributed to by doctors' prescribing antibiotics that are useless for certain conditions, and patients' stopping treatment once they feel better. When antibiotics are stopped before the course of treatment is complete, the bacteria will not only survive but will mutate into a resistant form.

ciprofloxacin

See Cipro*

cisapride

See Propulsid*

citalopram hydrobromide

See Celexa

clarithromycin

See Biaxin*

Brand Name
Claritin* (also Claritin-D 12 Hour*, Claritin-D 24 Hour)

Generic Name

loratadine (loratadine and pseudoephedrine sulfate)

Type of Drug

Antihistamine. These drugs counteract the effect of histamine, a chemical released in the body that can cause itching and swelling. Loratadine is commonly used by people who cannot tolerate the sedative side effects of other antihistamines.

For

Symptoms of seasonal and other allergies.

Availability and Dosage

Tablets: 10 mg. Extended release tablets: loratidine and pseudo-ephedrine. Should be taken on an empty stomach, 1 hour before or 2 hours after meals. Extended-release tablets (Claritin-D 12 HR and Claritin-D 24 HR) are taken twice a day; the 24-hour formula is taken once a day. Do not take more of this medicine than is prescribed.

Side Effects

More common include dry mouth, fatigue, drowsiness, and headache. Others include sore throat, dizziness, cough, fatigue, nausea, nervousness, and dysmenorrhea (painful menstrual cramps).

Drug Interactions

Loratadine may interact with antianxiety drugs, some antidepressants, pain relievers, and other antihistamines. Loratadine and pseudoephedrine (Claritin-D Extended Release forms) may interact with all of the above plus cimetidine, erythromycin, monoamine oxidase (MAO) inhibitor antidepressants, antifungals, central nervous systems (CNS) depressants, digoxin, beta-blockers, antimigraines, and methyldopa. Always inform your doctors of every medication you are taking, including nonprescription medicines, vitamins, herbal remedies, and dietary supplements. *Do not take any over-the-counter medications unless approved by your doctor.*

Food/Alcohol Interactions

When taking loratadine/pseudoephedrine (Claritin-D), avoid alcohol and caffeine.

Pregnancy/Nursing

Not recommended. Bottle-feed your baby if you must take this drug.

Seniors

Side effects may be more frequent or severe in patients taking the extended release form (loratadine/pseudoephedrine). Your doctor may prescribe a low dose.

Warning

Do not take any over-the-counter medications for coughs, colds, allergies, sinus problems, or appetite suppression while on this drug. Combining them with either loratadine or loratadine/pseudoephedrine may cause dizziness, nervousness, and difficulty in sleeping.

Comments

In addition to prescription antihistamines, there are dozens of over-the-counter antihistamines. Many people self-medicate with antihistamines for everything from hay fever to hives to insomnia. Both prescription and nonprescription antihistamines have the potential to interact with many different drugs, including those taken for heart disease, diabetes, and other conditions. Always check with your doctor or your pharmacist before combining over-the-counter antihistamines with any prescription drug. Follow package directions carefully and notify your doctor if you have any problems.

Climara

See Estrace*

Brand Name
Clomid (also Milophene, Serophene)

Generic Name

clomiphene

Type of Drug

Fertility. This drug stimulates ovulation in women who are not ovulating but have normal levels of estrogen.

For

Infertility in women.

Availability and Dosage

Tablets: 50 mg. The treatment lasts 5 days. Follow your doctor's instructions exactly.

Side Effects

More common include insomnia, dizziness, headache, hot flashes, depression, irritability, bleeding between periods, nausea, fatigue, and breast discomfort.

Drug Interactions

No special warnings, although all drugs have the ability to interact with other drugs. Report any problems to your doctor or your pharmacist.

Food/Alcohol Interactions

No special warnings.

Pregnancy/Nursing

Not recommended. You may need to take a pregnancy test to make sure you are not pregnant before starting treatment.

Seniors

Not usually prescribed.

Warning

Make sure your doctor has your complete medical history before starting fertility treatments, including a history of ovarian cysts, depression, unexplained vaginal bleeding, a blood-clotting disorder, or liver disease. This drug is usually used for 6 to 9 months. If you still haven't conceived, discuss other options with your doctor.

Comments

Unlike other fertility drugs, clomiphene has a 90% rate in producing single births where other drugs have an 80% rate. Clomiphene produces twins in 5% to 10% of cases; and triplets or more in only 1%. Other drugs produce twins in 15% to 20% of cases; triplets or more in 3% to 5% This is important if you are apprehensive about multiple births—understandable, given the physical risks and the emotional issues involved in delivering three or more babies and the decision to undergo selective reduction. This procedure, also called multifetal pregnancy reduction, involves terminating a specified number of embryos in the uterus because you want to increase survival chances for those remaining, or because you simply may not want to have quadruplets, quintuplets, or more. More than 100,000 women a year undergo fertility treatments.

clomiphene

See Clomid

clonazepam

See Klonopin

clorazepate dipotassium

See Tranxene

Brand Name
Cognex

Generic Name

tacrine hydrochloride

Type of Drug

Cholinesterase inhibitor (chemical nerve-muscle coordinator). This drug works in basically the same way as donepezil (Aricept)—by breaking down acetylcholine, a brain chemical essential for nerve cells to communicate with one another. This drug is not a cure for Alzheimer's, but it can produce improvement in mild to moderate symptoms: loss of memory, language skills, alertness, and the ability to perform simple activities.

For

Alzheimer's disease.

Availability and Dosage

Capsules: 10 mg, 20 mg, 30 mg, 40 mg. Should be taken on an empty stomach, 1 hour before or 2 hours after meals. Do not abruptly stop taking this drug without telling your doctor, as doing so may worsen the symptoms of Alzheimer's.

Side Effects

Side effects are numerous, and a high incidence of patient intolerance is reported both in studies and in practical use. They include liver inflammation, nausea, diarrhea, dizziness, changes in blood pressure, fainting, convulsions, nervousness, joint pain, sinus inflammation, weight gain, swelling of the face, feet, or legs, angina, cardiac abnormalities, migraine, difficulty in swallowing, anemia, respiratory problems, hair loss, shingles, psoriasis, vaginal bleeding. itching, dry eyes, ringing in ears, and changes in taste.

Drug Interactions

Tacrine may interact with some antiasthmatics, cimetidine, and presurgical muscle relaxants. Always inform your doctors of every medication you are taking, including nonprescription medicines, vitamins, herbal remedies, and dietary supplements. *Do not take any over-the-counter medications unless approved by your doctor.*

Food/Alcohol Interactions

Avoid alcohol.

Pregnancy/Nursing

No special warnings, although all drugs during pregnancy should be avoided if possible. Before taking this drug, discuss with your doctor the benefits versus the potential risks. Bottle-feed your baby if you must take this drug.

Seniors

No special warnings unless there is impaired liver function, which will result in increased side effects.

Warning

Patients on this drug must be regularly monitored with periodic blood tests to check liver function; tacrine can cause serious liver abnormalities. Avoid smoking, as it may lessen the drug's effectiveness.

Comments

Although research and studies continue to aggressively address this devastating illness (which affects 4 million Americans and will increase as the population ages), as of now tacrine and donepezil remain the only drugs that may help to slow disease progression in patients. Neither drug works for every Alzheimer's patient. Women are harder hit by Alzheimer's on two fronts: they live longer than men do, and so are affected in greater numbers, and they represent 80% of caregivers for family members who have Alzheimer's. A seven-minute word-and-picture test—designed to differentiate among people who have normal age-associated memory loss and those who have more serious problems—is 90% accurate in identifying early Alzheimer's. The test uses four recall and thinking quizzes and can be administered by a trained technician.

Brand Name
CombiPatch

Generic Name

estradiol and norethindrone acetate

Type of Drug

Estrogen. This drug is a combination of estrogen and progestin. The addition of progestin to estrogen in studies has shown to reduce the risk of endometrial cancer associated with estrogen-replacement therapy (ERT) alone.

For

Relief of menopausal symptoms, including hot flashes, mood changes, night sweats, and vaginal dryness.

Availability and Dosage

Extended release transdermal patch in various dosages. Follow package instructions for application. You may be prescribed an estrogen-only (estradiol) patch for some days; and a combination (estradiol and norethindrone) patch for other days. Use the patches exactly as instructed by your health care provider.

Side Effects

More common include breast pain, menstrual cramps, skin irritation at the patch site, irregular bleeding and spotting. Others include nausea, headache, fluid retention, back pain, flu-like symptoms, vaginitis, and rhinitis.

Drug Interactions

This drug may interact with cimetidine, oral antidiabetics, methotrexate, corticosteroids, phenytoin, thyroid drugs, tricyclic antidepressants, and anticoagulants (blood thinners). Always inform your doctors of every medication you are taking, including nonprescription medicines, vitamins, herbal remedies, and dietary supplements. *Do not take any over-the-counter medications unless approved by your doctor.*

Food/Alcohol Interactions

Avoid drinking grapefruit juice while on this medication.

Pregnancy/Nursing

A woman must never become pregnant while on this drug. If you think you may be pregnant, remove the patch immediately and contact your doctor. Bottle-feed your baby if you must take this drug.

Seniors

No special warnings. Take as prescribed and immediately inform your doctor of any persistent or troublesome side effects.

Warning

When using hormone-replacement therapy (HRT), if you experience leg, arm, groin, or chest pain, vision problems, severe headache, or abdominal pain, seek emergency medical treatment. Tell your doctor if you have a history of diabetes, hysterectomy, elevated blood calcium levels, high cholesterol, edema, migraine, depression, stroke, uterine fibroids, endometriosis, heart disease, or cancer. You may need to stop this drug prior to surgery. Smoking increases your risk of blood clots and stroke.

Comments

In our youth-oriented Western culture, menopause carries not only physiological ramifications for women but psychological ones as well. Negative perceptions of what is a natural stage of life can be difficult to overcome—fears of aging and chronic illness and feelings of worthlessness. Women entering menopause (between ages 45 and 55, when estrogen levels decline) should gain as much knowledge about the subject as possible, formulate with their gynecologists a personal health profile (and get second and third opinions if necessary), and decide if the benefits of hormone-replacement therapy (HRT) outweigh the risks. Many women also explore alternative methods to use in conjunction with drug therapies, including yoga, meditation, biofeedback, acupressure, and massage.

Combivir

*See **Retrovir***

Brand Name
Condylox

Generic Name

podofilox

Type of Drug

Antimitotic; chemical remover.

For

External genital and perianal warts (external condylomata acuminata).

Availability and Dosage

Topical gel or solution: 0.5%. Usual dosage is twice a day for 3 consecutive days, then no treatment for 4 days. Follow your doctor's instructions for repeating this cycle as necessary.

Side Effects

More common include itching, pain, burning, inflammation, and stinging at the application site. Others include blisters, swelling, and bleeding at the application site.

Drug Interactions

No special warnings, although all drugs have the ability to interact with other drugs. Report any problems to your doctor or your pharmacist.

Food/Alcohol Interactions

No special warnings.

Pregnancy/Nursing

No special warnings, although all drugs during pregnancy and breast-feeding should be avoided if possible. Before taking this drug, discuss with your doctor the benefits versus the potential risks.

Seniors

No special warnings. Take as prescribed and immediately inform your doctor of any persistent or troublesome side effects.

Warning

This drug is for external use only and not to be inserted in the vagina or the rectum. Avoid contact with eyes. This drug is not a cure for external genital and perianal warts. New warts may appear during therapy. Do not have sexual intercourse at any time while this drug is on the skin. To help protect further spread of this disease, use condoms.

Comments

Genital human papillomavirus (HPV) is one of the most common sexually transmitted diseases (STDs) in the United States. More than 700,000 new cases are diagnosed each year. Women with HPV should get an annual Pap smear; some forms of HPV have been associated with an increased risk of cervical cancer.

conjugated estrogens

See Premarin*

conjugated estrogens (synthetic)

See Cenestin

Cotrim

See Bactrim

Brand Name
Coumadin*

Generic Name
warfarin

Type of Drug
Anticoagulant (blood thinner). This type of drug is used in the treatment of stroke, abnormal blood clotting, and heart disease. It is also used to prevent a blood clot from traveling and lodging in the heart, lungs, or brain, a potentially life-threatening condition.

For
Reducing the risk of blood clots.

Availability and Dosage
Tablets: 1 mg, 2 mg, 2.5 mg, 5 mg, 7.5 mg, 10 mg. Should be taken on an empty stomach, 1 hour before or 2 hours after a meal, preferably at the same time every day. Dosages must be determined by your doctor. Do not take more or less of this medicine than is prescribed.

Side Effects
More common include abnormal bleeding; notify your doctor immediately if you experience this. Other side effects include nausea, vomiting, diarrhea, anemia, abdominal pain, and rash.

Drug Interactions

The potential for numerous and serious drug interactions involving warfarin is significant. A partial list includes antiinflammatories, nonsteroidal antiinflammatory drugs (NSAIDs), cholesterol-lowering drugs, antibiotics, antifungals, aspirin, allopurinol, drugs for heart conditions, estrogen oral contraceptives, antihypertensives, diuretics, carbamazepine, thyroid drugs, anticonvulsants, some anticancer drugs, antiulcers, corticosteroids, and cimetidine. Do not take vitamins E and K or ginseng. Always inform your doctors of every medication you are taking, including nonprescription medicines, vitamins, herbal remedies, and dietary supplements. *Do not take any over-the-counter medications unless approved by your doctor.*

Food/Alcohol Interactions

Avoid alcohol. Your doctor may provide a list of foods rich in vitamin K to avoid or restrict: broccoli, cabbage, spinach, cauliflower, liver, and kale. These foods can interfere with the effectiveness of warfarin.

Pregnancy/Nursing

A woman must never become pregnant while taking this drug. If you become pregnant, contact your doctor. If you must take this drug, you will need to discuss with your doctor the benefits versus the potentially serious risks. Bottle-feed your baby if you must take this drug.

Seniors

Side effects may be more frequent and severe in older patients. Your doctor may prescribe a low dose.

Warning

When taking warfarin, it is essential that all of your doctors and your pharmacist have a complete list of all medications—both prescription and nonprescription—that you are taking, as potentially serious drug interactions are significantly increased. You must be carefully and regularly monitored while on this drug; periodic blood tests are required to check clotting time. *Do not change brands of warfarin without consulting your doctor or your pharmacist.* With the ability to order prescription drugs over the Internet, this is especially important to remember.

Comments

While on this drug, you should carry a card indicating that you are on warfarin (or any other anticoagulant) along with a list all of the other medications you are currently taking.

Brand Name
Cozaar*

Generic Name

losartan potassium

Type of Drug

Antihypertensive. This drug reduces abnormally high pressure of the blood against the walls of the blood vessels.

For

High blood pressure.

Availability and Dosage

Tablets: 25 mg, 50 mg. May be taken with or without food.

Side Effects

More common include headache, upset stomach, and diarrhea. Others include muscle aches, back pain, sinusitis, insomnia, and dizziness.

Drug Interactions

No special warnings, although any drug has the ability to interact with any other drug. Do not take nonprescription medications for coughs, colds, allergies, sinus problems, or appetite suppression. Always inform your doctors of every medication you are taking, including nonprescription medicines, vitamins, herbal remedies, and dietary supplements. *Do not take any over-the-counter medications unless approved by your doctor*.

Food/Alcohol Interactions

Avoid or limit alcohol; it can increase dizziness. Do not use salt substitutes.

Pregnancy/Nursing

Not recommended, especially during the second and third trimesters. Bottle-feed your baby if you must take this drug.

Seniors

No special warnings. Take as prescribed and immediately inform your doctor of any persistent or troublesome side effects. Your doctor may prescribe a low dose.

Warning

Hypertension can cause strokes and heart attacks as well as cause damage to the eyes and kidneys. Hypertension is often referred to as "the silent killer" because it has no symptoms, yet forces the heart to work harder. You must be regularly monitored while on this drug.

Comments

There is a version of losartan combined with hydrochlorothiazide, a diuretic. (See Hyzaar.)

Brand Name
Crixivan

Generic Name

indinavir sulfate

Type of Drug

Antiviral; protease inhibitor. This drug has been shown to help eliminate much of the human immunodeficiency virus (HIV) in the blood. This drug is not a cure, but studies indicate that lower levels of the virus can improve prognosis for patients.

For

HIV infection.

Availability and Dosage

Capsules: 200 mg, 333 mg, 400 mg. Drug management therapy for patients with HIV infection or AIDS is a complex process involving a combination of drugs in what is now commonly referred to as an "AIDS cocktail." There is no one "cocktail"— these combinations, including protease inhibitors and nucleoside analogs, are providing increased life expectancy and dramatic improvement in symptoms for some patients. For example, zidovudine is used in one of the newer drugs (brand name Retrovir), in combination with lamivudine in one tablet. Patients play a critical role in the management of this disease by taking medications for HIV and AIDS exactly as prescribed, in the proper dosages and at the proper times. Take this medication exactly as prescribed.

Side Effects

More common include diarrhea, nausea, weakness, and abdominal pain. Others include headache, vomiting, dry skin, dizziness, depression, abdominal bloating, and changes in taste.

Drug Interactions

Indinavir can interact with ketoconazole, fluconazole, dihydroergotamine, dexamethasone, ethinyl estradiol, triazolam, carbamazepine, and phenytoin. Always inform your doctors of every medication you are taking, including nonprescription medicines, vitamins, herbal remedies, and dietary supplements. *Do not take any over-the-counter medications unless approved by your doctor.*

Food/Alcohol Interactions

Avoid alcohol. Do not take this drug with high-fat foods; they may interfere with absorption. Drink plenty of water while on this medication.

Pregnancy/Nursing

The decision to take this drug during pregnancy must be discussed with your doctor. Pregnant women should use indinavir only when the benefits outweigh the risks. Bottle-feeding is recommended to reduce any possible risk of infection from an HIV-positive mother.

Seniors

No special warnings. Take as prescribed and immediately inform your doctor of any persistent or troublesome side effects.

Warning

Taking this or any drug to treat HIV or AIDS does not affect the possibility of transmission of the virus. You must use preventive precautions when engaging in any form of sexual contact.

Comments

Although overall deaths from AIDS are on the decline, the disease is increasing faster among women than men and still affects minorities disproportionately. Women with HIV often have difficulty accessing proper health care, and the prohibitive cost of the drugs involved (up to $16,000 or more a year) often excludes those who need them. Given the rise in heterosexually transmitted HIV, more prevention efforts—namely, insisting that a partner use latex condoms—are being aimed at women. Although there is presently no cure for this disease, new drug trials and research continue. See the Women's Resource Directory at the back of this book for the names of organizations that have the latest information on treatments.

cromolyn sodium

See Intal

cyclobenzaprine

See Flexeril

cyclophosphamide

See Cytoxan

cyclosporine

See Sandimmune

Cycrin*

*See Provera**

cyproheptadine

See Periactin

Brand Name
Cytotec

Generic Name

misoprostol

Type of Drug

Antiulcer.

For

Prevention of stomach ulcers caused by nonsteroidal antiinflammatory drugs (NSAIDs) for arthritis; also used for treatment (not prevention) of duodenal ulcers.

Availability and Dosage

Tablets: 0.1 mg, 0.2 mg. Should be taken on an empty stomach, 1 hour before or 2 hours after a meal. Do not take more of this medicine than is prescribed.

Side Effects

More common include diarrhea and abdominal or stomach pain. These may subside as your body adjusts to the drug. Others include constipation, nausea, vaginal bleeding, painful menstrual cramps, and menstrual disorders.

Drug Interactions

Misoprostol may interact with nonsteroidal antiinflammatory drugs (NSAIDs) and with antacids that contain magnesium. Always inform your doctors of every medication you are taking, including nonprescription medicines, vitamins, herbal remedies, and dietary supplements. *Do not take any over-the-counter medications unless approved by your doctor.*

Food/Alcohol Interactions

Avoid alcohol; it can aggravate ulcers.

Pregnancy/Nursing

A woman must never become pregnant while on this drug. Misoprostol can cause uterine contractions and spontaneous miscarriage. If you become pregnant while on this drug, stop taking it immediately and notify your doctor. Within two weeks of starting misoprostol, you must have a blood test (not an over-the-counter home pregnancy test) to rule out pregnancy. Use effective contraception the entire time you are taking this drug. Bottle-feed your baby if you must take this drug.

Seniors

Because of its serious implications for women of childbearing age, misoprostol may be more suited to seniors who have shown a low tolerance for other types of antiulcer medications. However, there may be a higher absorption rate. Your doctor may prescribe a low dose.

Warning

Prescription medicines should never be shared, and this drug poses special risks. Do not share this medication with any woman of childbearing age (see Pregnancy/Nursing, above). Smoking can aggravate ulcers.

Comments

It may take several days before you experience noticeable improvement in ulcer symptoms. Ulcers caused by NSAIDs (for example, ibuprofen and aspirin) can develop when the thick, protective stomach lining is disturbed or weakened by the use of these medications. This can lead to bleeding, gastritis (stomach-lining inflammation), and perforation.

Brand Name
Cytoxan

Generic Name

cyclophosphamide

Type of Drug

Anticancer (antineoplastic). This chemotherapy drug helps to prevent the growth of multiplying cancer cells.

For

Breast, ovarian, lung, and other types of cancer.

Availability and Dosage

Tablets: 25 mg, 50 mg. Should be taken on an empty stomach, 1 hour before or 2 hours after a meal, but may be taken with food if stomach upset occurs.

Side Effects

More common include nausea, vomiting, hair loss (temporary), and fatigue. Others include darkening of skin, diarrhea, dizziness, and rapid pulse. Side effects can continue after the course of treatment is finished.

Drug Interactions

Cyclophosphamide may interact with anticoagulants (blood thinners), allopurinol, insulin, some diuretics, cimetidine, some anticonvulsants, and heart drugs. Always inform your doctors of every medication you are taking, including nonprescription medicines, vitamins, herbal remedies, and dietary supplements. *Do not take any over-the-counter medications unless approved by your doctor.*

Food/Alcohol Interactions

Avoid or limit alcohol. Drink plenty of water while on this drug.

Pregnancy/Nursing

Not recommended. Birth defects can result during therapy and for up to 4 months after stopping this drug. Bottle-feed your baby if you must take this drug.

Seniors

Older patients may experience more side effects. Your doctor may prescribe a low dose.

Warning

You must have periodic blood tests while on this drug and after completing treatment. Do not take any vaccinations without consulting your doctor. If you experience fever, sore throat, chills, unusual bleeding, or bruising, contact your doctor immediately. Do not self-medicate with over-the-counter drugs. Avoid contact with people who have colds, flu, or bronchitis. This drug can cause slow wound healing; try to avoid injury, including damage to teeth and gums.

Comments

Cyclophosphamide can cause changes in both female eggs and male sperm, which can result in birth defects even after the drug is stopped. If you or your male partner are on this drug, discuss its effects on the reproductive system with your doctor.

Brand Name
Darvocet-N 100 (also Propacet 100)

Generic Name

propoxyphene napsylate and acetaminophen

Type of Drug

Narcotic analgesic.

For

Pain relief.

Availability and Dosage

Tablets: 650 mg acetaminophen and 100 mg propoxyphene napsylate. Darvocet-N 50 tablet: 325 mg acetaminophen and 50 mg propoxyphene napsylate. May be taken with or without food. Do not take more of this medicine than is prescribed.

Side Effects

More common include drowsiness, dizziness, constipation, and nausea. Others include fatigue, vomiting, stomach pain, headache, euphoria, dry mouth, nightmares, insomnia, blurred vision, unsteadiness, skin flushing, and increased sweating.

Drug Interactions

This drug has the potential to interact with a wide variety of medications, including central nervous system (CNS) depressants, anticonvulsants, antihypertensives, muscle relaxants, cimetidine, and anticoagulants (blood thinners). Do not take any over-the-counter drugs containing acetaminophen; possible overdose may result. Other nonprescription medications to avoid are antihistamines, decongestants, sleep aids, medicines for coughs or colds, and antacids. Always inform your doctors of every medication you are taking, including nonprescription medicines, vitamins, herbal remedies, and dietary supplements. *Do not take any over-the-counter medications unless approved by your doctor.*

Food/Alcohol Interactions

Avoid alcohol. It can result in sedation, confusion, and respiratory distress. Acetaminophen should not be taken by people who drink more than 3 alcoholic beverages a day.

Pregnancy/Nursing

Not recommended. This drug has been shown to cause birth defects. This drug passes into breast milk, but its effects are unknown. You may wish to bottle-feed your baby if you must take this drug.

Seniors

Older adults may be more susceptible to adverse side effects. Your doctor may prescribe a low dose.

Warning

This combination drug carries an increased risk of physical or psychological addiction. Make sure your doctor has your complete medical history, including a history of alcohol or substance abuse, suicidal thoughts, or severe depression. Propoxyphene has been implicated in numerous suicides or suicide attempts, especially when combined with alcohol.

Comments

This combination drug has numerous brand names with the same ingredients (acetaminophen and propoxyphene). Darvon and Dolene are two brand names for propoxyphene alone. There are also dozens of prescription pain relievers that use acetaminophen in combination with other narcotics and/or caffeine. Any narcotic should be used with caution. Never share this type of drug with others.

Brand Name
Daypro*

Generic Name

oxaprozin

Type of Drug

Nonsteroidal antiinflammatory drug (NSAID). Drugs in this group reduce pain, inflammation, and stiffness associated with a wide range of conditions that affect bones, joints, and muscles. NSAIDs do not cure a disease; they are used for relief of symptoms. Your physician may routinely prescribe a variety of NSAIDs in order to find the one best suited for you.

For

Relief of symptoms of rheumatoid arthritis and osteoarthritis, including joint pain, inflammation, stiffness, and swelling.

Availability and Dosage

Tablets: 600 mg. Should be taken with food.

Side Effects

More common include nausea, constipation, diarrhea, upset stomach, and heartburn. Others include dizziness, drowsiness, depression, and ringing in the ears.

Drug Interactions

This drug may interact with aspirin and other NSAIDs, antifungals, phenytoin, lithium, methotrexate, antihypertensives, and anticoagulants (blood thinners). Always inform your doctors of every medication you are taking, including nonprescription medicines, vitamins, herbal remedies, and dietary supplements. *Do not take any over-the-counter medications unless approved by your doctor.*

Food/Alcohol Interactions

Avoid alcohol; it can increase stomach irritation. Tell your doctor if you drink more than 3 alcoholic beverages a day.

Pregnancy/Nursing

This drug is not recommended during pregnancy, especially during the last trimester. NSAIDs, including flurbiprofen, may pass into breast milk. Bottle-feed your baby if you must take this drug.

Seniors

Older people may be at increased risk for side effects, especially gastrointestinal problems. Your doctor may prescribe a low dose.

Warning

NSAIDs can cause several potentially serious side effects, including gastrointestinal disorders, dizziness, and gastric bleeding. Seek immediate medical treatment if you experience vomiting, diarrhea, rapid heartbeat, confusion, or abdominal pain. Make sure your doctor has your complete medical history, especially a history of ulcers, anemia, asthma, kidney or liver disease, or lupus.

Comments

When using any of the numerous over-the-counter NSAIDs, follow package directions carefully. Women may have a higher risk of developing ulcers while taking NSAIDs, particularly if they smoke, drink alcohol, are over age 60, or use corticosteroid drugs.

Brand Name
Deltasone* (also Orasone, Liquid Pred, Meticorten)

Generic Name

prednisone

Type of Drug

Corticosteroid. These drugs are most often used to treat many types of inflammatory diseases.

For

Relief of inflammation and symptoms associated with rheumatoid arthritis, severe asthma, systemic lupus erythematosus (SLE), multiple sclerosis, and skin diseases.

Availability and Dosage

Deltasone tablets: 2.5 mg, 5 mg, 10 mg, 20 mg, 50 mg. Orasone tablets: 1 mg, 5 mg, 20 mg, 50 mg. Liquid Pred oral syrup: 5 mg per 5 ml. Meticorten tablets: 1 mg. Should be taken with food. Do not abruptly stop taking this drug without consulting your doctor.

Side Effects

More common include stomach upset, increased or decreased appetite, restlessness, and insomnia. Others include headache, round face, nausea, menstrual problems, muscle weakness, cataracts, osteoporosis, and abdominal swelling.

Drug Interactions

Corticosteroids can interact with a wide variety of medications, including carbamazepine, anticoagulants (blood thinners), oral antidiabetics, insulin, oral contraceptives, phenytoin, digitalis drugs, and medications containing potassium or sodium. Always inform your doctors of every medication you are taking, including nonprescription medicines, vitamins, herbal remedies, and dietary supplements. *Do not take any over-the-counter medications unless approved by your doctor.*

Food/Alcohol Interactions

Avoid alcohol. Your physician may recommend a special diet if you are taking prednisone daily.

Pregnancy/Nursing

Not recommended, especially during the first trimester. Consult your doctor about breast-feeding; safety may be determined by dosage and length of treatment.

Seniors

Increased side effects can be more likely in older adults, including hypertension. Your doctor may prescribe a low dose.

Warning

For women, a potential and significant side effect of prednisone is osteroporosis. Use caution with long-term steroid use, as bone loss increases with the dose and duration of steroid treatment. The bones in the spine, ribs, and wrists are most susceptible to the effects of steroids. Bone mass must be carefully monitored during treatment with these medications. Make sure your doctor has your complete medical history before you take any corticosteroid.

Comments

Lupus, an autoimmune disease, is one of the many conditions treated with corticosteroids. Systemic lupus erythematosus (SLE) can be one of the more severe forms, causing inflammation in multiple organs or sites—lungs, kidneys, blood, skin, and joints. Lupus occurs 10 times more frequently in women than in men and is more prevalent among female African Americans, Latinas, Native Americans, and Asians. Its cause is unknown, but some research suggests that hormonal factors (particularly estrogen) may influence the immune system; flare-ups often occur during pregnancy or when taking oral contraceptives.

Demulen

See Oral Contraceptives

Brand Name
Depakote*

Generic Name
divalproex sodium

Type of Drug
Anticonvulsant.

For
Seizure disorders including epilepsy; manic-depression (bipolar disorder); migraine.

Availability and Dosage
Capsules: 250 mg. Enteric-coated tablets: 125 mg, 250 mg, 500 mg. Oral syrup: 250 mg per 5 ml. Sprinkle capsules: 125 mg. Tablet and capsule forms should be taken on an empty stomach, unless stomach upset occurs. Oral syrup may be taken with uncarbonated liquids. The sprinkle capsules may be mixed with applesauce or pudding.

Side Effects
More common include nausea, vomiting, drowsiness, and dizziness. Others include changes in appetite, weight loss or gain, tremor, excitability, constipation, irritability, hair loss, confusion, unsteadiness, and heartburn.

Drug Interactions

This drug can interact with a wide variety of drugs, including other anticonvulsants, anticoagulants (blood thinners), central nervous system (CNS) depressants, aspirin, nonsteroidal antiinflammatory drugs (NSAIDs), monoamine oxidase (MAO) inhibitors, and tricyclic antidepressants. Always inform your doctors of every medication you are taking, including nonprescription medicines, vitamins, herbal remedies, and dietary supplements. *Do not take any over-the-counter medications unless approved by your doctor.*

Food/Alcohol Interactions

Avoid alcohol.

Pregnancy/Nursing

A woman must never become pregnant while taking this drug. Divalproex is known to cause birth defects. But seizures during pregnancy also pose risks to the fetus. You and your doctor will have to weigh the benefits against the potential risks. This drug passes into breast milk. Bottle-feed your baby if you must take this drug.

Seniors

Side effects may be more pronounced in older adults due to decreased kidney and liver function. Your doctor may prescribe a low dose.

Warning

In some cases, the generic equivalent of this drug is not recommended. Verify this with your doctor or your pharmacist. This drug increases the risk of spina bifida (a birth defect involving the incomplete closure of the spinal column) from 1 in 1,000 births in the general population to 1 to 2 in 100 for pregnant women who take this drug.

Comments

If you have a seizure disorder, you should wear a medical identification tag and carry an ID card listing the type of disorder and a list of your current medications.

Brand Name
Depo-Provera (contraceptive injection)

Generic Name
medroxyprogesterone acetate

Type of Drug
Progestin; contraceptive injection. This drug is a synthetic steroid that mimics the effects of progesterone, a naturally occurring hormone essential to the female reproductive system.

For
Birth control.

Availability and Dosage
Injection by a health practitioner: Usual injection schedule is once every three months. When taken regularly and properly, this method of birth control is more than 99 percent effective. Women who wish to become pregnant usually do so within one year of stopping the injections.

Side Effects
More common include weight gain and irregular menstrual bleeding. Others include nervousness, dizziness, stomach pain, headache, and fatigue. This drug may also cause bone loss, a risk factor in osteoporosis.

Drug Interactions
This drug may interact with some anticonvulsants, troglitazone, and carbamazepine. Always inform your doctors of every medication you are taking, including nonprescription medicines, vitamins, herbal remedies, and dietary supplements.

Food/Alcohol Interactions
No special warnings.

Pregnancy/Nursing
A woman must not become pregnant while on this drug. To guarantee this, the first injection is usually given during the first 5 days of your menstrual period. If you are breast-feeding, the first injection will not be given until the sixth week.

Seniors

Older adults would be more likely to take this drug for conditions other than birth control. No special warnings. Immediately inform your doctor of any persistent or troublesome side effects.

Warning

Make sure your doctor has your entire medical history, including a history of blood clots in your legs, stroke, cancer, or heart, liver, or kidney disease. If you experience numbness in your arms or legs, unexpected flow of breast milk, skin rash, severe headache, shortness of breath, or changes in speech or vision, *seek emergency medical treatment*.

Comments

Progestins are also prescribed for menstrual irregularities, including amenorrhea (cessation of menstrual periods) and endometriosis. The oral tablet form of medroxyprogesterone acetate can be used to treat hormonal imbalances, abnormal menstrual or uterine bleeding, endometriosis, and premenstrual syndrome (see Provera).

Desogen

See Oral Contraceptives

desogestrel and ethinyl estradiol

See Oral Contraceptives

Brand Name
Desyrel

Generic Name

trazodone*

Type of Drug

Antidepressant

For

Depression; panic disorder

Availability and Dosage

Tablets: 50 mg, 100 mg, 150 mg, 300 mg. Should be taken with food. Do not take more of this medicine than prescribed. Do not suddenly stop taking this medication without consulting your doctor.

Side Effects

More common include drowsiness, dizziness, light-headedness, dry mouth, headache, and insomnia. Others include nervousness, nausea, vomiting, fatigue, constipation, blurred vision, and muscle aches.

Drug Interactions

This drug may interact with antihypertensives and other medications for depression, particularly monoamine oxidase (MAO) inhibitors. Do not take trazodone within 14 days of taking an MAO inhibitor. Trazodone may also interact with digoxin, central nervous system (CNS) depressants, muscle relaxants, antiseizures, and antihistamines. Over-the-counter medications containing alcohol should be avoided, as well as any herbal medications containing kava kava, St. John's wort, or valerian. Always inform your doctors of every medication you are taking, including nonprescription medicines, vitamins, herbal remedies, and dietary supplements. *Do not take any over-the-counter medications unless approved by your doctor.*

Food/Alcohol Interactions

Avoid alcohol. It may increase the sedative effect.

Pregnancy/Nursing

A woman must never take this drug during pregnancy, or if she is trying to become pregnant. There is a risk of damage to the fetus. This drug passes into breast milk. Bottle-feed your baby if you must take this drug.

Seniors

Older adults may be more sensitive to trazodone. Your doctor may prescribe a low dose.

Warning

You will need to be monitored by a health care professional while on trazodone or any antidepressant. Make sure your physician has your entire medical history, including a history of suicidal thoughts, irregular heartbeat, manic-depressive illness (bipolar disorder), or heart, kidney, or liver disease. Do not self-medicate with nonprescription medications while taking trazodone; some of their ingredients have the potential to interact with this drug.

Comments

Trazodone is chemically unrelated to tricyclic or other known antidepressants. It is often used when depression does not respond to other antidepressants or when the patient has experienced intolerable side effects from them. Trazodone works by helping to balance levels of serotonin, a brain chemical known to affect mood and emotions.

Brand Name
Detrol

Generic Name

tolterodine tartrate

Type of Drug

Anticholinergic; bladder sedative. This drug helps to control abnormal bladder contractions that result in frequent, strong, sudden urges to urinate.

For

Overactive bladder.

Availability and Dosage

Tablets: 1 mg, 2 mg.

Side Effects

More common include dry mouth, constipation, dry eyes, headache, and indigestion. Others include dizziness, blurred vision, and inability to urinate.

Drug Interactions

Dosages of this drug may need to be adjusted if you are taking erythromycin, clarithromycin, itraconazole, ketoconazole, or fluoxetine. Use caution when taking any over-the-counter remedies for coughs or colds. Always inform your doctors of every medication you are taking, including nonprescription medicines, vitamins, herbal remedies, and dietary supplements. *Do not take any over-the-counter medications unless approved by your doctor.*

Food/Alcohol Interactions

No special interaction warnings, although alcohol and caffeine should be avoided or restricted as they can act as diuretics.

Sugar, spicy foods, and carbonated drinks can also irritate the bladder.

Pregnancy/Nursing

No special warnings, although all drugs during pregnancy and breast-feeding should be avoided if possible. Before taking this drug, discuss with your doctor the benefits versus the potential risks.

Seniors

Studies of this drug included patients up to age 91. Generally, no dosage adjustment is required except in cases of potential interaction with other drugs or if there is impaired liver function.

Warning

Make sure your doctor has your entire medical history, including a history of bladder blockage, gastrointestinal blockage, narrow-angle glaucoma, or liver or kidney disease.

Comments

An estimated 17 million Americans, primarily women, are affected by overactive bladder. Symptoms include the need to urinate at least 8 times in 24 hours, getting up more than twice a night to urinate, frequent, sudden urges to urinate, and wetting accidents. Stress incontinence (passing urine when coughing, sneezing, or laughing) often occurs in postmenopausal women whose pelvic muscles have been weakened by pregnancy. Many women are reluctant to discuss this problem with their gynecologists or urologists due to embarrassment, but medication and lifestyle changes can often help once a proper diagnosis is made.

diazepam*

See Valium

dicyclomine hydrochloride

See Bentyl

diethylpropion

See Tenuate

Brand Name
Diflucan*

Generic Name

fluconazole

Type of Drug

Antifungal. This drug was the first of its type to treat vaginal yeast infections systemically with a single oral dose. Some doctors prescribe it in conjunction with a topical antifungal to provide immediate relief of uncomfortable burning and itching.

For

Vaginal yeast infections due to candida; thrush (infections of the mouth or the throat); infections of the central nervous system.

Availability and Dosage

Tablets: 150 mg. A single oral tablet is the full course of therapy for most vaginal yeast infections. May be taken with or without food. Doses for other uses of fluconazole may vary depending on the condition being treated.

Side Effects

More common include headache, nausea, and stomach pain. Others include diarrhea, indigestion, dizziness, and changes in taste.

Drug Interactions

This drug may interact with certain oral contraceptives, cimetidine, oral antidiabetics, some antiasthmatics, anticoagulants (blood thinners), phenytoin, zidovudine, and antacids. Always inform your doctors of every medication you are taking, including nonprescription medicines, vitamins, herbal remedies, and dietary supplements. *Do not take any over-the-counter medications unless approved by your doctor.*

Food/Alcohol Interactions

If you suffer from repeated, persistent vaginal yeast infections, your doctor, nutritionist, or other health care provider may supply a list of foods to avoid or restrict.

Pregnancy/Nursing

Not recommended. Bottle-feed your baby if you must take this drug.

Seniors

No special warnings unless you have impaired kidney function. Take as prescribed and immediately inform your doctor of any persistent or troublesome side effects.

Warning

If symptoms persist, notify your doctor. Women receiving fluconazole in studies experienced relief in 1 to 2 days. Women who are diabetic, pregnant, using oral contraceptives, or taking antibiotics are more susceptible to vaginal yeast infections.

Comments

An overgrowth of the fungus *candida albicans* results in a vaginal yeast infection, a common condition that affects up to 75 percent of women at some point in their lives. This fungus lives naturally in the body until something upsets the balance—an antibiotic designed to treat another infection, for example, that also wipes out the "good" bacteria in the vagina, and a yeast infection follows. Nonprescription intravaginal treatments for yeast infections should be used for *recurrent* infections only; do not attempt to self-medicate using over-the-counter products without a proper diagnosis. Some doctors recommend that women refrain from sexual intercourse during treatment.

digoxin

See Lanoxin

dihydroergotamine mesylate

See Migranal

Dilacor SR

See Cardizem CD*

Brand Name
Dilantin*

Generic Name

phenytoin

Type of Drug

Anticonvulsant. This drug does not cure epilepsy. It works only to control symptoms. If you have epilepsy, you should wear a medical identification tag at all times and carry an ID card that lists all the medications you are currently taking.

For

Certain types of epileptic seizures.

Availability and Dosage

Capsules: 30 mg, 100 mg. Chewable tablets: 50 mg. Oral suspension: 30 mg, 125 mg per 5 ml. Should be taken with food, not milk. Do not abruptly stop taking this drug without your doctor's approval.

Side Effects

More common include dizziness, constipation, drowsiness, growth of gums, and rapid or uncontrolled eye movements (nystagmus). Others include twitching, fatigue, depression, tremor, and excessive growth of body or facial hair.

Drug Interactions

Phenytoin has the potential to interact with a wide variety of medications, including central nervous system (CNS) depressants, anticoagulants (blood thinners), cimetidine, fluconazole, tricyclic antidepressants, fluoxetine, corticosteroids, estrogens, oral contraceptives, sulfa drugs, divalproex, and antacids. Always inform your doctors of every medication you are taking, including nonprescription medicines, vitamins, herbal remedies, and dietary supplements. *Do not take any over-the-counter medications unless approved by your doctor.*

Food/Alcohol Interactions

Avoid alcohol and caffeine. Avoid or limit foods or beverages high in calcium; they can interfere with the absorption of this drug.

Pregnancy/Nursing

Not recommended. Birth defects have been reported. However, if a woman has seizures during pregnancy, that can also pose a risk to the fetus. Discuss with your doctor the risks versus the benefits of taking this drug. Bottle-feed your baby if you must take this drug.

Seniors

Side effects may be increased in older adults. Your doctor may prescribe a low dose.

Warning

Dental care including regular teeth cleaning is essential while on this drug. If you experience swelling or bleeding of your gums, notify your doctor or your dentist.

Comments

Discuss with your doctor how much calcium you can take while on this drug. Although this is an essential mineral for women, it may interfere with absorption of phenytoin.

diltiazem, hydrochloride

See Cardizem CD*

Brand Name
Diovan* (also Diovan HCT)

Generic Name

valsartan; valsartan and hydrochlorothiazide (Diovan HCT)

Type of Drug

Antihypertensive; angiotensin-receptor blocker. Antihypertensives do not cure high blood pressure; they control the condition for as long as the drugs are taken. Diovan HCT is used for patients who need both an angiotensin-receptor blocker and a diuretic to control hypertension.

For

High blood pressure.

Availability and Dosage

Capsules: 80 mg, 160 mg.

Side Effects

More common include headache, dizziness, fatigue, and abdominal pain. More common with Diovan HCT include headache, dizziness, fatigue, sore throat, cough, and diarrhea.

Drug Interactions

No special warnings, although all drugs have the ability to interact with other drugs. Report any problems to your doctor or your pharmacist. Always inform your doctors of every medication you are taking, including nonprescription medicines, vitamins, herbal remedies, and dietary supplements.

Food/Alcohol Interactions

Avoid salt substitutes. Your doctor may suggest a diet low in sodium to help control high blood pressure.

Pregnancy/Nursing

Not recommended, especially during the second and third trimesters. Bottle-feed your baby if you must take this drug.

Seniors

No special warnings. Take as prescribed and immediately inform your doctor of any persistent or troublesome side effects.

Warning

This drug may cause dizziness. Do not drive, operate machinery, or perform any task that requires alertness until you know how this drug affects you.

Comments

Heart disease is the leading cause of death in women, although hypertension is more common in men than in women. However, African American women have the highest incidence of the disease. Stroke—which is linked to hypertension—is also higher in African American women than in white women. Signs of stroke, according to the American Heart Association, include sudden, severe headache, sudden loss or dimming of vision, loss of speech, and sudden weakness or numbness of the face, arm, or leg on one side of the body.

divalproex sodium

See Depakote*

donepezil

See Aricept

Brand Name

Doryx (also Vibramycin)

Generic Name

doxycycline hyclate

Type of Drug

Antibiotic. This large class of drugs is among the most commonly prescribed. Some antibiotics work against a limited number of microorganisms. Broad-spectrum antibiotics are effective against a variety of bacteria. Your doctor will prescribe the correct antibiotic depending on the type of infection. Antibiotics are useless against viral infections such as colds and flu. Doxycycline is a tetracycline antibiotic.

For

Various bacterial infections including urinary-tract infections (UTIs); sexually tranmitted diseases (STDs) including chlamydia; fevers caused by ticks and lice, including Lyme disease and Rocky Mountain spotted fever.

Availability and Dosage

Tablets: 50 mg, 100 mg. Capsules: 50 mg, 100 mg. Oral suspension: 25 mg per 5 ml. Oral syrup: 50 mg per 5 ml. Take with a full glass of water, either with or without food. It is essential to take the complete course of antibiotics prescribed. If you fail to do so, increased drug resistance by any leftover bacteria is likely to occur.

Side Effects

More common include stomach cramps, diarrhea, nausea, and increased sun sensitivity. Others include vomiting, rash, sore throat, loss of appetite, tongue irritation, and genital itching.

Drug Interactions

Tetracycline antibiotics have the potential to interact with other antibiotics, oral contraceptives, anticonvulsants, antivirals, and lithium; multivitamins that contain calcium, zinc, and magnesium; antacids, and calcium supplements. Do not take iron supplements or sodium bicarbonate within 3 hours of taking tetracycline antibiotics. Always inform your doctors of every medication you are taking, including nonprescription medicines, vitamins, herbal remedies, and dietary supplements. *Do not take any over-the-counter medications unless approved by your doctor.*

Food/Alcohol Interactions

Avoid or limit alcohol. Do not consume dairy products and iron-fortified cereals within 2 hours of taking this drug. Drink plenty of water while on this medication.

Pregnancy/Nursing

Not recommended. Doxycycline passes into breast milk. Bottle-feed your baby if you must take this drug.

Seniors

Side effects may be increased in older adults, including genital itching. Your doctor may prescribe a low dose.

Warning

Women who take a combination of birth control pills and tetra-cycline have become pregnant. Use an additional method of contraception while on this course of treatment.

Comments

Chlamydia is the most common sexually transmitted disease (STD), but is asymptomatic in as many as 75 percent of infected women. Symptoms include lower abdominal pain, bleeding or pain during intercourse, a bleeding or swollen cervix, and vaginal discharge. It can lead to pelvic inflammatory disease (PID) and infertility.

Brand Name
Dovonex

Generic Name

calcipotriene

Type of Drug

Antipsoriatic. This drug—a synthetic form of vitamin D—is used to relieve symptoms of psoriasis: patches of inflamed, red skin covered by silvery scales. There is no cure; drug therapy is used only to relieve symptoms.

For

Plaque psoriasis.

Availability and Dosage

Topical cream, ointment, and solution: 0.005%. The solution is used for psoriatic scalp conditions. Follow package insert for application instructions.

Side Effects

More common include rash, burning and stinging (temporary), and skin peeling. Others include dry skin, thinning skin, headache, and worsening of symptoms.

Drug Interactions

No special warnings, although all drugs have the ability to interact with other drugs. Report any problems to your doctor or your pharmacist. Ask your doctor about taking products that contain vitamin D.

Food/Alcohol Interactions

No special warnings.

Pregnancy/Nursing

Not recommended. It is unknown whether this drug passes into breast milk. Discuss the benefits versus the risks with your doctor.

Seniors

Side effects may be more likely in older adults, including side effects involving the skin.

Warning

Make sure your doctor has your entire medical history, including a history of high levels of calcium in the urine (hypercalciuria), high blood levels of calcium (hypercalcemia), high blood levels of vitamin D, and kidney stones.

Comments

You may see improvement as soon as 2 weeks, but the maximum benefit of this drug may take up to 8 weeks.

doxazosin

See Cardura

doxycycline hyclate

See Doryx

Brand Name
Dyazide*

Generic Name

hydrochlorothiazide (HCTZ) and triamterene

Type of Drug

Diuretic. This drug contains two diuretics in combination to promote the loss of water and salt from the body, which results in the lowering of blood pressure. There are many combination drugs containing hydrochlorothiazide. Your doctor will tell you which type of diuretic you are using and whether any dietary changes are needed.

For

High blood pressure; edema; elimination of excess water from the body.

Availability and Dosage

Tablets: 25 mg, 50 mg, 100 mg. Oral solution: 50 mg per 5 ml. Intensol oral solution: 100 mg per ml. May be taken with or without food.

Side Effects

More common include headache, stomach upset, loss of appetite, and drowsiness. Others include dizziness, increased sun sensitivity, burning tongue and diarrhea. There may be increased urination, which may subside as your body adjusts to this drug.

Drug Interactions

This drug can interact with digitalis drugs, allopurinol, anticoagulants (blood thinners), some chemotherapy drugs, oral antidiabetics, insulin, lithium, and indomethacin. Always inform your doctors of every medication you are taking, including nonprescription medicines, vitamins, herbal remedies, and dietary supplements. *Do not take any over-the-counter medications unless approved by your doctor.*

Food/Alcohol Interactions

Avoid alcohol. Your doctor may provide you with a list of foods high in potassium to avoid or restrict.

Pregnancy/Nursing

Not recommended. This drug may pass into breast milk. You may wish to bottle-feed your baby while on this drug.

Seniors

Side effects may be more likely in older adults, including increased dizziness when rising abruptly from a sitting or reclining position.

Warning

Do not drive or operate machinery until you know how this drug will affect you. If you experience weakness, nausea, vomiting, rapid heartbeat, dizziness, or rash, notify your doctor immediately.

Comments

Both diuretics in this combination drug cause loss of body water, but triamterene has the ability to hold potassium in the body. Do not take any potassium supplements while on this drug.

E-Mycin

See Ery-Tab*

E.E.S.

See Ery-Tab*

Brand Name
Easprin (also ZORprin)

Generic Name

aspirin

Type of Drug

Nonsteroidal antiinflammatory drug (NSAID). Aspirin, in use since 1899, is the original and most well-known NSAID.

For

Relief of pain and inflammation; reduction of fever; relief of symptoms of arthritis; prevention of blood-clot formation.

Availability and Dosage

Tablets, capsules, caplets, chewable tablets: aspirin comes in numerous dosages in both prescription and nonprescription strength, in plain or buffered, and is also an ingredient widely used in combination with other drugs. Your doctor will determine the appropriate dose. When used for arthritic conditions, you may be prescribed up to 5400 mg a day in divided doses. Wait 30 minutes before you lie down to reduce irritation of the esophagus. Should be taken with food to reduce stomach upset.

Side Effects

More common include stomach upset and ringing in the ears. Others include diarrhea, nausea, reduction in urine output, and rash.

Drug Interactions

Anticoagulants (blood thinners) should not be combined with aspirin. Interactions can occur with corticosteroids, oral antidiabetics, methotrexate, antiarthritics, anticonvulsants, and other NSAIDs. Always inform your doctors of every medication you are taking, including nonprescription medicines, vitamins, herbal remedies, and dietary supplements. *If you take high doses for arthritis, do not take any over-the-counter medications unless approved by your doctor.*

Food/Alcohol Interactions

Avoid or limit alcohol, as it may increase the risk of stomach irritation and bleeding. Aspirin carries a label warning for people who drink 3 or more alcoholic beverages a day. Caffeine can heighten aspirin's pain-relieving effect. Drink plenty of water when taking large doses for arthritis or rheumatoid arthritis.

Pregnancy/Nursing

Not recommended, especially during the last trimester. It can cause fetal bleeding, low birth weight, and an increased risk of bleeding for the mother. Reports differ regarding the use of aspirin during breast-feeding; consult your doctor.

Seniors

Older adults may have an increased risk of gastrointestinal bleeding and stomach irritation.

Warning

Do not give aspirin to children. It can cause Reye's syndrome, a rare but potentially fatal condition. If you are going to have surgery, you will need to stop this drug. Tell your doctor if you have a history of asthma, diabetes, ulcers, hemophilia, hypertension, thyroid disease, or kidney or liver disease. If you experience hearing loss, blood in the urine, rapid breathing, swelling, or dizziness, *seek emergency medical treatment*.

Comments

Aspirin's blood-thinning properties play an important role in reducing the risk of complications or death from heart attack if taken at the first signs of an attack, preventing recurrent attacks with regular use of low doses, and reducing the risk of recurring stroke. Do not self-medicate for cardiovascular problems without consulting your doctor. If you are self-medicating for pain or fever using one of the many nonprescription brands of aspirin or aspirin combinations, read package instructions carefully and notify your doctor if you experience any unpleasant side effects or if your symptoms do not improve. Do not combine nonprescription aspirin medications with other pain relievers including ibuprofen, naproxen, acetaminophen, and ketoprofen.

Brand Name
Effexor*

Generic Name

venlafaxine

Type of Drug

Antidepressant. This drug is used to treat symptoms in patients experiencing major depression who have not responded to other antidepressants. A major depressive episode suggests a persistent depressed mood that interferes with normal functioning.

For

Depression.

Availability and Dosage

Tablets: 25 mg, 37.5 mg, 75 mg, 100 mg. Should be taken with food at regularly spaced intervals. It may take 2 weeks before you see an improvement in symptoms. Do not abruptly stop taking this drug. Your dosage will have to be gradually decreased.

Side Effects

More common include drowsiness, dry mouth, dizziness, changes in taste, nausea, weakness, sweating, constipation, and loss of appetite. Others include abnormal dreams, anxiety, blurred vision, headache, prickling sensation, and tremors.

Drug Interactions

This drug has the potential to interact with drugs that affect the central nervous system, including narcotic painkillers, tranquilizers, weight-loss drugs, sleep aids, and the herbal remedy St. John's wort. The most serious interactions occur with monoamine oxidase MAO inhibitors. Never take these drugs together; dosing should be separated by a minimum of 14 days. Always inform your doctors of every medication you are taking, including nonprescription medicines, vitamins, herbal remedies, and dietary supplements. *Do not take any over-the-counter medications unless approved by your doctor.*

Food/Alcohol Interactions

Avoid alcohol.

Pregnancy/Nursing

There have been no adequate studies of venlafaxine during pregnancy. All drugs during pregnancy and breast-feeding should be avoided if possible. Before taking this drug, discuss with your doctor the benefits versus the potential risks.

Seniors

No special warnings. Take as prescribed and immediately inform your doctor of any persistent or troublesome side effects.

Warning

The use of venlafaxine within 14 days of taking a monoamine oxidase (MAO) inhibitor antidepressant can cause severe and potentially fatal reactions. If you experience difficulty in breathing, rapid heartbeat, seizures, muscle spasms or rigidity, or high fever, seek emergency medical treatment immediately. This drug should be used with caution if you have a history of heart, liver, or kidney disease, hypertension (high blood pressure), hypotension (low blood pressure), suicidal tendencies, or seizures.

Comments

This drug is unlike other types of antidepressants. It works by helping to maintain the balance of serotonin and norepinephrine levels in the brain. In 1999, venlafaxine was the first antidepressant to be approved for general anxiety disorder (GAD).

Brand Name
Elavil (also Endep)

Generic Name
amitriptyline*

Type of Drug
Tricyclic antidepressant. These drugs increase the levels of norepinephrine and serotonin in the brain, may have a mild sedative effect, and generally work to correct a chemical imbalance believed to be the basis for certain types of depression. Your physician may prescribe one of several tricyclics based on your particular symptoms.

For
Depression; migraines; chronic pain; bulimia.

Availability and Dosage
Tablets: 10 mg, 25 mg, 50 mg, 75 mg, 100 mg, 150 mg. Some doctors recommend taking this drug at bedtime to minimize side effects. Do not take more of this medicine than is prescribed. Do not abruptly stop taking this medication. Your dose will have to be gradually reduced.

Side Effects
More common include daytime drowsiness, dizziness, dry mouth, anxiety, and nausea. Others include numbness and tingling in hands or feet, fluid retention, changes in sex drive, constipation, diarrhea, dry eyes, blurred vision, and urine colored bright green.

Drug Interactions
Amitriptyline has the potential to interact with a wide variety of medications, including amphetamines, appetite suppressants, antidiabetics, antipsychotics, cimetidine, other central nervous system (CNS) depressants, thyroid drugs, muscle relaxants, oral contraceptives, and some blood-pressure–lowering medications. The most serious interactions occur with monoamine oxidase (MAO) inhibitor antidepressants. The use of MAO inhibitors and amitriptyline must be separated by a minimum of 14 days. Always inform your doctors of every medication you are taking, in-

cluding nonprescription medicines, vitamins, herbal remedies, and dietary supplements. *Do not take any over-the-counter medications unless approved by your doctor.*

Food/Alcohol Interactions

Avoid alcohol; it will increase the sedative effect. Amitriptyline can cause significant weight gain in some patients (up to 30 pounds or more), although it is unclear whether this is caused by the drug itself or by an increase in appetite.

Pregnancy/Nursing

Not recommended.

Seniors

Older patients may be more susceptible to side effects, including drowsiness, dizziness, and confusion.

Warning

The use of amitriptyline within 14 days of taking a monoamine oxidase (MAO) inhibitor antidepressant can cause severe and potentially fatal reactions. If you experience difficulty in breathing, rapid heartbeat, seizures, muscle spasms or rigidity, or high fever, seek emergency medical treatment immediately. This drug should be used with caution if you have a history of heart, liver, or kidney disease, glaucoma, asthma, alcohol abuse, suicidal tendencies, or seizures.

Comments

Tricyclics were much more commonly prescribed before the development of newer antidepressants such as fluoxetine (Prozac). They are often used for other conditions including migraine, nerve pain, ulcers, and interstitial cystitis. Amitriptyline has also been shown to be effective in relieving the symptoms of fibromyalgia, a chronic, debilitating condition marked by constant muscular pain, fatigue, and insomnia. Fibromyalgia affects 6 million Americans, most of them women between age 20 and 40, most of whom were told that these symptoms were "all in their heads." In 1993, the American College of Rheumatology officially recognized fibromyalgia as a disease.

Brand Name
Eldepryl

Generic Name

selegiline

Type of Drug

Antiparkinsonian; monoamine oxidase (MAO) inhibitor.

For

Parkinson's disease. This drug is often used in combination with other antiparkinsonian drugs to help relieve the symptoms of the disease—trembling of head and limbs, muscular stiffness, and inability to control movement. They do not cure the disease.

Availability and Dosage

Tablets: 5 mg. Capsules: 5 mg. Take with food, usually during the daytime. Your physician will probably use the lowest effective dose to minimize the risk of side effects.

Side Effects

Side effects may be increased when selegiline is used in combination with levodopa or carbidopa. More common include nausea, anxiety, constipation, diarrhea, loss of appetite, stomach pain, dizziness, fainting, dry mouth, and insomnia. Others include increased tremors, vivid dreams, loss of coordination, weakness, hair loss, headache, confusion, back pain, itchy skin, ringing in the ears, taste changes, fatigue, and clenching or grinding of the teeth (with higher doses).

Drug Interactions

Selegiline is a monoamine oxidase (MAO) inhibitor and has an increased risk of potentially serious interactions. This drug may interact with narcotics, antidepressants, sumatriptan, nefazodone, paroxetine, sertraline, venlafaxine, and fluoxetine. Always inform your doctors of every medication you are taking, including nonprescription medicines, vitamins, herbal remedies, and dietary supplements. *Do not take any over-the-counter medications unless approved by your doctor.*

Food/Alcohol Interactions

Avoid alcohol. MAO inhibitors carry a high risk of food interactions. Avoid foods high in tyramine, such as aged cheeses (cheddar, Camembert, Stilton, and others), sauerkraut, chicken liver, chocolate, overripe avocados, fermented meats (salami, pepperoni), and yeast extracts. MAO inhibitor/food interactions can lead to dizziness, nausea, pounding headache, rapid heartbeat, and a dangerous rise in blood pressure. Your doctor or your pharmacist should supply you with a list of specific foods to avoid.

Pregnancy/Nursing

No special warnings, although all drugs during pregnancy and breast-feeding should be avoided if possible. Before taking this drug, discuss with your doctor the benefits versus the potential risks.

Seniors

No special warnings. Take as prescribed and immediately inform your doctor of any persistent or troublesome side effects.

Warning

If you experience chest pain, enlarged pupils, rapid or slow heartbeat, fever, stiff neck, muscle spasms, or severe headache, seek emergency medical treatment immediately.

Comments

Parkinson's disease is a degenerative disease caused by a loss of dopamine-producing cells in the brain, which help to convey information about movement to other parts of the brain. Symptoms include tremors, stiffness, difficulty in walking or moving, slowing of body movements, loss of balance and jerky movements. Research is now being conducted on at least a dozen additional drugs to treat this debilitating disease.

Brand Name
Elocon*

Generic Name

mometasone furoate

Type of Drug

Topical corticosteroid.

For

Relief of swelling, redness, itching, and other discomforts of various skin problems.

Availability and Dosage

Topical cream, ointment, lotion: 0.1%. Follow your doctor's instructions for application. You may experience a mild stinging when first applied. The topical forms of mometasone are for external use only. Do not use near the eyes.

Side Effects

More common include itching or burning, irritation, acne, redness, dryness, and scaling. Others include blurred vision, nausea, stretch marks, tearing of the skin, increase in hair growth, and fatigue.

Drug Interactions

No special warnings, although all drugs have the ability to interact with other drugs. Report any problems to your doctor or your pharmacist.

Food/Alcohol Interactions

No special warnings.

Pregnancy/Nursing

Not recommended. This drug may pass into breast milk. Bottle-feed your baby while on this drug.

Seniors

Topical corticosteroids present less risk of bone loss than do oral forms of the drug. Older adults should not use this medicine or any over-the-counter (hydrocortisone) products unless under a doctor's supervision.

Warning

If symptoms do not improve after 7 days of treatment, notify your doctor. If you have painful sores or blisters that are not healing, or severe burning or itching, contact your doctor at once.

Comments

Do not bandage or cover the affected area unless directed by your doctor. If you are to apply a bandage or wrap, make sure you understand the instructions for application. Wrapping the skin may increase the possibility of side effects, as it causes more of the drug to be absorbed into the skin. Symptomatic relief gained from these topical drugs may be temporary if the underlying cause of the skin condition is not found and treated.

enalapril maleate

See Vasotec*

Brand Name
Enbrel

Generic Name
etanercept

Type of Drug
Antirheumatic.

For
The relief of symptoms of rheumatoid arthritis, including pain, fatigue, and stiffness. This drug is usually prescribed for patients who have not responded adequately to other antirheumatic drugs. It is sometimes used in conjunction with methotrexate (Rheumatrex).

Availability and Dosage
Subcutaneous (under the skin) injection. Recommended dosage for adults: 25 mg twice weekly, 72 to 96 hours apart. Your doctor will administer the first injection. You may give yourself subsequent injections with proper instruction from a health care professional. Usual sites are the arms, stomach, and thighs.

Side Effects
More common include itching, pain, or swelling at the injection site, and upper respiratory infections. Others include dizziness, cough, headache, rhinitis, abdominal pain, rash, and sinusitis.

Drug Interactions
No known interactions with other drugs. However, etanercept may interact with live-virus vaccines. Notify your doctor before you get any vaccinations.

Food/Alcohol Interactions
Avoid alcohol.

Pregnancy/Nursing
No special warnings, although all drugs during pregnancy and breast-feeding should be avoided if possible. Before taking this

drug, discuss with your doctor the benefits versus the potential risks. This drug may pass into breast milk.

Seniors

No special warnings. Take as prescribed and immediately inform your doctor of any persistent or troublesome side effects.

Warning

In 1999, the FDA revealed that 30 of the estimated 25,000 adult users of this drug had developed serious infections, 6 of them fatal. These events occurred in patients who were prone to infections, such as those who had advanced or poorly controlled diabetes, or those whose immune systems were compromised. Do not take this drug if you have an infection of any type or if you have an allergy to etanercept or one of its components. Make sure your doctor has your complete medical history.

Comments

About 2 million Americans suffer from rheumatoid arthritis, 1.5 million of them women. The immune system, which normally protects the body from disease, attacks healthy joints of the body, resulting in pain, stiffness, and swelling. Etanercept, a breakthrough drug, was found in clinical trials to enable RA patients to improve performance in daily activities—62% of patients had at least a 20% improvement in study criteria that included pain and joint swelling. The effectiveness of this drug continues only for as long as it is taken. Studies indicate that you may see improvement in symptoms in as little as 2 weeks, with most people receiving maximum benefits within 3 months.

Endep

See Elavil

Endocet*

See Percocet

Brand Name
Entex

Generic Name

guaifenesin and phenylpropanolamine*

Type of Drug

Nasal decongestant/expectorant combination. Phenylpropanolamine constricts blood vessels to reduce nasal inflammation,
and guaifenesin loosens upper respiratory-tract mucus secretions to promote expectoration.

For

Relief of symptoms of allergy, the common cold, and other respiratory ailments.

Availability and Dosage

Capsules, oral syrup, and granules in various doses. Take as directed by your doctor or your pharmacist. Drink plenty of water
while on this product to promote liquefaction of mucus secretions.

Side Effects

More common include restlessness, nervousness, insomnia,
headache, tremors, and stomach upset. Others include heart arrhythmias, palpitations, irritability, loss of appetite, and skin pallor.

Drug Interactions

These two drugs, separately and together, have the potential to
interact with a wide variety of medications. Do not take this product if you are on monoamine oxidase (MAO) inhibitor antidepressants or antihypertensives. Always inform your doctors of
every medication you are taking, including nonprescription medicines, vitamins, herbal remedies, and dietary supplements. *Do
not take any over-the-counter medications unless approved by
your doctor.*

Food/Alcohol Interactions

Avoid alcohol. Drink plenty of water and other fluids while on this
medication. Caffeine may intensify the effects of phenylpropanolamine and can result in aggravation of some side effects. You may want to limit your intake of coffee, colas,
chocolate, and other caffeinated foods and beverages while on
this drug.

Pregnancy/Nursing

Not recommended. Bottle-feed your baby if you must take this
product.

Seniors

Older adults may be more susceptible to the side effects associated with this drug combination. Ask your doctor about taking the lowest possible effective dose to minimize adverse reactions.

Warning

Do not use this product within 14 days of taking a monoamine oxidase (MAO) inhibitor. Phenylpropanolamine can raise heart rate and blood pressure. Do not take this product if you have heart disease, high blood pressure, glaucoma, stomach ulcers, diabetes, or thyroid disease. If you experience tremors, confusion, seizures, hallucinations, heart arrhythmias, changes in blood pressure, vomiting, or lethargy, seek emergency medical treatment.

Comments

Entex is only one of hundreds of prescription and nonprescription allergy and cold medications in which guaifenesin is either the main ingredient or is used in combination with other active ingredients. Both guiafenesin and phenylpropanolamine are found in many over-the-counter medications used to self-medicate coughs, colds, bronchitis, sinus and throat infections, and other ailments. Phenylpropanolamine is also found in nonprescription diet pills. Generally speaking, these products should not be used by people with high blood pressure, diabetes, glaucoma, thyroid disease, stomach ulcers, heart disease, and other conditions as indicated. Follow package directions carefully, and consult your doctor if you have any problems.

Brand Name
Ery-Tab* (also E-Mycin, E.E.S.)

Generic Name

erythromycin (E.E.S. is erythromycin ethylsuccinate)

Type of Drug

Antibiotic.

For

Various infections including urinary-tract infections (UTIs), acne; chlamydia; gonorrhea; bacterial endocarditis; pelvic inflammatory disease (PID); respiratory-tract infections.

Availability and Dosage

(Ery-Tab) Delayed-release tablets: 250 mg, 333 mg, 500 mg. (E-Mycin) Delayed-release tablets: 250 mg, 333 mg. (E.E.S.) Oral suspension: 200 mg per 5 ml. (E.E.S.) Tablets: 400 mg. (E.E.S.) Chewable tablets: 200 mg. Should be taken on an empty stomach with a full glass of water, 1 hour before or 2 hours after a meal. Because the recommended dosage will vary depending on the individual infection, follow your doctor's directions and refer to the detailed instructions given by your pharmacist. This drug works best when taken at evenly spaced intervals. Take this medicine exactly as prescribed.

Side Effects

More common include nausea, stomach cramping, diarrhea, and colitis. Others include vaginal irritation, sore tongue, abdominal pains, loss of appetite, and rash.

Drug Interactions

Erythromycin has the potential to interact with a wide variety of medications. When taking this medication, it is especially important that you be careful with any and all other medications you are taking. The following is only a partial list of drugs that may interact with erythromycin: anticonvulsants, antiasthmatics, some other antibiotics, acetaminophen, anabolic steroids, thyroid drugs, hydroxychloroquine, promethazine, estrogens, oral contraceptives, gold salts, some antihistamines, digoxin, lovastatin, felodipine, cyclosporine, carbamazepine, anticoagulants (blood thinners), and methotrexate. Always inform your doctors of every medication you are taking, including nonprescription medicines, vitamins, herbal remedies, and dietary supplements. *Do not take any over-the-counter medications unless approved by your doctor.*

Food/Alcohol Interactions

Avoid or limit alcohol.

Pregnancy/Nursing

Not recommended. Erythromycin passes into breast milk. Bottle-feed your baby while on this drug.

Seniors

Older adults may be at increased risk for some side effects, including hearing loss, when taking higher doses of this drug. People who have liver disease or liver damage should be monitored regularly while on this drug.

Warning

Any antibiotics should be taken for the full course of treatment. It is especially important to do so when taking erythromycin for any streptococcal ("strep") infection. Failure to do so may result in potentially serious heart problems later.

Comments

Make sure your doctor knows your entire medical history if this drug is prescribed, especially a history of heart disease (including heart arrhythmias), liver disease, colitis, or hearing impairment. There are topical forms of erythromycin (brand names A/T/S, Erycette, T-Stat) that are used for acne.

Erycette

*See Ery-Tab**

erythromycin

*See Ery-Tab**

Brand Name
Esidrix (also HydroDIURIL)

Generic Name

hydrochlorothiazide (HCTZ)*

Type of Drug

Diuretic; antihypertensive. Diuretics promote the loss of water and salt from the body, which results in the lowering of blood pressure. Antihypertensives work to reduce abnormally high pressure of the blood against the walls of the blood vessels. Hypertension can cause strokes and heart attacks as well as cause damage to the eyes and kidneys. Antihypertensives do not cure high blood pressure; they control it only for as long as the drugs are taken.

For

High blood pressure, congestive heart failure, and edema, including fluid retention caused by diseases of the heart, liver, and kidneys.

Availability and Dosage

Tablets: 25 mg, 50 mg, 100 mg. Oral solution: 50 mg per 5 ml. oral solution: 100 mg per ml.

Side Effects

More common include dry mouth, increased thirst, heart arrhythmias, fatigue, weakness, drowsiness, muscle cramps, and stomach upset. Others include diarrhea, dizziness or light-headedness, and loss of appetite.

Drug Interactions

This drug has the potential to interact with many other drugs, including lithium, digoxin, anticoagulants (blood thinners), captopril and other blood-pressure–lowering drugs, adrenocortocosteroids, oral antidiabetics, allopurinol, other diuretics, some heart medications, nonsteroidal antiinflammatory drugs (NSAIDs), especially indomethacin and sulindac, and laxatives. Always inform your doctors of every medication you are taking, including nonprescription medicines, vitamins, herbal remedies, and dietary supplements. *Do not take any over-the-counter medications unless approved by your doctor.*

Food/Alcohol Interactions

Avoid or limit alcohol. This drug increases the chances of dehydration when combined with alcohol. Your doctor may recommend supplementing your diet with foods high in potassium, such as bananas or oranges, but do not change your diet on your own.

Pregnancy/Nursing

Not recommended. Bottle-feed your baby if you must take this drug.

Seniors

Older adults may be more susceptible to some of the side effects of this drug, particularly dizziness when rising too quickly from a seated or reclining position.

Warning

Thiazide diuretics can cause increased sensitivity to sunlight. You may experience skin rash, itching, redness, or severe sunburn. Wear protective clothing, a sunscreen with an SPF factor of at least 15 (including on your lips), a hat, and sunglasses. Avoid direct sunlight when possible. Do not use tanning lamps or tanning beds.

Comments

Regular and careful monitoring by your doctor is essential when taking any diuretic, as the loss of potassium, sodium, and other essential electrolytes from the body can lead to serious and possibly fatal reactions.

Brand Name
Eskalith (also Lithobid, Lithonate)

Generic Name

lithium

Type of Drug

Antimanic.

For

Treatment of the manic stage of manic depression (bipolar disorder).

Availability and Dosage

Capsule: 300 mg. Extended-release tablet: 450 mg. Should be taken with food to minimize stomach upset. Your physician will need to find a dose that is effective for you while keeping side effects to a minimum, as most adverse effects are related to the amount of lithium present in the blood. Take this medication exactly as prescribed. Do not abruptly stop taking this drug without consulting your doctor.

Side Effects

The potential for side effects increases with higher blood levels of this drug and in individuals who are especially sensitive to it. More common include nausea, vomiting, loss of appetite, diarrhea, and tremor. Others include drowsiness, fatigue, increased thirst, weight gain, increased urination, bloating, muscle twitching, blurred vision, unsteadiness, confusion, and slurred speech.

Drug Interactions

This drug has the potential to interact with a wide variety of medications, which can affect the levels of lithium in the blood and lead to adverse effects. These include nonsteroidal antiinflammatory drugs (NSAIDs), tetracycline antibiotics, carbamazepine, verapamil, metronidazole, angiotensin-converting enzyme (ACE) inhibitors, diuretics, sodium bicarbonate antacids, and some antidepressants. Always inform your doctors of every medication you are taking, including nonprescription medicines, vitamins, herbal remedies, and dietary supplements. *Do not take any over-the-counter medications unless approved by your doctor.*

Food/Alcohol Interactions

Drink a minimum of 8 glasses of water a day while on this drug. Avoid alcohol, as it can increase the sedative effect. Avoid caffeine in foods and beverages, as it can affect blood levels of lithium. Your body's balance of salt and fluids is essential while on this drug. Do not use salt substitutes. Do not attempt a weight-loss diet or make any changes in salt intake without discussing it with your physician.

Pregnancy/Nursing

Not recommended, especially during the first trimester. If treatment is required, discuss with your obstetrician the benefits versus the potential risks. Lithium passes into breast milk. Bottle-feed your baby if you must take this drug.

Seniors

Older adults are at a higher risk of lithium toxicity due to reduced kidney function. Your doctor will probably prescribe the lowest possible effective dose.

Warning

Because of the potential for lithium toxicity, you must be carefully and regularly monitored by a doctor while on this drug. Avoid overexertion and any activities (saunas, hot tubs) that may cause dehydration; diminished blood volume may lead to toxic levels of lithium in the blood. If you experience diarrhea, slurred speech, extreme drowsiness, confusion, muscle weakness, or twitching, *seek emergency medical treatment.* Make sure your doctors have your complete medical history, including a history of diabetes, schizophrenia, kidney disease, epilepsy, thyroid disease, psoriasis, heart disease, Parkinson's disease, or leukemia.

Comments

Manic-depressive illness (bipolar disorder) affects 2 million Americans. If left untreated, the suicide rate is 15%. Lithium—discovered by accident in 1949 when an Australian doctor used the drug to treat gout in hamsters and found that it calmed them—is one of the most-studied drugs to treat bipolar disorder. The manic phase of manic depression is marked by dramatic mood swings, hyperactivity, insomnia, grandiose thoughts, irritability, rapid speech, and poor judgment.

Brand Name

Estrace* (also Climara*, Estraderm*, FemPatch)

Generic Name

estradiol*

Type of Drug

Conjugated estrogens. Estradiol is used to replace the female hormone estrogen, which is naturally produced by the ovaries. After menopause, estrogen levels decrease; estrogen-replacement therapy maintains the proper level of this hormone necessary for normal female functions. Estrogen can help to ease postmenopausal symptoms, including hot flashes, sweating, vaginal dryness, aching joints, mood changes, and lapses in memory. It can also help to reduce the risk of postmenopausal osteoporosis and postmenopausal heart attacks. Estrogen is sometimes prescribed in conjunction with progestin, depending on your individual medical condition. This combination is usually prescribed for women who have not had a hysterectomy.

For

Relief of menopausal and postmenopausal symptoms; postmenopausal osteoporosis, ovarian failure.

Availability and Dosage

(Estrace) Vaginal cream: 0.01% strength. Tablets: 0.5 mg, 1 mg, 2 mg. (Climara) Transdermal patch: 0.025 mg/24 hours, 0.05 mg/24 hours, 0.075 mg/24 hours, 0.1 mg/24 hours. (Estraderm) Transdermal patch: 0.05 mg/24 hours, 0.1 mg/24 hours. (FemPatch) 0.025 mg/24 hours. Estrogen-therapy regimens are highly individualized. Follow all directions carefully for dosage and administration.

Side Effects

More common include stomach upset, bloating, mood changes, changes in appetite, fatigue, vaginal yeast infection, weight gain, and anxiety. Others include dizziness, diarrhea, headaches, contact-lens discomfort, increased sex drive, and vomiting.

Drug Interactions

Estrogens in their various forms have the potential for a wide variety of interactions. The following is a partial list: some antibiotics, anticoagulants (blood thinners), acetaminophen, oral contraceptives, HIV medications, some anticonvulsants, carbamazepine, cimetidine, antidiabetics, methotrexate, cortisone, raloxifene, tamoxifen, tricyclic antidepressants, other hormones, thyroid drugs, and some antimigraines. Taking estrogen with ginseng may enhance estrogen's effects, resulting in possible vaginal bleeding and breast pain. Always inform your doctors of every medication you are taking, including nonprescription medicines, vitamins, herbal remedies, and dietary supplements. *Do not take any over-the-counter medications unless approved by your doctor.*

Food/Alcohol Interactions

No alcohol warnings. Avoid drinking grapefruit juice while on this medication.

Pregnancy/Nursing

Not recommended. Estrogens have been proven to cause birth defects. Do not use this drug while nursing.

Seniors

No special warnings. Take as prescribed and immediately inform your doctor of any persistent or troublesome side effects.

Warning

Make sure that the doctor who prescribes your estrogen has your complete medical history. Estrogen must be used with extreme caution if you have breast cancer promoted by estrogen, if you have a family history of breast cancer, fibrocystic breast disease, or a blood-clotting disorder. If you have reason to believe you're pregnant, stop taking this drug immediately and consult your gynecologist. Smoking increases the risk of blood clotting when used concurrently with estradiol transdermal patches. If you are over age 35, it is strongly recommended that you quit smoking. If you experience persistent vaginal bleeding, notify your doctor at once.

Comments

The decision to take or not to take estrogen is by no means a simple one. Many women find the estrogen dilemma at best confusing and at worst frightening, having to carefully weigh the pros and cons of estrogen-replacement therapy. Studies indicate that estrogen protects the heart and the bones but may increase the risk of breast and other cancers. The subject of hormone-replacement therapy is very controversial, fraught with more questions than answers, and with no one solution that is right for every woman. The best course for a woman entering meno-pause (between age 45 and 55) is to gain as much knowledge about the subject as possible, formulate with her gynecologist a personal health profile (and get second and third opinions if nec-essary), and decide if the benefits of estrogen- or hormone-replacement therapy far outweigh the risks. Regular and careful monitoring by your gynecologist is essential while on any type of hormone-replacement therapy.

Estraderm*

See Estrace*

estradiol*

See Estrace*

estradiol/norethindrone acetate

See CombiPatch

estropipate

See Ogen

Estrostep

See Oral Contraceptives

etanercept

See Enbrel

ethynodial diacetate and ethinyl estradiol

See Oral Contraceptives

Brand Name
Evista

Generic Name
raloxifene HCl

Type of Drug
Selective estrogen receptor motivator (SERM).

For
Decrease of bone loss due to postmenopausal osteoporosis. This drug will not help with the symptoms of menopause such as hot flashes.

Availability and Dosage
Tablets: 60 mg.

Side Effects
More common include hot flashes, leg cramps, sweating, muscle or joint pain, depression, stomach upset, flatulence, vomiting, and weight gain. Others include abdominal pain, lung congestion, diarrhea, hoarseness, loss of appetite, nausea, weakness, and risk of blood clots.

Drug Interactions
Raloxifene can interact with injection estrogens, oral estrogens, transdermal estrogens, and anticoagulants (blood thinners). Always inform your doctors of every medication you are taking, including nonprescription medicines, vitamins, herbal remedies, and dietary supplements. *Do not take any over-the-counter medications unless approved by your doctor.*

Food/Alcohol Interactions
No special warnings.

Pregnancy/Nursing
If you are or can still become pregnant, do not take this drug. Bottle-feed your baby if you must take this drug.

Seniors
No special warnings. Take as prescribed and immediately inform your doctor of any persistent or troublesome side effects. This drug was tested only in postmenopausal women and was not shown to cause any different side effects.

Warning

Make sure your doctor has your complete medical history, especially a history of blood clot formation, pulmonary embolism, deep vein thrombosis, retinal embolism, liver disease, congestive heart failure, cancer, or tumors.

Comments

This drug mimics estrogen's bone-saving effects but without the risk of breast cancer. At present, there are studies using raloxifene as a means to prevent cancer recurrence. It is not used for treatment. In studies of up to 3 years, women taking raloxifene had no increased risk of breast or uterine cancer. An estimated ten million women currently have osteoporosis, a bone-thinning disease that can cause crippling, deformity, and fractures. Every year, more than 300,000 women suffer broken hips and 700,000 have fractured vertebrae. You may be at increased risk of osteoporosis if you are Caucasian or Asian, have a slender build, do not exercise, or have a family history of this disease.

famciclover

See Famvir

famotidine

See Pepcid*

Brand Name
Famvir

Generic Name

famciclovir

Type of Drug

Antiviral.

For

Herpes zoster (shingles); herpes simplex (genital herpes).

Availability and Dosage

Tablets: 124 mg, 250 mg, 500 mg. Dosages are different for herpes zoster (shingles) and herpes simplex (genital herpes). May be taken with or without food. Dosages should be evenly spaced and taken at the first sign of symptoms, including itching, tingling, or pain. Take the full course of treatment prescribed even if you begin to feel better. Drink plenty of water while on this medication.

Side Effects

More common include nausea, headache, diarrhea, dizziness, and fatigue. Others include vomiting, constipation, fever, and sore throat. Some side effects may subside as your body adjusts to this medication.

Drug Interactions

Famciclovir has the potential to interact with digoxin; it can increase the levels of digoxin in the blood. Always inform your doctors of every medication you are taking, including nonprescription medicines, vitamins, herbal remedies, and dietary supplements.

Food/Alcohol Interactions

No special warnings.

Pregnancy/Nursing

Not recommended. Bottle-feeding your baby is recommended while on this drug.

Seniors

Older adults with reduced kidney function may be started on a low dose of this drug.

Warning

This drug does not cure herpes, nor does it prevent the spread of infection. Genital herpes is easily spread by sexual contact, especially when there are sores and blisters on the vulva, the vaginal or anal area, or the cervix. Herpes can also be transmitted even when there no visible sores, as when viral particles may be shedding on the skin. The use of condoms by your partner is recommended at all times. Genital herpes can be transmitted to a newborn and increase his or her risk of brain damage and blindness. If you know or suspect you have herpes, make sure that you tell your ob/gyn.

Comments

There is no known cure for genital herpes, although patients now have better treatment options for this viral disease. Studies show that famciclovir appears to decrease recurrences of genital herpes outbreaks when taken continuously for a year. In drug trials, patients who took a twice-daily dose reported 80% fewer outbreaks. Clinical trials are now under way to develop a herpes vaccine, which some researchers predict will be available in 2003. The FDA is also expected to approve POCkit, a herpes blood test that can be taken anytime and shows results in six minutes instead of the traditional "swab tests" that can be done only when sores are present and take several days to provide results.

Brand Name
Fastin (also Adipex-P, Ionamin)

Generic Name
phentermine

Type of Drug
Appetite suppressant.

For
Obesity and short-term weight loss.

Availability and Dosage
(Fastin) Tablets and capsules: 8 mg to 37.5 mg. (Adipex-P) Capsules and tablets: 37.5 mg. (Ionamin) Extended-release capsules: 15 mg, 30 mg. Should be taken with water at least 30 minutes before meals.

Side Effects
More common include difficulty in sleeping, dry mouth, restlessness, nausea, and a sense of elation. Others include chest pain, dry cough, vomiting, dizziness, palpitations, tremors, headache, and unpleasant taste.

Drug Interactions
This drug may interact with antihypertensives or other blood-pressure–lowering medications, oral antidiabetics, and some antidepressants including monoamine oxidase (MAO) inhibitors. Always inform your doctors of every medication you are taking, including nonprescription medicines, vitamins, herbal remedies, and dietary supplements

Food/Alcohol Interactions
Avoid alcohol.

Pregnancy/Nursing

Not recommended. Notify your doctor if you are pregnant, or trying to become pregnant, while on this drug.

Seniors

This drug is not recommended for those who have atherosclerosis (hardening of the arteries), overactive thyroid, glaucoma, or high blood pressure.

Warning

Do not increase or otherwise change your dosage thinking that doing so will increase weight loss. Phentermine produces the best results when used in conjunction with a healthy diet and exercise plan. Phentermine will most likely be used only for short-term weight loss. If you experience shortness of breath during normal activities while on this medication, notify your doctor at once.

Comments

Phentermine was the "phen" half of the "fen-phen" combination weight-loss drug known as Redux, which was recalled in 1997 after being linked to serious heart-valve defects in women first discovered by doctors at the Mayo Clinic. The FDA then reviewed 291 patients at five national medical centers and found that 92 had developed problems with their aortic or mitral valves. The "fen" half (fenfluramine, sold under the brand name Pondimin) was also recalled. The drug described in this profile—phentermine—when taken alone, was never associated with any heart-valve damage and has stayed on the market as a short-term weight loss medication.

felodipine

See Plendil*

FemPatch

See Estrace*

fexofenadine hydrochloride

See Allegra*

Brand Name

Flagyl (also Protostat and MetroGel)

Generic Name

metronidazole

Type of Drug

Antibiotic; antiparasitic.

For

Bacterial infections, including vaginal infections, urinary-tract infections (UTIs), abdominal infections, and lower-respiratory-tract infections.

Availability and Dosage

Capsules: 375 mg. Tablets: 250 mg, 500 mg. Extended-release tablets: 750 mg. Topical gel: 0.75%. Oral forms may be taken with or without food. Dosages will vary depending on the particular infection being treated. Take the full course of treatment prescribed.

Side Effects

More common include diarrhea, dry mouth, headache, stomach cramps, dizziness or light-headedness, and loss of appetite. Others include metallic taste, numbness or tingling in hands or feet.

Drug Interactions

This drug has the potential to interact with cimetidine, some anticonvulsants, phenobarbital, and lithium. Also, this drug can increase the effect of anticoagulants such as warfarin.

Food/Alcohol Interactions

Avoid alcohol. Serious interactions can occur, including rapid heartbeat, flushing, abdominal pain, nausea, and vomiting. Also avoid over-the-counter medications containing alcohol (e.g., cough syrups).

Pregnancy/Nursing

Not recommended, especially during the first trimester. This drug passes into breast milk. Bottle-feeding your baby is recommended while on this drug.

Seniors

Your doctor may start you on a low dose, especially if you have decreased liver function.

Warning

If you are taking Antabuse (the drug used to maintain alcohol abstinence in alcoholics), do not take metronidazole. The combination of these two drugs can result in central nervous system (CNS) side effects including psychotic reactions. This drug may increase the risk of seizures in people who have CNS disorders.

Comments

Under treatment for trichomoniasis (a sexually transmitted disease affecting both men and women) women should ask their doctors' advice about treating any sexual partners as well, even if they have no symptoms. Men should use condoms to avoid repeatedly giving and getting this infection before treatment is completed and the infection has cleared up. The topical version of this drug is used to treat rosacea, a chronic and progressive facial skin disorder. There is also an intravaginal gel available (see MetroGel-Vaginal).

flavoxate hydrochloride

See Urispas

Brand Name
Flexeril

Generic Name

cyclobenzaprine*

Type of Drug

Muscle relaxant.

For

Relief of muscle spasms, muscular stiffness, and pain.

Availability and Dosage

Tablets: 10 mg.

Side Effects

More common include drowsiness, dizziness, dry mouth, fatigue, weakness, and nausea. Others include heartburn, constipation, headache, blurred vision, metallic taste, and restlessness.

Drug Interactions

This drug has the potential to interact with a wide variety of medications, including anticoagulants, anticonvulsants, estrogens, oral contraceptives, and thyroid drugs. Potentially serious interactions can occur between cyclobenzaprine and monoamine oxidase (MAO) inhibitor antidepressants, including convulsions and high fever. Do not take MAO inhibitor drugs within 14 days of taking cyclobenzaprine. Sedatives, tranquilizers, antihistamines, narcotic pain relievers, sleep aids, tricyclic antidepressants, and other drugs that cause drowsiness may intensify the sedative effects of cyclobenzaprine. Always inform your doctors of every medication you are taking, including nonprescription medicines, vitamins, herbal remedies, and dietary supplements. *Do not take any over-the-counter medications unless approved by your doctor.*

Food/Alcohol Interactions

Avoid alcohol.

Pregnancy/Nursing

Not recommended. This drug passes into breast milk. You may want to bottle-feed your baby while on this drug.

Seniors

Drowsiness may be increased in older adults. Take as prescribed and immediately inform your doctor of any persistent or troublesome side effects.

Warning

This drug may impair your ability to drive, operate machinery, or perform tasks that require mental alertness. Do not drive until you know how this medication will affect you.

Comments

This drug is mainly used in short-term therapy of painful symptoms caused by injury, in conjunction with physical therapy, bed rest, and other treatments as prescribed by your doctor. It is not used for muscle pain or spasms associated with chronic illnesses or spinal cord injuries.

Brand Name
Flonase* (also Flovent*)

Generic Name
fluticasone propionate

Type of Drug
Corticosteroid nasal spray; corticosteroid inhalation aerosol. These drugs work by reducing nasal-passage inflammation. In allergic rhinitis it decreases the allergic response to allergens. In asthmatic patients, it reduces inflammation in the lining of the airways.

For
Relief of seasonal or chronic allergies and allergic rhinitis. Flovent is used to preventively treat bronchial asthma (not to be used for acute asthma).

Availability and Dosage
Flonase nasal spray: 50 mcg per spray. Usual dose is 2 sprays in each nostril once daily, or 1 spray in each nostril twice daily, for treatment of seasonal and year-round allergies. Flovent oral inhalation: 44 mcg, 110 mcg, and 220 mcg per metered dose. For asthma, use Flovent inhalation aerosol as directed by your physician. In asthmatic patients, the lowest effective dose of Flovent is generally used once asthma stability has been achieved. Do not abruptly stop taking this type of drug without consulting your doctor.

Side Effects
More common (Flonase nasal spray) include nosebleed, nasal irritation or burning, sore throat, and headache. More common (Flovent inhalation aerosol) include white patches in mouth or throat, sore throat, and hoarseness.

Drug Interactions
Few interactions have been reported with this medication. Inform all your doctors if you are taking oral corticosteroids (including other inhalation forms of corticosteroid) or any drugs that suppress the immune system.

Food/Alcohol Interactions
No special warnings.

Pregnancy/Nursing

No special warnings, although all drugs during pregnancy and breast-feeding should be avoided if possible. Before taking this drug, discuss with your doctor the benefits versus the potential risks.

Seniors

No special warnings. Take as prescribed and immediately inform your doctor of any persistent or troublesome side effects.

Warning

In rare instances, deaths have occurred in asthmatic patients who switched from oral (systemic) corticosteroids to inhaled corticosteroids too quickly. Your doctor will be able to adjust and monitor your transition from oral corticosteroids to inhalation forms. You should carry a medical identification tag and an ID card indicating that you may need supplementary systemic corticosteroids during periods of stress or severe asthma attacks. Seek emergency treatment immediately.

Comments

Unlike antihistamines, fluticasone does not cause drowsiness. The effectiveness of this drug depends on regular use, as it does not treat the symptoms of nasal allergies but the underlying cause—inflammation. You may begin to see improvement within 12 hours. Maximum relief may take several days. People who take drugs that suppress the immune system are more susceptible to infections than others are. Chicken pox and measles can have a serious or even fatal course in adults who take corticosteroids. If you think you have been exposed to either of these diseases, contact your doctor immediately.

Flovent*

*See Flonase**

Brand Name
Floxin

Generic Name

ofloxacin

Type of Drug

Antibiotic. This large class of drugs is among the most commonly prescribed, resulting in such widespread use that the bacteria they were developed to kill have become resistant to them. These "resistant" forms are then passed from person to person, further causing the spread of infections that become even more difficult to treat. Your doctor will prescribe the correct antibiotic depending on the type of infection. Antibiotics are useless against viral infections such as colds and flu.

For

Various bacterial infections including sexually transmitted diseases (STDs) such as chlamydia and gonorrhea; chronic bronchitis and pneumonia; urinary-tract infections (UTIs); pelvic inflammatory disease (PID).

Availability and Dosage

Tablets: 200 mg, 300 mg, 400 mg. Take with a full glass of water on an empty stomach, 1 hour before or 2 hours after a meal. It is essential to take the complete course of antibiotics prescribed. If you fail to do so, increased drug resistance by any leftover bacteria is likely to occur. Drink plenty of water while on this medication.

Side Effects

More common include diarrhea, nausea, insomnia, stomach pain, headache, dizziness, drowsiness, increased sensitivity to sunlight, dry mouth, and itching. Others include restlessness, vaginal irritation, and changes in taste.

Drug Interactions

Some antibiotics can interfere with the effectiveness of oral contraceptives. Women who take a combination of birth control pills and certain antiinfectives—tetracycline, sulfa, and penicillin—have become pregnant. Other interactions can occur with anticancer drugs, anticoagulants (blood thinners), and some bronchodilators such as theophylline. Antacids, iron supplements, and multivitamins containing iron, calcium, magnesium salts, manganese, or zinc may interfere with ofloxacin absorption. Always inform your doctors of every medication you are taking, including nonprescription medicines, vitamins, herbal remedies, and dietary supplements.

Food/Alcohol Interactions

Avoid or limit alcohol. Avoid or restrict caffeine, including coffee, colas, chocolate, and other caffeinated foods or beverages.

Pregnancy/Nursing

Not recommended. May cause birth defects. This drug passes into breast milk. You may want to bottle-feed your baby while on this drug.

Seniors

Your doctor may start you on a low dose if you have reduced kidney function. Use caution when rising abruptly from a sitting or reclining position to minimize dizziness.

Warning

Severe side effects can occur even after only one dose. If you experience extreme dizziness, nausea, convulsions or seizures, cardiovascular symptoms (shortness of breath, heart arrhythmia, chest pain), hallucinations, or swelling of the face or extremities, seek emergency treatment immediately.

Comments

Frequent UTIs may indicate another underlying problem. Kidney or bladder damage can result from frequent, untreated UTIs. If your doctor is unable to find a cause for chronic UTIs, you may need to consult a urologist or a urogynecologist. In 1997, ofloxacin was approved for treating pelvic inflammatory disease (PID), the symptoms of which include pain in the lower abdomen, increased vaginal discharge, bleeding between periods, and painful sexual intercourse. When ofloxacin was taken twice daily for 2 weeks, studies showed that 98% of patients with PID were cured.

fluconazole

See Diflucan*

fluoxetine

See Prozac*

fluoxymesterone

See Halotestin

flurbiprofen

See **Ansaid**

fluticasone phosphate

See **Flonase***

fluvastatin

See **Lescol***

fluvoxamine

See **Luvox**

Brand Name
Fosamax*

Generic Name

alendorate sodium

Type of Drug

Aminobiphosphonate (bone resorption inhibitor).

For

Postmenopausal osteoporosis.

Availability and Dosage

Tablets: 5 mg, 10 mg, 40 mg. This drug must be taken on an empty stomach with a full glass (8 ounces) of water upon arising in the morning. Do not eat or drink anything for at least 30 minutes after you take this medicine; it is effective only on an empty stomach. Do not take with coffee, tea, juice, or mineral water. Do not lie down for at least 30 minutes. Failure to take this drug as prescribed can result in inflammation or bleeding ulcers in the esophagus.

Side Effects

More common include abdominal or stomach pain, nausea, heartburn, and irritation or pain in the esophagus. Others include difficulty in swallowing, vomiting, constipation, bloating, diarrhea, and gas.

Drug Interactions

Taking nonsteroidal antiinflammatory drugs (NSAIDs) including aspirin with this drug can result in increased risk of stomach or intestinal irritation. Do not take any other medication within 30 minutes of taking alendorate, as other drugs can interfere with absorption and decrease the drug's effectivenes.

Food/Alcohol Interactions

If you take this drug with food, beverages, antacids, calcium supplements, or vitamins, they will interfere with the effectiveness of this drug. Alcohol restriction is recommended.

Pregnancy/Nursing

Not recommended. This drug is for use by women after menopause.

Seniors

No special warnings. Take as prescribed and immediately inform your doctor of any persistent or troublesome side effects.

Warning

The most serious side effect of alendorate was first discovered in 1996 at the Mayo Clinic, when three elderly women developed an inflamed or ulcerated esophagus after taking the drug. Dosage instructions need to be followed carefully to avoid this type of damage. If you experience pain or difficulty when swallowing, call your doctor at once.

Comments

Alendorate was the first nonhormonal treatment for osteoporosis, a progressive disease of the skeleton that leads to brittle bones and affects more than 25 million Americans, 80% of them women. Women should have their risk for osteoporosis assessed by their doctors after menopause and may need a bone-density test to determine bone loss. Risks are increased among women of Caucasian or Asian descent who are thin, had insufficient calcium intake, smoke, had or have an eating disorder, and who experienced early menopause.

fosinopril

See Monopril*

fosfomycin tromethamine

See Monurol

furosemide

See Lasix*

gabapentin

See Neurontin*

Brand Name

Gantrisin

Generic Name

sulfisoxazole

Type of Drug

Antibacterial; sulfa.

For

Urinary-tract infections (UTIs), kidney infections; cystitis.

Availability and Dosage

Tablets: 500 mg. Oral syrup: 500 mg per 5 ml. Should be taken on an empty stomach with a full glass of water, 1 hour before or 2 hours after a meal. Drink plenty of fluids while on this medication. Be sure to finish the complete course of treatment.

Side Effects

More common include diarrhea, headache, itching, nausea, and stomach pain. Others include drowsiness, dizziness, loss of appetite, disorientation, and excessive fatigue.

Drug Interactions

Interactions can occur with oral contraceptives, some oral antidiabetics, blood thinners (anticoagulants), other antibiotics, anticonvulsants, and methotrexate. Always inform your doctors of every medication you are taking, including nonprescription medicines, vitamins, herbal remedies, and dietary supplements.

Food/Alcohol Interactions

No special warnings. Drink plenty of water while on this medication to reduce the possibility of kidney problems.

Pregnancy/Nursing

Not recommended, especially late in pregnancy. Sulfisoxazole may cause jaundice in newborns. The drug can pass into breast milk. You may want to bottle-feed your baby if you must take this drug.

Seniors

The potential for side effects is increased in older people. Contact your doctor immediately if you have any type of allergic reaction: difficulty in breathing, increased thirst, lower back pain, pain or difficulty in urinating.

Warning

This drug should be used cautiously by people who have kidney or liver disease or any kind of blood disorder (including AIDS patients). It can result in anemia or other serious blood disorders. If you experience unusual bleeding or bruising, bluish nails or lips, fever, chills, jaundice, or sore throat, seek immediate medical help.

Comments

If you must take this drug for a long time, it is important that your doctor do periodic blood tests to check for folic-acid deficiency, among other problems. Wear protective clothing when outdoors, and apply sunscreen with an SPF factor of at least 15 to exposed areas, including your lips. Do not use tanning beds or tanning lamps.

gemfibrozil*

See Lopid

Genora

See Oral contraceptives

glimepiride

*See Amaryl**

glipizide

See Glucotrol

Brand Name
Glucophage*

Generic Name

metformin hydrochloride

Type of Drug

Antidiabetic. When combined with dietary changes and exercise habits, antidiabetic drugs provide relief of symptoms and enable most diabetics to lead healthy and productive lives. You should wear a medical identification tag at all times along with an ID card that lists your medications. Regular monitoring by your doctor is essential if you have diabetes.

For

Type II (non-insulin–dependent) diabetes mellitus (NIDDM).

Availability and Dosage

Tablets: 500 mg, 850 mg, 1000 mg. May be taken with food. Your doctor will determine initial dosage and subsequent increases. Follow dosage instructions carefully.

Side Effects

Most common are diarrhea, nausea, and upset stomach, which usually subside after the first few weeks. Metformin does not cause weight gain, as do other oral antidiabetic drugs.

Drug Interactions

If you have congestive heart failure and are taking digoxin or furosemide, do not take metformin. Always provide your doctors with a complete and current list of prescription and nonprescription drugs you are taking. *Do not take any over-the-counter medications unless approved by your doctor.*

Food/Alcohol Interactions

If you drink alcohol excessively (either long-term or binge drinking), do not take this drug. Any use of alcohol can increase the possibility of adverse side effects.

Pregnancy/Nursing

As with other oral glucose-control medications, metformin is not recommended during pregnancy. This drug passes into breast milk.

Seniors

Because of the usual decline in kidney function that occurs with age, you may be started on a low dose. People who have chronic kidney or liver problems should not take this drug, nor should people age 80 or over without first testing kidney function. If you are going to have surgery, this drug will have to be stopped temporarily.

Warning

The most serious side effect of this drug is a condition called lactic acidosis, a buildup of lactic acid in the blood that occurs when kidney function is impaired. This condition is rare (1 in 33,000 patients), but can be fatal in up to half the cases. Symptoms include extreme weakness, unusual muscle pain, feeling cold, dizzy, or light-headed, and slow and/or irregular heartbeats. *Seek emergency medical attention immediately.*

Comments

Type II diabetes affects women and men equally, but a disproportionate number of minorities: More than 33% of Hispanics and nearly 25% of African Americans develop this disease by age 65 to 74. Gestational diabetes occurs only during pregnancy. Women over age 35 who have a family history of diabetes, are overweight, or have had gestational diabetes during a previous pregnancy are at greatest risk. *Remember that regular monitoring by your doctor is essential if you have diabetes and are taking any antidiabetic drugs.*

Brand Name
Glucotrol (also Glucotrol XL*)

Generic Name

glipizide

Type of Drug

Antidiabetic. When combined with dietary changes and exercise habits, antidiabetic drugs provide relief of symptoms and enable most diabetics to lead healthy and productive lives. You should wear a medical identification tag at all times along with an ID card that lists your medications. Regular monitoring by your doctor is essential if you have diabetes.

For

Type II (non-insulin–dependent) diabetes mellitus (NIDDM).

Availability and Dosage

Tablets: 5 mg, 10 mg. Should not be taken with food. Your doctor will determine initial dosage and subsequent increases. Follow dosage instructions carefully.

Side Effects

Most common include nausea, vomiting, stomach upset, and increased sensitivity to sunlight. Others include excessive thirst, tingling in hands or feet, jaundice, itching, and rash. If any side effects persist or become severe, contact your doctor.

Drug Interactions

Glipizide has the ability to interact with a number of medications, including beta-blockers, aspirin, and other nonsteroidal antiinflammatory drugs (NSAIDs), some antibiotics, fenfluramine, corticosteroids, thyroid drugs, oral contraceptives, blood thinners (anticoagulants), antiulcer drugs including those for gastroesophageal reflux disease (GERD), and tricyclic antidepressants, among others. Always provide your doctors with a complete and current list of prescription and nonprescription drugs you are taking. *Do not take any over-the-counter medications unless approved by your doctor.*

Food/Alcohol Interactions

If you drink alcohol excessively (either long-term or binge drinking), do not take this drug. Any use of alcohol can increase the possibility of adverse side effects.

Pregnancy/Nursing

Not recommended. Glipizide can cause birth defects and cause abnormally low blood sugar in the newborn. This drug passes into breast milk. Bottle-feed your baby if you must take this drug.

Seniors

Because of the usual decline in kidney function that occurs with age, you may be started on a low dose. The potential for side effects is greater because of the slower elimination of this drug. If you are going to have surgery, this drug will have to be stopped temporarily.

Warning

People who have chronic kidney or liver problems should not take this drug. Mild symptoms of low blood sugar (hypoglycemia) may be alleviated by drinking fruit juice or other food containing sugar. However, if severe symptoms occur (seizures, convulsions, faintness, chest pains, low blood pressure, sweating), do not eat or drink anything, as choking could result. *Seek emergency medical attention immediately.*

Comments

Type II diabetes affects women and men equally, but a disproportionate number of minorities: More than 33% of Hispanics and nearly 25% of African Americans develop this disease by age 65 to 74. Gestational diabetes occurs only during pregnancy. Women over age 35 who have a family history of diabetes, are overweight, or have had gestational diabetes during a previous pregnancy are at greatest risk. *Remember that regular monitoring by your doctor is essential if you are taking any antidiabetic drugs.*

guaifenesin/phenylpropanolamine*

See Entex

Brand Name
Halcion

Generic Name

triazolam

Type of Drug

Benzodiazepine sedative. These drugs are central nervous system (CNS) depressants and work on the part of the brain that controls emotions by slowing nervous-system transmissions.

For

Treatment of short-term insomnia or frequent nighttime awakening.

Availability and Dosage

Tablets: 0.125 mg, 0.25 mg. May be taken with or without food, at bedtime. The lowest effective dose is usually used. Do not take more of this drug than your doctor has prescribed. The FDA has restricted the number of pills to 10 per prescription so that patients cannot increase their dosage. Do not abruptly stop taking this drug without consulting your physician.

Side Effects

More common are light-headedness, dizziness, daytime drowsiness, headache, increase in strange dreams, and nausea. Others include behavior problems, loss of concentration, depression, anxiety, confusion, increased pulse rate, and menstrual cramps.

Drug Interactions

Like other benzodiazepine drugs, triazolam can interact with antihistamines, tranquilizers, antianxiety drugs, erythromycin, digoxin, some antidepressants including monoamine oxidase (MAO) inhibitors, oral contraceptives, and anticonvulsants. Always inform your doctors of every medication you are taking, including nonprescription medicines, vitamins, herbal remedies, and dietary supplements.

Food/Alcohol Interactions

Do not drink alcohol while taking triazolam. The sedative effect is increased. Avoid grapefruit juice, as it may increase the level of this drug in the bloodstream.

Pregnancy/Nursing

A woman must never take this drug during pregnancy, or if she is trying to become pregnant. Studies show that triazolam causes fetal damage. The drug is present in breast milk. Bottle-feed your baby while on this medication.

Seniors

A risk of side effects, particularly confusion, memory loss, and impaired coordination, may be higher in older adults. Your doctor will probably start you on a low dose. If you must take this drug, notify your doctor at once of any persistent or troublesome side effects.

Warning

Psychotic behavior changes have been reported in connection with triazolam, including violent behavior, hallucinations, and severe memory loss.

Comments

It is imperative that you take this medicine exactly as prescribed. There have been ongoing investigations of the safety of this drug, but at the time of publication this drug is still on the market. Regular and careful monitoring by your doctor is essential while on this drug.

Brand Name
Halotestin

Generic Name

fluoxymesterone

Type of Drug

Androgen (male hormone).

For

Certain types of advanced breast cancer or for women who have breast tumors promoted by female hormones.

Availability and Dosage

Tablets: 2 mg, 5 mg, 10 mg. May be taken with food if stomach upset occurs.

Side Effects

Because androgens are involved in the normal growth of male sex organs, the most common side effects in women include the development of male sex characteristics such as deepening of the voice, excessive hairiness (hirsutism), enlargement of the clitoris, and absence of or irregularities in menstrual periods. Other side effects include acne, depression, fluid retention, headache, a tingling feeling, hair loss, and rash. If you have painful or swollen breasts, this drug may aggravate that condition.

Drug Interactions

This drug may interact with blood thinners (anticoagulants), some antibiotics, insulin, and some antidepressants. Always inform your doctors of every medication you are taking, including nonprescription medicines, vitamins, herbal remedies, and dietary supplements.

Food/Alcohol Interactions

No special warnings.

Pregnancy/Nursing

Not recommended for use during pregnancy, as it may affect a female embryo. Not recommended for use during breast-feeding.

Seniors

No special warnings for women (older men may be at a higher risk of prostate cancer). Take as prescribed and immediately inform your doctor of any persistent or troublesome side effects.

Warning

Notify your doctor immediately if you develop jaundice (yellowing of the skin) or swelling of the ankles. An excess of blood calcium may result from taking this drug. Liver problems, such as hepatitis, and cancer may develop.

Comments

This type of drug must be used only under the close supervision of your doctor. The greatest risk of long-term use is the increased risk of liver cancer.

Brand Name
Humalin 70/30* (also Humalin N*, Humalin R*)

Generic Name

insulin

Type of Drug

Antidiabetic.

For

Type I (insulin-dependent) diabetes. When combined with dietary changes and exercise habits, antidiabetic drugs provide relief of symptoms and enable most diabetics to lead healthy and productive lives. You should wear a medical identification tag at all times along with an ID card that lists your medications.

Availability and Dosage

There are many types of insulin preparations, including daily subcutaneous (under the skin) injections and insulin pens with premeasured dosages. A new insulin delivery system, the Humalin Pen, is a lightweight, disposable, pocket-sized device that comes prefilled with the most commonly prescribed insulin. Your doctor will prescribe and monitor insulin dosages to keep your blood-glucose level as normal as possible. Take this medicine exactly as prescribed—your dosage and schedule has been individualized for you. Follow directions for usage and storage carefully. Never share insulin cartridges, pens, or needles, and never change the brand or type of insulin without checking with your health care practitioner.

Side Effects

Too little glucose in the blood (hypoglycemia) is a common side effect among insulin users. Mild to moderate symptoms include palpitations, tremor, restlessness, tingling in hands, feet, lips, or tongue, anxiety, headache, and unsteady movement. Occasionally there may be itching or swelling at the site of the injection.

Drug Interactions

You may need to reduce your dose of insulin if you are taking large doses of aspirin, some antibiotics, monoamine oxidase (MAO) inhibitors, or oral antidiabetic drugs. If you are taking corticosteroids, oral contraceptives, thiazide diuretics, or thyroid-replacement drugs, you may need more insulin. Always inform your doctors of every medication you are taking, including nonprescription medicines, vitamins, herbal remedies, and dietary supplements. *Do not take any over-the-counter medications unless approved by your doctor.*

Food/Alcohol Interactions

Diabetics must follow a special diet and avoid alcohol and products that contain alcohol and/or sugar.

Pregnancy/Nursing

Insulin poses no risk to the fetus during pregnancy or to the baby during breast-feeding. However, you should be monitored closely during pregnancy.

Seniors

No special warnings. Take as prescribed and immediately inform your doctor of any persistent or troublesome side effects.

Warning

Symptoms of severe hypoglycemia—seizures, disorientation, loss of consciousness—warrant emergency treatment. Symptoms of low blood sugar (hypoglycemia) may be alleviated by drinking fruit juice or other food containing sugar. However, if severe symptoms occur (seizures, convulsions, faintness, chest pains, low blood pressure, sweating), do not eat or drink anything, as choking could result. *Seek emergency medical attention immediately.*

Comments

You should not smoke within 30 minutes of injecting insulin. Changes in your exercise regimen may result in dosage adjustment. *Remember that regular monitoring by your doctor is essential if you have diabetes and are receiving insulin injections.*

Humalin N*

*See Humalin 70/30**

Humalin R*

*See Humalin 70/30**

hydrochlorothiazide (HCTZ)*

See Esidrix

hydrochlorothiazide (HCTZ) and triamterene

*See Dyazide**

HydroDIURAL

See Esidrix

hydroxychloroquine

See Plaquenil

Brand Name
Hytrin*

Generic Name

terazosin HCL

Type of Drug

Antihypertensive. These drugs work to reduce abnormally high pressure of the blood against the walls of the blood vessels.

They do not cure high blood pressure; they control the condition for as long as the medication is taken.

For

Mild to moderate high blood pressure.

Availability and Dosage

Tablets: 1 mg, 2 mg, 5 mg, 10 mg. May be taken with or without food. Taking your first doses with food may reduce the severity of initial side effects.

Side Effects

More common include dizziness, drowsiness, and fainting. These are more likely to occur when you start taking the drug and should diminish as your body adjusts to the medication. Others include constipation, headache, nausea, unusual weakness, and fatigue. To minimize dizziness, stand up slowly when rising from a seated or reclining position.

Drug Interactions

This drug can interact with diuretics (water pills) and beta-blockers and other drugs to lower blood pressure. Estrogens and nonsteroidal antiinflammatory drugs (NSAIDs) may decrease the effectiveness of terazosin. Always inform your doctors of every medication you are taking, including nonprescription medicines, vitamins, herbal remedies, and dietary supplements. *Do not take any over-the-counter medications unless approved by your doctor.*

Food/Alcohol Interactions

Avoid alcohol, as it may increase the sedative effect of terazosin. Caffeine may decrease the effectiveness of this medication.

Pregnancy/Nursing

No special warnings, although all drugs during pregnancy and breast-feeding should be avoided if possible. Before taking this drug, discuss with your doctor the benefits versus the potential risks.

Seniors

No special warnings. Take as prescribed and immediately inform your doctor of any persistent or troublesome side effects.

Warning

The adverse reactions of dizziness, drowsiness, and unsteadiness are more likely to occur if you stand for long periods of time, do strenuous exercise, or during hot weather. Avoid getting overheated while taking this drug. If you experience severe dizziness, heart arrhythmias, chest pain, shortness of breath, blurred vision, or swelling of the legs or ankles, notify your doctor immediately.

Comments

Heart disease is the number-one killer of women in the United States. Hypertension is often referred to as "the silent killer" because it has no symptoms. It forces the heart to work harder, which can bring about heart attacks and strokes as well as cause damage to the eyes and kidneys. People who have hypertension should be regularly monitored by health care practitioners to keep track of their blood pressure.

Brand Name
Hyzaar*

Generic Name
losartan potassium/hydrochlorothiazide (HCTZ)

Type of Drug
Antihypertensive. This drug is a combination of an antihypertensive (losartan) and a diuretic (HCTZ). They do not cure high blood pressure; they control the condition for as long as the medication is taken.

For
High blood pressure.

Availability and Dosage
Tablets: 12.5 mg, 50 mg. May be taken with or without food. Although women have a tendency to absorb higher amounts than do men, usually no adjustments to dosage are needed. Take exactly as prescribed by your doctor.

Side Effects
More common include cough, diarrhea, nausea, fatigue, headache, nasal congestion, and muscle aches and pains. Others include weakness, abdominal pain, and sore throat.

Drug Interactions
Interactions can occur with other blood-pressure–lowering medications, diuretics (water pills), antidiabetic drugs, potassium sup-

plements, and nonsteroidal antiinflammatory drugs (NSAIDs). Always inform your doctors of every medication you are taking, including nonprescription medicines, vitamins, herbal remedies, and dietary supplements. *Do not take any over-the-counter medications unless approved by your doctor.*

Food/Alcohol Interactions

Avoid salt substitutes. If you are diabetic, this drug may affect your blood-glucose level.

Pregnancy/Nursing

Women should never take this drug during the last six months of pregnancy. Fetal injury and death have been proven in connection with this drug. Not recommended for nursing mothers.

Seniors

No special warnings. Take as prescribed and immediately inform your doctor of any persistent or troublesome side effects.

Warning

Tell your doctor if you have cirrhosis of the liver before taking this drug. Dehydration is also a danger with this drug because of the addition of the diuretic; you may lose too much fluid. Notify your doctor immediately if you experience severe diarrhea, nausea and/or vomiting, or excessive sweating.

Comments

Heart disease is the number-one killer of women in the United States. Hypertension is often referred to as "the silent killer" because it has no symptoms. It forces the heart to work harder, which can bring about heart attacks and strokes as well as cause damage to the eyes and kidneys. People who have hypertension should be regularly monitored by health care practitioners to keep track of their blood pressure.

ibuprofen*

See Motrin

imipramine hydrochloride

See Tofranil

imiquimod

See Aldara

Brand Name
Imdur*

Generic Name
isosorbide mononitrate

Type of Drug
Antianginal. These drugs treat the type of chest pain known as angina by increasing the amount of oxygen to the heart muscle.

For
Recurrent angina.

Availability and Dosage
Sustained-release tablets: 30 mg, 60 mg, 120 mg. Usual dose for sustained-release tablets is once each morning, on an empty stomach, 1 hour before or 2 hours after meals. Do not crush sustained-release tablets. This medicine must be taken regularly to prevent angina attacks; the drug does not relieve chest pain once it has started. Do not stop taking this drug without consulting your doctor.

Side Effects
More common—which should subside after your body adjusts to the drug—include headache, flushing of the face or neck, dizziness or unsteadiness especially when rising suddenly from a sitting or reclining position, rapid pulse and restlessness. Others include skin rash, weakness, and nausea.

Drug Interactions
Interactions may occur with other heart drugs, including beta-blockers, antihypertensives, and diuretics. Always inform your doctors of every medication you are taking, including nonprescription medicines, vitamins, herbal remedies, and dietary supplements. *Do not take any over-the-counter medications unless approved by your doctor.*

Food/Alcohol Interactions
Avoid alcohol.

Pregnancy/Nursing

No special warnings, although all drugs during pregnancy and breast-feeding should be avoided if possible. Before taking this drug, discuss with your doctor the benefits versus the potential risks.

Seniors

Older adults may be especially susceptible to side effects, especially dizziness when rising abruptly from a sitting or reclining position.

Warning

If you are allergic to nitroglycerin, do not use this medication. If you experience blurred vision, dry mouth, prolonged or severe headache, bluish lips or fingernails, low blood pressure, palpitations or heart arrhythmias, excessive head pressure, or extreme fatigue, seek emergency medical treatment immediately.

Comments

This drug is a nitrate, one of the oldest and most common class of drugs used to prevent angina and heart attacks. You should be monitored regularly by your physician while you are on this medication.

Brand Name
Imitrex*

Generic Name

sumatriptan

Type of Drug

Antimigraine. Migraines are the most common neurological disease, with an estimated 28 million sufferers in the United States, 18 million of them women. About half of all women's migraine headaches are believed to be linked to estrogen; in these cases, migraines can disappear entirely after menopause. Doctors often prescribe calcium channel blockers, beta-blockers, and tricyclic antidepressants to prevent frequent migraines.

For

Acute migraine headaches.

Availability and Dosage

Tablets: 25 mg, 50 mg. Subcutaneous (beneath the skin) injections: single-dose (6 mg per 0.5 ml) prefilled syringes with autoinjector device. Nasal spray (sumatriptan succinate): 5 mg, 10 mg, 20 mg per metered spray. If you do not get relief or there is no improvement in symptoms after several weeks of use, contact your doctor.

Side Effects

More common are nausea, drowsiness, dizziness, numbness, feeling faint, tingling, and feelings of warmth or cold. Some side effects are difficult to distinguish from the migraine itself. Injection: Pain or burning at injection site. Nasal spray: Bad or unusual taste.

Drug Interactions

Potentially serious interactions can occur with monoamine oxidase (MAO) inhibitors and selective serotonin reuptake inhibitor (SSRI) antidepressants. Do not take any other antimigraine drug within 24 hours of taking sumatriptan. Always inform your doctors of every medication you are taking, including nonprescription medicines, vitamins, herbal remedies, and dietary supplements.

Food/Alcohol Interactions

Avoid alcohol and caffeine. Do not skip meals or fast. Your doctor should provide you with a list of foods, drinks, and additives that may trigger a migraine.

Pregnancy/Nursing

Not recommended. Before taking this drug, discuss with your doctor the benefits versus the potential risks. The drug also passes into breast milk.

Seniors

No special warnings. Take as prescribed and immediately inform your doctor of any persistent or troublesome side effects.

Warning

Sumatriptan can cause constriction of blood vessels and a slight increase in blood pressure. This drug is not recommended for patients who have heart disease, previous heart attacks, angina, high cholesterol, obesity, high blood pressure, or diabetes.

Comments

Migraine is a complex, debilitating disease and not just another name for headache. Migraine "triggers" are different in each case and include certain foods, bright lights, excessive noise, stress, lack of sleep, changes in temperature, and many more. The migraine is often preceded by an "aura" of flashing lights followed by intense pain, vision disturbances, nausea, and vomiting. Over-the-counter medications specifically formulated for migraine are now available, but always check with your doctor or your pharmacist before self-medicating. There is no cure, and many people are finding nondrug therapeutic relief in biofeedback, massage, and acupuncture.

Brand Name
Inderal

Generic Name

propranolol

Type of Drug

Beta-blocker. These drugs block the response of the heart and blood vessels, lower pulse rate, and reduce the force of the heartbeat, thereby reducing the workload of the heart. They are sometimes prescribed after a heart attack to help prevent future attacks.

For

High blood pressure; angina pectoris; irregular heartbeats.

Availability and Dosage

Tablets: 10 mg, 20 mg, 40 mg, 60 mg, 80 mg, 90 mg. Extended-release capsules: 60 mg, 80 mg, 120 mg, 160 mg. Should be taken without food on an empty stomach. Do not stop taking this medicine without consulting your doctor; stopping the drug suddenly could have serious effects on your heart.

Side Effects

More common include dizziness, drowsiness, nausea, hair loss, weakness, lethargy, and cold hands and feet. These may subside as your body adjusts to the medication. This drug may aggravate the symptoms of lupus.

Drug Interactions

This drug has the potential to interact with a wide variety of medications, including aspirin and other nonsteroidal antiinflammatory drugs (NSAIDs), oral antidiabetics, blood-pressure–lowering drugs, estrogens, certain migraine medications known as ergot alkaloids, calcium channel blockers, anticonvulsants, and monoamine oxidase (MAO) inhibitor antidepressants. Always inform your doctors of every medication you are taking, including nonprescription medicines, vitamins, herbal remedies, and dietary supplements. *Do not take any over-the-counter medications unless approved by your doctor.*

Food/Alcohol Interactions

Avoid alcohol.

Pregnancy/Nursing

Not recommended. Propranolol has been shown to reduce birth weight.

Seniors

Your doctor may start you on a low dose in order to minimize adverse effects.

Warning

Notify your doctor immediately if you experience difficulty in breathing, skin rash, easy bruising or bleeding, confusion, depression, fast or slow heartbeat, or fainting. If you are going to have any kind of surgery, tell your doctor or dentist that you are taking this drug.

Comments

This drug was introduced in 1968, the first beta-blocker to be available in the United States. Like all beta-blockers, this drug can affect the level of blood sugar in the body. Diabetics should use this drug with caution.

indinavir sulfate

See Crixivan

Brand Name
Indocin

Generic Name

indomethacin

Type of Drug

Nonsteroidal antiinflammatory drug (NSAID). Drugs in this group reduce pain, inflammation, and stiffness associated with a wide range of conditions that affect the bones, joints, and muscles. These drugs do not cure a disease; they are used for relief of symptoms.

For

Relief of symptoms associated with arthritis: inflammation, pain, stiffness, and swelling.

Availability and Dosage

Capsules: 25 mg, 50 mg. Extended-release capsules: 75 mg. Oral suspension: 25 mg per 5 ml, with 1% alcohol. Rectal suppositories: 50 mg. When taking the oral forms of this medication, take with food or immediately after meals with a full glass of water. To minimize adverse effects on your esophagus and stomach, do not take this drug right before lying down.

Side Effects

More common include stomach upset and irritation, heartburn, light-headedness, headache, nausea, diarrhea, constipation, and drowsiness. Others include gastrointestinal bleeding, stomach ulcers, dry nose and mouth, heart palpitations, ringing in the ears, and tingling in hands or feet.

Drug Interactions

Indomethacin has the potential to interact with a wide variety of medications, including anticoagulants (blood thinners), corticosteroids, aspirin and other NSAIDs (especially diflunisal), beta-blockers and other heart drugs, antidiabetics, anticonvulsants, and lithium. Do not take other painkillers while on this drug. Always inform your doctors of every medication you are taking, including nonprescription medicines, vitamins, herbal remedies, and dietary supplements.

Food/Alcohol Interactions

Avoid alcohol, as it may increase the potential for gastric bleeding.

Pregnancy/Nursing

Most NSAIDs are not recommended for pregnancy or for nursing mothers. Indomethacin should not be used after the first trimester because of possible adverse effects on the fetal heart.

Seniors

Older adults may be more susceptibile to the side effects of this drug, particularly stomach ulcers or gastrointestinal bleeding.

Warning

NSAIDs can cause several potentially serious side effects, including gastrointestinal disorders, dizziness, and gastric bleeding. Indomethacin can have a highly toxic effect on the kidneys. If you have impaired kidney function, ulcers, anemia, asthma, or lupus, you should use this drug with caution. Symptoms of gastric bleeding include severe abdominal cramps, diarrhea, or black tarry stools, and vomiting of blood. *Seek emergency medical treatment immediately.*

Comments

Your physician may routinely prescribe a series of different NSAIDs in order to find the one best suited for you. Some, like indomethacin, are available only by prescription, but many NSAIDs can be obtained without a prescription and are routinely used in self-medication. Side effects and interactions remain the same with nonprescription NSAIDs. When using any nonprescription NSAID, follow package directions carefully. If you are going to have surgery, you may need to discontinue this drug temporarily.

indomethacin

See Indocin

Brand Name
Intal

Generic Name

cromolyn sodium

Type of Drug

Antiallergy; antiasthmatic.

For

Allergic rhinitis; chronic asthma. Not for use in an acute asthma attack.

Availability and Dosage

Metered aerosol. Inhalation: 0.8 mg per inhalation. Inhalation solution: 20 mg per ml. Capsules: 100 mg. Inhalation solution is for use only in a nebulizer with an appropriate face mask or mouthpiece. Follow your health care practitioner's or pharmacist's directions for use. Do not take this medicine more often than is necessary, and do not discontinue it even if your symptoms improve. Cromolyn must be taken regularly for chronic asthma.

Side Effects

More common include cough and hoarseness and irritation of the mouth or tongue. Others include nausea, wheezing, and breathlessness.

Drug Interactions

No interactions are known. Always inform your doctors of every medication you are taking, including nonprescription medicines, vitamins, herbal remedies, and dietary supplements.

Food/Alcohol Interactions

No special warnings.

Pregnancy/Nursing

No special warnings, although all drugs during pregnancy and breast-feeding should be avoided if possible. Before taking this drug, discuss with your doctor the benefits versus the potential risks.

Seniors

No special warnings. Take as prescribed and immediately inform your doctor of any persistent or troublesome side effects.

Warning

Side effects of this drug are rare. However, if you have difficulty in swallowing, hives, swelling of the face, lips, or eyes, uncontrollable coughing or wheezing, or any other allergic-type reaction, notify your doctor at once. Do not use this medication for an acute asthma attack.

Comments

You may need to take this medicine for a while before you notice significant improvement in symptoms—up to 1 week for short-term allergies, up to 4 weeks for long-term allergies. There is a nonprescription nasal-spray version of cromolyn called Nasal-crom, used for seasonal allergies and allergic rhinitis. Follow package directions carefully and consult your doctor if you have any questions.

Intercon

See Oral Contraceptives

interferon beta 1-a

See Avonex

Ionamin

See Fastin

ipratropium

See Atrovent*

Isoptin

See Calan SR

isosorbide mononitrate

See Imdur*

isotretinoin

See Accutane

itraconazole

See Sporanox

Jenest-28

See Oral Contraceptives

Brand Name
K-Dur 20* (also K-Dur 10, Micro-K Extencaps, Klor-Con, Kato)

Generic Name
potassium chloride*

Type of Drug
Potassium replacement.

For
Mild hypertension; replaces depleted potassium levels.

Availability and Dosage
Potassium chloride comes in many different strengths and forms under a variety of brand names. K-Dur 20, K-Dur 10, and Micro-K Extencaps are available in controlled-release tablets and capsules. Klor-Con and Kato are oral powders. Other forms are effervescent tablets, enteric-coated tablets, and oral liquids. Do not attempt to self-medicate using potassium replacements. *Use of any form of potassium replacement must be closely monitored by your physician.*

Side Effects
More common include nausea, diarrhea, and indigestion. Others include rash, dizziness or light-headedness, muscle weakness, and extreme fatigue.

Drug Interactions
Potassium replacement drugs can interact with a variety of medications, including diuretics (water pills), drugs for high blood pressure, nonsteroidal antiinflammatory drugs (NSAIDs), drugs for Parkinson's disease, and digoxin. Always inform your doctors of every medication you are taking, including nonprescription medicines, vitamins, herbal remedies, and dietary supplements. *Do not take any over-the-counter medications unless approved by your doctor.*

Food/Alcohol Interactions

Avoid salt substitutes and low-sodium milk; they are high in potassium and may interact with this drug. You may need to change your diet while taking this drug, as many foods are high in potassium: bananas, broccoli, molasses, watermelon, orange juice, prunes, raisins, dates, potatoes, spinach, yams, and others. Your doctor or health care practitioner may provide you with a list of restricted foods.

Pregnancy/Nursing

No special warnings, although all drugs during pregnancy should be avoided if possible. You may want to bottle-feed your baby while taking this drug because of possible adverse effects on the newborn. Before taking this drug, discuss with your doctor the benefits versus the potential risks.

Seniors

No special warnings. Take as prescribed and immediately inform your doctor of any persistent or troublesome side effects.

Warning

If you have heart or kidney disease, heart arrhythmias, diarrhea, or dehydration, use this drug with extreme caution, and report any persistent or troublesome side effects immediately. Your blood pressure should be monitored regularly while on this drug. If you experience a feeling of heaviness in your muscles, muscle twitching, confusion, weak pulse, chest pain, or stools that are tarry or black, call your doctor at once.

Comments

Potassium is an essential ingredient of body fluids and has a major effect on the kidneys, heart, and all muscles. An excess of potassium can be as dangerous (hyperkalemia) as a potassium deficiency (hypokalemia). Potassium replacement therapy should be done only under the supervision of a physician.

Kato

See K-Dur 20*

Keflet

See Keflex

Brand Name
Keflex (also Keflet)

Generic Name
cephalexin*

Type of Drug
Antibiotic. These drugs are among the most commonly prescribed, resulting in such widespread use that the bacteria they were developed to kill have become resistant to them. These "resistant" forms are then passed from person to person, further causing the spread of infections that become even more difficult to treat. Some antibiotics work against a limited number of microorganisms. Broad-spectrum antibiotics are effective against a variety of bacteria. Your doctor will prescribe the correct antibiotic depending on the type of infection.

For
Various bacterial infections including urinary-tract infections (UTIs) and respiratory-tract infections; skin and bone infections.

Availability and Dosage
Tablets: 250 mg, 500 mg. Capsules: 250 mg, 500 mg. Oral suspension: 125 mg, 250 mg per 5 ml. May be taken with or without food. It is essential to take the complete course of antibiotics prescribed. If you fail to do so, increased drug resistance by any leftover bacteria is likely to occur.

Side Effects
More common include nausea, mild diarrhea, stomach cramps, and heartburn. Others include vaginal discharge or itching, headache, and dizziness.

Drug Interactions
This drug can interact with erythromycin and tetracycline antibiotics. It can also decrease the effectiveness of certain oral contraceptives. You may want to use an additional method of birth control while on this drug.

Food/Alcohol Interactions
Avoid or limit alcohol.

Pregnancy/Nursing

No special warnings, although all drugs during pregnancy and breast-feeding should be avoided if possible. Before taking this drug, discuss with your doctor the benefits versus the potential risks. You may want to bottle-feed your baby while on this drug.

Seniors

No special warnings, although reduced kidney function in older adults can be a factor in increasing side effects. Take as prescribed and immediately inform your doctor of any persistent or troublesome side effects.

Warning

Inform your doctor if you have ever had an allergic reaction to penicillin. If you experience difficulty in breathing, itching, swelling, rash, or severe vomiting or diarrhea, call your doctor at once.

Comments

Cephalexin is a "first-generation" cephalosporin antibiotic and is not as effective as broad-spectrum antibiotics. It usually is used for treating bronchitis, cystitis, and some skin and bone infections. It is usually given for short courses of treatment only (10 to 14 days). Prolonged use may result in a secondary infection of the vagina.

ketoconazole

See Nizoral

ketoprofen

See Orudis

Brand Name
Klonopin

Generic Name

clonazepam

Type of Drug

Anticonvulsant; benzodiazepine. It is important to take anticonvulsants exactly as prescribed, as the level of the drug in the body needs to be constant to be the most effective in preventing seizures. Benzodiazepines are central nervous system (CNS) depressants and work on the part of the brain that controls emotions by slowing nervous-system transmissions. They are also used as sedatives and muscle relaxants.

For

Convulsive disorders such as epilepsy including petit mal seizures; panic attacks; schizophrenia.

Availability and Dosage

Tablets and orally disintegrating tablets: 0.125 mg, .25 mg, 0.5 mg, 1 mg, 2 mg. Dosages vary depending on whether the drug is used for seizures or as an antianxiety agent. May be taken with or without food. Do not take antacids within 1 hour of taking clonazepam, as it may reduce the drug's effectiveness. Do not abruptly stop taking this drug; withdrawal symptoms may occur. Your doctor will need to gradually reduce your dose. This drug has the potential for physical or psychological dependence. Do not take more than is prescribed.

Side Effects

More common include daytime drowsiness, dizziness or unsteadiness, light-headedness, and headache. Others include nausea, fatigue, changes in sex drive, changes in weight and appetite, indigestion, mood or behavior changes, and dry mouth. Side effects may subside as your body adjusts to this medication.

Drug Interactions

Anticonvulsant and benzodiazepine drugs have the potential to interact with a wide variety of medications, including monoamine oxidase (MAO) inhibitor antidepressants, antihistamines, oral contraceptives, narcotic pain relievers, ketoconazole, fluoxetine, tricyclic antidepressants, other anticonvulsants (especially valproic acid), and other benzodiazepines. Always inform your doctors of every medication you are taking, including nonprescription medicines, vitamins, herbal remedies, and dietary supplements. *Do not take any over-the-counter medications unless approved by your doctor.*

Food/Alcohol Interactions

Avoid alcohol.

Pregnancy/Nursing

Not recommended. Women who have grand mal epilepsy may find that their seizures become more frequent during pregnancy; petit mal episodes are rare. During pregnancy, you must be consistently monitored by your doctor to control the amount and type of medication you are taking.

Seniors

The risk of side effects, particularly drowsiness, dizziness, and loss of coordination, is higher in older adults. Notify your doctor immediately of any persistent adverse effects.

Warning

This drug should be used with caution if you have kidney or liver disease or a history of alcohol or drug abuse, depression, sleep apnea, or stroke. Use caution when driving or operating machinery. Clonazepam can affect mental alertness and coordination.

Comments

Epilepsy is caused by brain and central nervous system disturbances resulting from a wide range of causes. If you have a seizure disorder, you should wear a medical identification tag and carry an ID card listing the type of disorder and a list of your current medications.

Klor-Con

See K-Dur 20*

Brand Name
Lamisil

Generic Name

terbinafine HCl

Type of Drug

Antifungal.

For

Nail and skin infections.

Availability and Dosage

Tablets: 250 mg. Topical gel, cream, solution: 1%. Tablets may be taken with or without food. Usual dose is once daily. Take the full prescribed treatment of both the oral and the topical forms, even if your symptoms improve. Do not wrap or cover the affected area when using the topical form.

Side Effects

Oral form: More common include headache, diarrhea, upset stomach, and changes in taste. Others include nausea, abdominal pain, flatulence, rash, itching, hives, and liver abnormalities. Topical form: More common include irritation, burning, itching, and dryness.

Drug Interactions

Oral form: This drug may interact with antituberculosis drugs, cimetidine, and some antiasthmatics. Topical form: No known interactions, but you should not use any other topical medications, hand creams, or cosmetics at the same affected area.

Food/Alcohol Interactions

No special warnings.

Pregnancy/Nursing

Not recommended. This drug passes into breast milk. Bottle-feed your baby if you must take this drug.

Seniors

No special warnings. Take as prescribed and immediately inform your doctor of any persistent or troublesome side effects.

Warning

With the oral form of terbinafine, make sure your doctor knows if you have a history of any immunodeficiency disease or liver or kidney disease. Abnormal blood counts and liver abnormalities have been reported. If you develop jaundice, dark urine, pale stools, persistent nausea, or fatigue, contact your doctor immediately.

Comments

Nail fungus (onychomycosis) is not just an unsightly cosmetic problem. It can spread from one site to another or from person to person and can permanently deform nails. Do not use acrylic or "press-on" type nails during treatment, and when you get manicures or pedicures, make sure that the soaking solutions are fresh and the instruments sterilized. In tablet form, terbinafine travels to the infected area under the nail and continues to work after the course of treatment. The nonprescription version of topical terbinafine is Lamisil AT Cream, used for athlete's foot. Follow package directions carefully and contact your doctor or your pharmacist with any questions.

Lanoxicaps

See Lanoxin*

Brand Name

Lanoxin* (also Lanoxicaps)

Generic Name

digoxin

Type of Drug

Digitalis. This type of drug is used to control heart rate and rhythm and to improve heart efficiency and blood circulation.

For

Heart arrhythmias; congestive heart failure.

Availability and Dosage

Tablets: 0.125 mg, 0.25 mg, 0.5 mg. Lanoxicap capsules: 0.05 mg, 0.1 mg, 0.2 mg. Should be taken on an empty stomach, 1 hour before or 2 hours after a meal, at the same time every day.

Side Effects

More common include nausea and changes in vision. Others include headache, drowsiness, weakness, tingling sensation, vomiting, loss of appetite, apathy, confusion, rash, anxiety, and depression.

Drug Interactions

Digoxin has the potential to interact with a wide variety of drugs, including bronchodilators, anticancer drugs, phenytoin, some antibiotics, cholesterol-lowering drugs, indomethacin, benzodiazepines, spironolactone, ibuprofen, verapamil, diuretics, triamterene, thyroid drugs, antacids, and drugs for any type of heart disease. Always inform your doctors of every medication you are taking, including nonprescription medicines, vitamins, herbal remedies, and dietary supplements. *Do not take any over-the-counter medications unless approved by your doctor.*

Food/Alcohol Interactions

Your doctor may recommend a special diet. Avoid taking this drug with high-fiber food (such as bran), as it may interfere with absorption. Avoid licorice, as it may cause arrhythmia.

Pregnancy/Nursing

No special warnings, although all drugs during pregnancy and breast-feeding should be avoided if possible. Before taking this drug, discuss with your doctor the benefits versus the potential risks. Bottle-feed your baby if you must take this drug.

Seniors

The risk of side effects may be increased in older adults who have impaired kidney function. Your doctor may prescribe a low dose.

Warning

Do not change brands of digoxin without consulting your doctor or your pharmacist. With the ability to order prescription drugs over the Internet, this is especially important to remember. Different brands of digoxin may not produce the same results and proper dosage is essential. If you experience dizziness, palpitations, or "halos" of color surrounding objects, contact your doctor immediately.

Comments

You must be regularly monitored by your doctor or other health care professional while on this drug, to check for irregular or slow heartbeat. You should wear a medical identification tag at all times along with an ID card that lists all the medications you are currently taking.

lansoprazole

See Prevacid

Brand Name
Lasix*

Generic Name

furosemide

Type of Drug

Diuretic; antihypertensive. Diuretics promote the loss of water and salt from the body, which results in the lowering of blood pressure. Antihypertensives work to reduce abnormally high pressure of the blood against the walls of the blood vessels. Hypertension can cause strokes and heart attacks as well as damage to the eyes and kidneys. Antihypertensives do not cure high blood pressure; they control it for as long as the medication is taken.

For

High blood pressure; congestive heart failure; kidney dysfunction; accumulation of fluid in the lungs.

Availability and Dosage

Tablets: 20 mg, 40 mg, 80 mg. Should be taken on an empty stomach, 1 hour before or 2 hours after meals, but may be taken with food if it irritates your stomach. Daytime dosage is recommended; if you take it at night you may have to get up to urinate frequently.

Side Effects

More common include increased thirst, dry mouth, weakness, lethargy, and drowsiness. Others include muscle pain or cramping, palpitations, nausea, vomiting, ringing in ears, loss of appetite, changes in blood sugar, and increased sun sensitivity.

Drug Interactions

Furosemide may interact with some antibiotics, nonsteroidal antiinflammatory drugs (NSAIDs), corticosteroids, digitalis drugs, lithium, oral antidiabetics, phenytoin, other diuretics, other blood-pressure–lowering drugs, and some anticancer drugs. Always inform your doctors of every medication you are taking, including nonprescription medicines, vitamins, herbal remedies, and dietary supplements. *Do not take any over-the-counter medications unless approved by your doctor.*

Food/Alcohol Interactions

Avoid alcohol. Your doctor may recommend a diet with foods high in potassium (bananas, orange juice, figs, prunes) to offset the loss caused by this drug, but do not make any dietary changes without consulting your doctor.

Pregnancy/Nursing

No special warnings, although all drugs during pregnancy and breast-feeding should be avoided if possible. Before taking this drug, discuss with your doctor the benefits versus the potential risks. Bottle-feed your baby if you must take this drug.

Seniors

Older adults may experience dizziness or light-headedness as a result of excessive potassium loss. Your doctor may prescribe a low dose.

Warning

Make sure your doctor has your complete medical history, including a history of diabetes, gout, systemic lupus erythematosus (SLE), or kidney or liver disease.

Comments

Furosemide is a very strong loop diuretic that may cause excessive loss of water or potassium, chloride, sodium, calcium, and magnesium. You should be carefully and regularly monitored with blood and electrolyte tests while on this drug.

latanoprost

See Xalatan*

leflunomide

See Arava

Brand Name

Lescol*

Generic Name

fluvastatin

Type of Drug

Cholesterol-lowering. These drugs are usually prescribed after dietary and lifestyle changes have failed to lower cholesterol, but they do not take the place of those changes. You still need to incorporate lifestyle changes, if indicated, including quitting smoking, reducing saturated fats, and getting adequate aerobic exercise as recommended by your physician. Drugs in this class are designed to work in different ways on different substances: total cholesterol, LDL (the "bad" cholesterol), HDL (the "good" cholesterol), and triglycerides. Your doctor will prescribe the one best suited to you based on the results of your blood tests.

For

High blood cholesterol, to be used with a diet and exercise program.

Availability and Dosage

Capsules: 20 mg, 40 mg. May be taken with or without food, usually in the evening.

Side Effects

More common include diarrhea, constipation, dizziness, and heartburn. Others include difficulty in sleeping, gas, muscle cramps, rash, abdominal pain, sore throat, vomiting, elevation of liver enzymes and fatigue.

Drug Interactions

This drug may interact with gemfibrozil, some antibiotics, cimetidine, digoxin, erythromycin, niacin, omeprazole, ranitidine, antifungals. Always inform your doctors of every medication you are taking, including nonprescription medicines, vitamins, herbal remedies, and dietary supplements. *Do not take any over-the-counter medications unless approved by your doctor.*

Food/Alcohol Interactions

Avoid alcohol.

Pregnancy/Nursing

A woman must never become pregnant while taking this drug. If you think you are pregnant, stop taking it immediately and contact your doctor. Bottle-feed your baby if you must take this drug.

Seniors

No special warnings. Take as prescribed, and immediately inform your doctor of any persistent or troublesome side effects.

Warning

You will need to be regularly monitored while on this drug, especially to test for liver function.

Comments

Heart attack is the leading cause of death for women in the United States. Every year 1.5 million Americans have heart attacks; one-third of those die, and one-half of those are women. Stroke kills another 88,000. Much attention is given to breast cancer (and early detection has proven to be key to successful treatment), but heart attacks claim the lives of more than six times as many women.

Brand Name
Levaquin*

Generic Name

levofloxacin

Type of Drug

Antibiotic. These drugs are among the most commonly prescribed, resulting in such widespread use that the bacteria they were developed to kill have become resistant to them. These "resistant" forms are then passed from person to person, further causing the spread of infections that become even more difficult to treat.

For

Various infections including those of the respiratory tract and the urinary tract.

Availability and Dosage

Tablets: 250 mg, 500 mg. May be taken with or without food. It is essential to take the complete course of antibiotics prescribed. If you fail to do so, increased drug resistance by any leftover bacteria is likely to occur.

Side Effects

More common include increased sun sensitivity. Others include constipation, diarrhea, insomnia, dizziness, headache, drowsiness, upset stomach, nausea, and dry mouth.

Drug Interactions

Levofloxacin may interact with iron, zinc, calcium, manganese, and magnesium salts. If you are taking a multivitamin or multimineral containing any of these ingredients, do not take it within

2 hours of taking levofloxacin. Do not take antacids within 2 hours of taking levofloxacin. Always inform your doctors of every medication you are taking, including nonprescription medicines, vitamins, herbal remedies, and dietary supplements. *Do not take any over-the-counter medications unless approved by your doctor.*

Food/Alcohol Interactions

Avoid or limit alcohol. Avoid or limit caffeine. As with any antibiotic, drink plenty of water while you are on this drug.

Pregnancy/Nursing

Not recommended. Bottle-feed your baby if you must take this drug.

Seniors

No special warnings. Take as prescribed, and immediately inform your doctor of any persistent or troublesome side effects.

Warning

Some antibiotics interfere with the effectiveness of oral contraceptives. Always check with your doctor to see if you need to use an additional method of birth control while taking an antibiotic.

Comments

This drug may also be prescribed for the following conditions as directed by your doctor: chronic bronchitis, sexually transmitted diseases (STDs), sinusitis, pneumonia, skin infections, and cystitis.

Levlen

See Oral Contraceptives

Levlite

See Oral Contraceptives

levofloxacin

See Levaquin*

levonorgestrel

See Plan B

levonorgestrel and ethinyl estradiol

See Preven

Levora

See Oral Contraceptives

Levothroid

See Synthroid*

levothyroxine

See Synthroid*

Levoxine

See Synthroid*

Levoxyl*

See Synthroid*

Brand Name
Librium

Generic Name
chlordiazepoxide

Type of Drug
Benzodiazepine sedative. These drugs are central nervous system (CNS) depressants and work on the part of the brain that controls emotions by slowing nervous-system transmissions. They are often the drug of choice to relieve the symptoms of anxiety but do not address the underlying cause.

For
Anxiety disorders.

Availability and Dosage
Tablets: 25 mg. Capsules: 5 mg, 10 mg, 25 mg. Should be taken on an empty stomach, 1 hour before or 2 hours after meals, but may be taken with food if stomach upset occurs. Do not take

more of this medicine than is prescribed. If you have been on this drug for 4 weeks or more, do not abruptly stop taking it without consulting your doctor; severe adverse reactions may result.

Side Effects

More common include drowsiness, dizziness, and clumsiness. Others include constipation, euphoria, nausea, vomiting, changes in sex drive, dry mouth, slurred speech, headache, tremor, irregular menstrual periods, arrhythmia, and liver abnormalities.

Drug Interactions

Chlordiazepoxide has the potential to interact with a wide variety of medications, including any central nervous system (CNS) depressant, narcotics, antihistamines, oral contraceptives, monoamine oxidase (MAO) inhibitors, digoxin, cimetidine, erythromycin, antifungals, levodopa, phenytoin, and some drugs for psychosis or depression. Do not take antacids within 1 hour of taking this drug. Always inform your doctors of every medication you are taking, including nonprescription medicines, vitamins, herbal remedies, and dietary supplements. *Do not take any over-the-counter medications unless approved by your doctor.*

Food/Alcohol Interactions

Avoid alcohol. This drug is also prescribed for acute withdrawal symptoms in alcoholics.

Pregnancy/Nursing

Not recommended. Bottle-feed your baby if you must take this drug.

Seniors

Some side effects may be more severe in older adults. Your doctor may prescribe a low dose.

Warning

This drug has a high risk of physical or psychological dependence. Tell your doctor of any history of alcohol or substance abuse, depression, or suicidal thoughts. Make sure your doctor has your complete medical history.

Comments

Chlordiazepoxide is sometimes used to treat irritable bowel syndrome (IBS), a condition that affects twice as many women as men, especially during menstrual periods. Symptoms include chronic diarrhea, abdominal pain, gas, constipation, and bloating, and can be triggered by stress or changes in diet.

Brand Name
Lipitor*

Generic Name
atorvastatin calcium

Type of Drug
Cholesterol-lowering. These drugs are usually prescribed after dietary and lifestyle changes have failed to lower cholesterol, but they do not take the place of those changes. You still need to incorporate lifestyle changes, if indicated, including quitting smoking, reducing saturated fats, and getting adequate aerobic exercise as recommended by your physician.

For
High cholesterol.

Availability and Dosage
Tablets: 10 mg, 20 mg, 40 mg. May be taken with or without food at any time of the day.

Side Effects
More common include headache, flu-like symptoms, back pain, and flatulence. Others include constipation, dizziness, heartburn, diarrhea, sore throat, and muscle weakness.

Drug Interactions
Atorvastatin may interact with erythromycin, antifungals, gemfibrozil, digoxin, immunosuppressants, spironolactone, niacin, and antacids. Always inform your doctors of every medication you are taking, including nonprescription medicines, vitamins, herbal remedies, and dietary supplements. *Do not take any over-the-counter medications unless approved by your doctor.*

Food/Alcohol Interactions
No special warnings.

Pregnancy/Nursing
A woman must never become pregnant while taking this drug. If you think you are pregnant, stop taking it immediately and contact your doctor. Bottle-feed your baby if you must take this drug.

Seniors

No special warnings. Take as prescribed and immediately inform your doctor of any persistent or troublesome side effects.

Warning

You must be regularly monitored while you are taking this drug. If you experience muscle weakness, muscle pain, or muscle tenderness accompanied by fever and fatigue, contact your doctor immediately.

Comments

Atorvastatin was found in clinical studies to reduce LDL ("bad") cholesterol by 39% to 60% (in conjunction with appropriate diet and exercise). It is the only statin drug approved for the reduction of triglycerides as well as total and LDL cholesterol. It also raises HDL ("good") cholesterol by up to 10%.

Liquid Pred

See Deltasone*

lisinopril

See Zestril*

lisinopril/HCTZ

See Zestoretic*

lithium

See Eskalith

Lithobid

See Eskalith

Lithonate

See Eskalith

Lo-Ovral 28*

See Oral Contraceptives

Brand Name
Lopid

Generic Name
gemfibrozil*

Type of Drug
Cholesterol-lowering. This drug is used for people whose triglyceride levels are very high. It is usually prescribed after dietary and lifestyle changes have failed to lower triglycerides, a fatty substance in the blood that contributes to dangerous buildup in the arteries. You still need to incorporate lifestyle changes, if indicated, including quitting smoking, reducing saturated fats, and getting adequate aerobic exercise as recommended by your physician.

For
High levels of blood triglycerides.

Availability and Dosage
Tablets: 600 mg. Should be taken on an empty stomach, usually in the morning and evening in divided doses.

Side Effects
More common include stomach pains, gas, nausea, and diarrhea. Others include vomiting, changes in sex drive, headache, weight gain, flu-like symptoms, muscle aches, constipation, dry mouth, ringing in the ears, heartburn, and anemia.

Drug Interactions
Gemfibrozil may interact with any of the statin drugs (atorvastatin, fluvastatin, lovastatin, pravastatin, simvastatin), anticoagulants (blood thinners), oral antidiabetics, and niacin. Always inform your doctors of every medication you are taking, including nonprescription medicines, vitamins, herbal remedies, and dietary supplements. *Do not take any over-the-counter medications unless approved by your doctor.*

Food/Alcohol Interactions
Avoid alcohol. Follow a healthy diet as recommended by your doctor or other health care provider to reduce the risk of heart disease.

Pregnancy/Nursing

Not recommended. Discuss with your doctor the likelihood of your triglyceride levels increasing during pregnancy; in some cases the increase is significant. Bottle-feed your baby if you must take this drug.

Seniors

Side effects may be increased in older patients who have impaired kidney function. Your doctor may prescribe a low dose.

Warning

Tell your doctor if you have a history of diabetes or gallbladder, kidney, or liver disease. You must be regularly monitored while on this drug, with periodic blood tests to check for abnormalities in the liver, gallbladder, and pancreas.

Comments

It may take up to 4 weeks before you see any improvement in blood triglyceride levels. Ask your doctor what triglyceride levels are normal for you; the usual range is between 50 and 200 mg. If other risk factors are present (obesity, smoking), you may be prescribed drug therapy even if your triglyceride levels are normal.

Brand Name
Lopressor (also Toprol XL*)

Generic Name

metoprolol tartrate*

Type of Drug

Beta-blocker. These drugs block the response of the heart and blood vessels, lower the pulse rate, and reduce the force of the heartbeat, thereby reducing the workload of the heart. They are sometimes prescribed after a heart attack to help prevent future attacks.

For

Angina pectoris; high blood pressure; heart attack; migraine headaches; anxiety.

Availability and Dosage

Tablets: 50 mg, 100 mg. The drug also comes in extended-release form. Should be taken on an empty stomach, 1 hour before or 2 hours after meals. Do not abruptly stop taking this drug without consulting your doctor.

Side Effects

More common include dizziness, sexual dysfunction, and drowsiness. Others include weakness, fatigue, irritability, loss of short-term memory, anxiety, nightmares, tingling in the hands, feet, or scalp, sweating, nausea, cramps, skin rash, hair loss, and back pain.

Drug Interactions

Metoprolol may interact with oral antidiabetics, insulin, calcium channel blockers, aspirin, indomethacin, estrogens, benzodiazepines, and thyroid drugs. Do not take metoprolol within 2 weeks of taking a monoamine (MAO) inhibitor antidepressant. Always inform your doctors of every medication you are taking, including nonprescription medicines, vitamins, herbal remedies, and dietary supplements. *Do not take any over-the-counter medications unless approved by your doctor.*

Food/Alcohol Interactions

Avoid alcohol; it can cause a rapid drop in blood pressure. Your doctor or other health care provider may recommend a special diet to control high blood pressure.

Pregnancy/Nursing

Not recommended. Bottle-feed your baby if you must take this drug.

Seniors

Side effects may be more frequent and severe in older patients. Your doctor may prescribe a low dose.

Warning

Make sure your doctor knows if you have a history of systemic lupus erythematosus (SLE), as metoprolol may aggravate this condition. You may need to stop taking metoprolol prior to surgery, as it can interact with anesthetics and increase the risk of heart problems during surgery.

Comments

For women overall, smoking is the greatest risk factor for heart attack and stroke. For women between age 65 and 74, hypertension is the greatest risk factor for heart attacks, just slightly ahead of obesity. However, "central obesity"—having a waist larger than your hips—is a risk factor for all women (to calculate this, divide your waist measurement by your hip measurement; it should be lower than 0.85).

Brand Name
Lorabid*

Generic Name
loracarbef

Type of Drug
Antibiotic. These types of drugs are among the most commonly prescribed. Some antibiotics work against a limited number of microorganisms. Broad-spectrum antibiotics are effective against a variety of bacteria. Your doctor will prescribe the correct antibiotic depending on the type of infection. Antibiotics are useless against viral infections such as colds and flu

For
Bacterial infections including those of the middle ear, upper and lower respiratory tract, and skin; urinary-tract infections (UTIs); streptococcal pharyngitis, "strep throat."

Availability and Dosage
Capsules: 200 mg, 400 mg. Oral suspension: 100 mg, 200 mg per 5 ml. Should be taken on an empty stomach, 1 hour before or 2 hours after meals. Take this drug exactly as prescribed, and at evenly spaced intervals. It is essential to take the complete course of loracarbef prescribed. If you fail to do so, serious heart-related problems may develop. Do not miss any doses.

Side Effects
More common include nausea, vomiting, diarrhea, stomach pain, abdominal pain, and gas. Others include headache, drowsiness, dizziness, loss of appetite, and vaginal itching or discharge.

Drug Interactions
Loracarbef may interact with erythromycin. Always inform your doctors of every medication you are taking, including nonprescription medicines, vitamins, herbal remedies, and dietary supplements.

Food/Alcohol Interactions

Avoid or limit alcohol. Drink plenty of water while on this drug.

Pregnancy/Nursing

No special warnings, although all drugs during pregnancy should be avoided if possible. Before taking this drug, discuss with your doctor the benefits versus the potential risks. Bottle-feed your baby if you must take this drug.

Seniors

No special warnings. Take as prescribed and immediately inform your doctor of any persistent or troublesome side effects.

Warning

Tell your doctor if you have a history of allergies to any antibiotics. If you experience severe diarrhea, do not self-medicate with over-the-counter remedies. Contact your doctor.

Comments

Repeated urinary-tract infections (UTIs) may be a symptom of an underlying disorder, including menopausal changes or kidney stones. They are extremely common among women; most will have at least one or two during their lifetimes and probably more. Symptoms include urgency, burning, pain, decreased urinary output, dark urine, and blood in the urine. Your health care provider will culture a urine specimen to determine the correct antibiotic. Further tests may be required.

loracarbef

*See Lorabid**

loratadine

*See Claritin**

loratadine and pseudoephedrine

*See Claritin-D**

lorazepam*

See Ativan

Lorcet

See Vicodin

Lortab

See Vicodin

losartan potassium/HCTZ

See Hyzaar*

losartan potassium

See Cozaar*

Brand Name
Lotensin*

Generic Name

benazepril

Type of Drug

Angiotensin-converting enzyme (ACE) inhibitor. ACE inhibitors are antihypertensives used to treat high blood pressure (hypertension). They work by blocking an enzyme in the body that is required to produce a substance that causes blood vessels to tighten. When this enzyme is blocked, blood vessels are relaxed, blood pressure is lowered, the workload of the heart and arteries is reduced, and blood and oxygen supplies are increased.

For

High blood pressure.

Availability and Dosage

Tablets: 5 mg, 10 mg, 20 mg, 40 mg. May be taken with or without food.

Side Effects

More common in women is a dry, hacking cough. Others include fatigue, headache, dizziness, fainting, indigestion, heart palpitations, difficulty in sleeping, abdominal pain, nausea, vomiting, constipation, and tingling in the hands and feet.

Drug Interactions

Benazepril may interact with lithium, oral capsaicin, nonsteroidal antiinflammatory drugs (NSAIDs), other antihypertensives, potassium supplements, diuretics, allopurinol, and digoxin. Do not take antacids within 2 hours of taking benazepril. Always inform your doctors of every medication you are taking, including nonprescription medicines, vitamins, herbal remedies, and dietary supplements. *Do not take any over-the-counter medications unless approved by your doctor.*

Food/Alcohol Interactions

Avoid alcohol. Do not use salt substitutes.

Pregnancy/Nursing

Not recommended, especially during the second and third trimesters. Birth defects or fetal death may result. Bottle-feed your baby while taking this drug.

Seniors

Side effects may be more frequent or severe in older patients who have impaired kidney function. Your doctor may prescribe a low dose.

Warning

If you experience swelling of the face, tongue, or larynx, have a rapid pulse, difficulty in breathing, or become severely dizzy or faint, *seek emergency medical treatment.*

Comments

In a study published in the American Heart Association's journal *Circulation* in 1996, researchers found that a test used to evaluate the risk of death among patients who have had a heart attack is less accurate for women than for men. The test shows how the left ventricle—the heart's main pumping chamber—is functioning by measuring the amount of blood the heart pumps out with each beat. For men, a low number indicates a high risk of death, but the test is not as accurate in predicting the risk of death for women. The study concluded that doctors need to look for factors other than pumping efficiency when evaluating female heart patients. Heart attacks kill nearly 250,000 women each year.

Brand Name

Lotrel*

Generic Name

amlodipine/benazepril

Type of Drug

Antihypertensive. Calcium channel blocker and angiotensin-converting enzyme (ACE) inhibitor combination. Calcium channel blockers are used to correct certain heart arrhythmias (irregular heartbeats) and to lower blood pressure by blocking or slowing the flow of blood into the two chambers of the heart. Amlodipine increases the supply of blood and oxygen to the heart and reduces its workload. ACE inhibitors work by blocking an enzyme in the body required to produce a substance that causes blood vessels to tighten. When this enzyme is blocked, blood vessels are relaxed, blood pressure is lowered, the workload of the heart and arteries is reduced, and blood and oxygen supplies are increased.

For

High blood pressure.

Availability and Dosage

Capsules: 2.5 mg amlodipine and 10 mg benazepril; 5 mg amlodipine and 10 mg benazepril; 5 mg amlodipine and 20 mg benazepril. Should be taken on an empty stomach 1 hour before or 2 hours after meals.

Side Effects

More common include cough, dizziness, and headache. Others include fatigue, dry mouth, swelling, nausea, constipation, decreased blood potassium, anxiety, decreased sex drive, hot flashes, and tremors.

Drug Interactions

This drug may interact with lithium, triamterene, and spironolactone. Always inform your doctors of every medication you are taking, including nonprescription medicines, vitamins, herbal remedies, and dietary supplements. *Do not take any over-the-counter medications unless approved by your doctor.*

Food/Alcohol Interactions

Avoid alcohol.

Pregnancy/Nursing

Not recommended. ACE inhibitors are known to cause fetal damage, especially in the second and third trimesters. Bottle-feed your baby if you must take this drug.

Seniors

No special warnings. Take as prescribed and immediately inform your doctor of any persistent or troublesome side effects.

Warning

If you experience swelling of the face, tongue, or larynx, have a rapid pulse or difficulty in breathing, or become severely dizzy or faint, seek emergency medical treatment.

Comments

Heart disease is the leading cause of death in women, although hypertension is more common in men than in women. Hypertension has no symptoms and can lead to stroke. Signs of stroke, according to the American Heart Association, include sudden, severe headache, sudden loss or dimming of vision, loss of speech, and sudden weakness or numbness of the face, arm, or leg on one side of the body.

Brand Name
Lotrisone*

Generic Name

betamethasone and clotrimazole

Type of Drug

Topical corticosteroid; antifungal.

For

Fungal infection; rash.

Availability and Dosage

Topical cream: 0.05% betamethasone dipropionate and 1% clotrimazole.

Side Effects

More common include irritation or burning upon application. Others include itching, redness, swelling, dry skin, and acne.

Drug Interactions

No special warnings, although all drugs have the ability to interact with other drugs. Report any problems to your doctor or your pharmacist.

Food/Alcohol Interactions

No special warnings.

Pregnancy/Nursing

Not recommended.

Seniors

No special warnings. Take as prescribed and immediately inform your doctor of any persistent or troublesome side effects.

Warning

Do not use this drug in or near your eyes. Tell your doctor if you have a history of allergic reactions to other corticosteroids, including cortisone, dexamethasone, methylprednisolone, and prednisone.

Comments

Clotrimazole is an antifungal that prevents the growth of a wide variety of fungi and yeast. The corticosteroid betamethasone treats skin inflammation. It may take up to a week to see improvement in your symptoms. It is important to take the complete prescribed course of treatment, as stopping the drug too soon may result in fungi continuing to grow and becoming resistant.

lovastatin

See Mevacor*

Brand Name
Luvox

Generic Name

fluvoxamine

Type of Drug

Selective serotonin reuptake inhibitor (SSRI). This drug belongs to a newer class of antidepressants that work by raising the brain's level of serotonin, a chemical associated with mood and mental alertness. It can also help to relieve the repetitive rituals and anxiety associated with obsessive-compulsive disorder.

For

Obsessive-compulsive disorder (OCD); depression.

Availability and Dosage

Tablets: 50 mg, 100 mg. May be taken with or without food, usually at bedtime. Do not take more of this medicine than is prescribed. Do not abruptly stop taking this drug. Your dose may have to be gradually decreased.

Side Effects

More common include insomnia, drowsiness, nausea, weakness, nervousness, dry mouth, and constipation. Others include loss of appetite, heartburn, headache, yawning, sweating, tremor, and decreased sex drive.

Drug Interactions

Fluvoxamine can interact with a wide variety of medications, including alprazolam, beta-blockers, carbamazepine, lithium, diazepam, tricyclic antidepressants, and anticoagulants (blood thinners). The most serious interactions occur with monoamine oxidase (MAO) inhibitor antidepressants (selegiline, phenelzine, tranylcypromine). These drugs and fluvoxamine should never be taken together or within 2 weeks of each other. Always inform your doctors of every medication you are taking, including nonprescription medicines, vitamins, herbal remedies, and dietary supplements. *Do not take any over-the-counter medications unless approved by your doctor.*

Food/Alcohol Interactions

Avoid alcohol.

Pregnancy/Nursing

Not recommended. Fluvoxamine passes into breast milk. Bottle-feed your baby if you must take this drug.

Seniors

Side effects may be more severe in older adults. Your doctor may prescribe a low dose.

Warning

You must be regularly monitored by a physician while on this drug. Tell your doctor if you smoke, as smoking can affect how this drug is metabolized. Make sure your doctor has your complete medical history, including a history of alcohol or substance abuse, suicidal thoughts, seizures, or mania.

Comments

Obsessive-compulsive disorder (OCD) is characterized by recurrent, disturbing thoughts and/or compulsive behaviors. Compulsions manifest as repetitive, ritualistic behaviors that the person feels driven to perform. This drug is also used to treat bulimia. In one study of 20 bulimic women, fluvoxamine significantly reduced the frequency of binge eating episodes.

Brand Name
Macrobid* (also Macrodantin)

Generic Name

nitrofurantoin

Type of Drug

Antiinfective. These antibacterial drugs are similar to antibiotics in practice, but are of chemical origin instead of botanical. Athough they have been largely overshadowed by antibiotics, there are instances in which antiinfectives are prescribed.

For

Urinary-tract infections (UTIs).

Availability and Dosage

Capsules: 25 mg, 50 mg, 75 mg, 100 mg. Should be taken with food to minimize stomach upset. It is essential to take the complete course of antiinfectives prescribed. If you fail to do so, increased drug resistance by any leftover bacteria is likely to occur.

Side Effects

More common include nausea, diarrhea, vomiting, and abdominal pain. Others include cough, chest pain, itching, arthriticlike symptoms, headache, dizziness, and changes in blood cell counts. Dark yellow or brownish urine can occur.

Drug Interactions

Nitrofurantoin may interact with oral antidiabetics, methyldopa, carbamazepine, lithium, phenytoin, antacids, and some antibiotics, and other antiinfectives. Always inform your doctors of every medication you are taking, including nonprescription medicines, vitamins, herbal remedies, and dietary supplements. *Do not take any over-the-counter medications unless approved by your doctor.*

Food/Alcohol Interactions

Avoid or limit alcohol. Avoid dairy products. Avoid caffeine, carbonated beverages, or spicy foods, as they can aggravate symptoms. Drink plenty of water while on this drug.

Pregnancy/Nursing

Not recommended, especially during the last month of pregnancy. Nitrofurantoin passes into breast milk. Bottle-feed your baby if you must take this drug.

Seniors

Side effects may be more frequent in older adults who have impaired kidney function. Your doctor may prescribe a low dose.

Warning

Make sure your doctor has your complete medical history, including a history of diabetes, vitamin B deficiency, dehydration, nerve damage, kidney or lung disease, or a glucose-6-phosphate dehydrogenase (G6PD) deficiency, which can lead to hemolytic anemia. Frequent, severe, or untreated UTIs can lead to potentially serious kidney infections. Symptoms of kidney infection include fever, chills, nausea, and back pain. Contact your doctor immediately.

Comments

At least 1 in 5 women experience a urinary-tract infection (UTI) at some point in their lives, and of those, another 4 out of 5 will have a recurrence within 18 months. Symptoms are a burning feeling when urinating, urgency, low abdominal pain, cloudy or bloody urine, and pain in the lower back or under the ribs.

Macrodantin

See Macrobid

Brand Name
Maxalt

Generic Name

rizatriptan benzoate

Type of Drug

Antimigraine.

For

Short-term treatment of acute migraine headaches. This drug is not for migraine prevention, other types of headaches, hemiplegic migraine, or basilar migraine.

Availability and Dosage

Tablets: 5 mg, 10 mg. Orally disintegrating tablets: 5 mg, 10 mg. The disintegrating tablets contain aspartame; notify your health care provider if you have ever had an allergic reaction to aspartame. Should be taken at the first sign of migraine attack. You may take another dose after 2 hours after consulting your doctor. Do not take more than 30 mg within 24 hours.

Side Effects

More common include dizziness, drowsiness, feelings of heat or cold, hot flashes, tremor, euphoria. Others include difficulty in swallowing, nausea, fatigue, and weakness.

Drug Interactions

Do not take rizatriptan within 24 hours of taking dihydroergotamine, methysergide, or other ergot-type drugs, or sumatriptan, zolmitriptan, or naratriptan. Do not take rizatriptan within 2 weeks of taking a monoamine oxidase (MAO) inhibitor antidepressant. Other interactions can occur with selective serotonin reuptake inhibitors (SSRIs) including fluvoxamine, fluoxetine, paroxetine, and sertraline. Always inform your doctors of every medication you are taking, including nonprescription medicines, vitamins, herbal remedies, and dietary supplements. *Do not take any over-the-counter medications unless approved by your doctor.*

Food/Alcohol Interactions

Avoid alcohol. Your health care provider can supply you with a list of foods and beverages to avoid, including ripened cheeses, chocolate, fermented foods, bananas, nuts, monosodium glutamate, and citrus fruits.

Pregnancy/Nursing

No special warnings, although all drugs during pregnancy and breast-feeding should be avoided if possible. Before taking this drug, discuss with your doctor the benefits versus the potential risks.

Seniors

Not recommended, especially if you have heart disease or impaired kidney function.

Warning

Make sure your doctor has your complete medical history, including a history of angina, diabetes, heart disease, hypertension, arrhythmia, stroke, vascular disease, obesity, or kidney or liver disease. Smoking increases the risk of side effects.

Comments

Migraine affects three times as many women as men. Hormonal changes are suspected in the majority of these cases. From 60% to 70% of women who suffer from migraines report worse symptoms around the time of their menstrual periods. The majority of migraineurs (70% to 80%) have a family history of headache and/or migraine.

Brand Name
Mazanor (also Sanorex)

Generic Name

mazindol

Type of Drug

Appetite suppressant.

For

Appetite suppression; short-term treatment of obesity, to be used in conjunction with an appropriate diet and exercise program.

Availability and Dosage

Tablets: 1 mg, 2 mg. Usual dose is 1 mg three times a day an hour before meals, or 2 mg once a day an hour before lunch. Do not take more of this medicine than prescribed. Do not abruptly stop taking this drug without consulting your doctor.

Side Effects

More common include nervousness, irritability, pounding heart-beat, and insomnia. Others include headache, sweating, dry mouth, nausea, and constipation.

Drug Interactions

Do not take mazindol within 14 days of taking a monoamine oxidase (MAO) inhibitor antidepressant. Always inform your doctors of every medication you are taking, including nonprescription medicines, vitamins, herbal remedies, and dietary supplements. *Do not take any over-the-counter medications unless approved by your doctor.*

Food/Alcohol Interactions

Mazindol is designed to be used with a healthy, low-fat, reduced-calorie diet and appropriate exercise program.

Pregnancy/Nursing

A woman must never become pregnant while taking this drug. If you suspect you are pregnant during treatment, stop taking mazindol immediately and contact your doctor. Bottle-feed your baby if you must take this drug.

Seniors

Side effects may be more frequent in older patients. Your doctor may prescribe a low dose.

Warning

If you experience shortness of breath, chest pain, fainting, or swelling in the lower legs and feet, contact your doctor immediately. Tell your doctor if you have a history of alcohol or substance abuse, anorexia, bulimia, depression, hypertension, arrhythmia, diabetes, glaucoma, or migraine headaches.

Comments

As many as 40% of women are trying to lose weight at any given time. Appetite suppressants should not be used by people who are overweight by 10 pounds or less unless there are other risk factors present, including high cholesterol, diabetes, or hypertension. Mazindol is approved only for short-term use (a few weeks or months, as defined by the FDA), but your doctor may prescribe it for a longer period of time. Because there is little information on the safety and effectiveness of mazindol for more than 1 year, you should be regularly monitored by a physician.

meclizine

See Antivert

Brand Name
Medrol

Generic Name

methylprednisolone*

Type of Drug

Corticosteroid. The drugs in this group—often referred to as steroids—are most often used to treat inflammatory diseases.

For

Various types of inflammation.

Availability and Dosage

Tablets: 2 mg, 4 mg, 8 mg, 16 mg, 24 mg, 32 mg. Dosages vary according to the condition being treated. Should be taken with food to reduce stomach irritation or upset.

Side Effects

More common include indigestion, nervousness, increased appetite, and insomnia. Others include dizziness, weight gain, changes in mood, unusual growth of body hair, muscle cramps, headache, stomach ulcers, weakness, blurred vision, frequent urination, and increased thirst.

Drug Interactions

Methylprednisolone may interact with carbamazepine, phenytoin, oral antidiabetics, anticoagulants (blood thinners), some diuretics, oral contraceptives, aspirin, insulin, and digitalis drugs. Always inform your doctors of every medication you are taking, including nonprescription medicines, vitamins, herbal remedies, and dietary supplements. *Do not take any over-the-counter medications unless approved by your doctor.*

Food/Alcohol Interactions

Avoid or limit alcohol. Your doctor may recommend a special diet while you take this drug.

Pregnancy/Nursing

Not recommended, especially during the first trimester. Bottle-feed your baby if you must take this drug.

Seniors

Side effects may be more frequent and severe in older patients, particularly osteoporosis.

Warning

For women, a potential and significant side effect of this type of drug is osteoporosis. Use caution with long-term steroid use, as bone loss increases with the dose and duration of steroid treatment. The bones in the spine, ribs, and wrists are most susceptible to the effects of steroids. Bone mass is carefully monitored during treatment with these medications. Make sure your doctor has your complete medical history before taking any corticosteroid, including a history of allergies to this type of drug.

Comments

There are more than 100 different forms of inflammatory arthritis. Corticosteroid drugs are used to treat numerous conditions in addition to rheumatoid arthritis, including bursitis, chronic obstructive pulmonary disease, systemic lupus erythematosus, psoriasis, dermatitis, eczema, inflammatory bowel disease, allergic rhinitis, allergic reactions, multiple sclerosis, eye inflammation, and chronic active hepatitis. About 2 million Americans suffer from rheumatoid arthritis, 1.5 million of them women. The immune system, which normally protects the body from disease, attacks healthy joints of the body, resulting in pain, stiffness, and swelling.

medroxyprogesterone*

*See Provera**

medroxyprogesterone acetate

See Depo-Provera

Brand Name
Meridia

Generic Name
sibutramine hydrochloride monohydrate

Type of Drug
Appetite suppressant.

For
Obesity (at least 25 to 45 pounds overweight), to be used in conjunction with an appropriate diet and exercise program.

Availability and Dosage
Capsules: 5 mg, 10 mg, 15 mg. Do not take more of this medicine than is prescribed.

Side Effects
More common include dry mouth, constipation, and insomnia. Others include headache, increased sweating, increased blood pressure, and rapid pulse.

Drug Interactions
Sibutramine may interact with a wide variety of medications, including lithium, sumatriptan, phentermine, venlafaxine, bupropion, amitriptyline, antiparkinsonians, nefazodone, dihydroergotamine, ketoconazole, erythromycin, and selective serotonin reuptake inhibitor (SSRI) antidepressants. Do not take sibutramine within 14 days of taking a monoamine oxidase (MAO) inhibitor antidepressant. Do not combine sibutramine with any herbal or over-the-counter weight-loss preparations. Do not self-medicate with OTC cold, cough, or allergy medicines. Do not take the amino acid tryptophan. Always inform your doctors of every medication you are taking, including nonprescription medicines, vitamins, herbal remedies, and dietary supplements. *Do not take any over-the-counter medications unless approved by your doctor.*

Food/Alcohol Interactions
Avoid alcohol, as it may increase the sedative effects of this drug. Avoid excessive intake of caffeine. Sibutramine is designed to be used with a healthy, low-fat, reduced-calorie diet and appropriate exercise program.

Pregnancy/Nursing

A woman must never become pregnant while taking this drug. If you suspect you are pregnant during treatment, stop taking sibutramine immediately and contact your doctor. Bottle-feed your baby if you must take this drug.

Seniors

No special warnings. Take as prescribed and immediately inform your doctor of any persistent or troublesome side effects.

Warning

Sibutramine can substantially raise blood pressure in some individuals. This drug should not be taken by people who have heart disease, arrhythmias, congestive heart failure, or glaucoma.

Comments

This drug was the first obesity drug approved for use after the 1997 withdrawal of Redux and fenfluramine, drugs that were found to be the cause of heart valve damage. Although sibutramine is the only appetite suppressant drug approved for longer-term use in obese patients, its safety and effectiveness have not been determined beyond 1 year.

metformin HCl

See Glucophage*

methotrexate

See Rheumatrex

methylprednisolone*

See Medrol

Meticorten

See Deltasone*

metoprolol tartrate

See Lopressor

Brand Name
MetroGel (also MetroGel Vaginal)

Generic Name

metronidazole

Type of Drug

Oral and topical antibiotic; antiparasitic.

For

Treatment of rosacea, various bacterial infections, sexually transmitted diseases (STDs); trichomonas. The intravaginal form (MetroGel Vaginal) is for bacterial vaginosis.

Availability and Dosage

Tablets: 250 mg, 500 mg. Topical gel, cream, lotion: 0.75%. MetroGel Vaginal intravaginal gel: 0.75%. Oral form should be taken with food.

Side Effects

Oral form: More common include nausea, stomach cramps, loss of appetite, dizziness, and headache. Others include dry mouth, metallic taste in the mouth, and constipation. Topical gel form: skin irritation, dry skin, and red or watery eyes. Intravaginal gel: vaginal itching, irritation, and discharge, and burning upon urination.

Drug Interactions

The oral form of metronidazole can interact with a wide variety of medications, including lithium, anticoagulants (blood thinners), phenytoin, cimetidine, and drugs that affect the nervous system. The intravaginal gel form can interact with anticoagulants. Always inform your doctors of every medication you are taking, including nonprescription medicines, vitamins, herbal remedies, and dietary supplements. *Do not take any over-the-counter medications unless approved by your doctor.*

Food/Alcohol Interactions

Avoid alcohol, as serious interactions can occur.

Pregnancy/Nursing

Not recommended, especially during the first trimester. Metronidazole passes into breast milk. Bottle-feed your baby if you must take this drug.

Seniors

No special warnings, unless you have impaired liver function. Your doctor may prescribe a low dose. Take as prescribed and immediately inform your doctor of any persistent or troublesome side effects.

Warning

You must avoid alcohol while taking this drug and for at least 2 days following treatment. Serious adverse reactions may occur, including rapid pulse, vomiting, stomach pains, dizziness, and skin flushing. Do not take any over-the-counter medications that contain alcohol (cough or cold remedies).

Comments

Bacterial vaginosis is one of the most common vaginal infections, found in up to 25% of American women. The main symptom is a vaginal discharge that has a fishy odor, although many women found to have BV through diagnostic testing have no symptoms. Avoid sexual intercourse or use condoms until you have finished treatment. Topical metronidazole has been shown to maintain remission of moderate to severe rosacea, a chronic and progressive facial skin disorder characterized by skin flushing, redness, and spider veins (broken blood vessels). Rosacea affects more than 13 million adults and is diagnosed more often in women than in men. There is an oral form of this drug (see Flagyl).

metronidazole

See Flagyl, MetroGel

Brand Name

Mevacor*

Generic Name

lovastatin

Type of Drug

Cholesterol-lowering. These drugs are usually prescribed after dietary and lifestyle changes have failed to lower cholesterol, but they do not take the place of those changes. You still need to incorporate lifestyle changes, if indicated, including quitting smoking, reducing saturated fats, and getting adequate aerobic exercise as recommended by your physician.

For

High blood cholesterol.

Availability and Dosage

Tablets: 10 mg, 20 mg, 40 mg. Should be taken with food.

Side Effects

More common include nausea, headache, constipation, diarrhea, and heartburn. Others include stomach pain, dizziness, and elevation of liver enzymes.

Drug Interactions

Lovastatin may interact with erythromycin, anticoagulants (blood thinners), antifungals, gemfibrozil, and niacin. Always inform your doctors of every medication you are taking, including nonprescription medicines, vitamins, herbal remedies, and dietary supplements. *Do not take any over-the-counter medications unless approved by your doctor.*

Food/Alcohol Interactions

Avoid or limit alcohol. Avoid grapefruit juice. Foods high in fiber may interfere with absorption. Lovastatin should be used as part of a complete cholesterol-management program that includes a healthy diet and appropriate exercise.

Pregnancy/Nursing

A woman must never become pregnant while taking this drug. If you think you are pregnant, stop taking it immediately and contact your doctor. Bottle-feed your baby if you must take this drug.

Seniors

No special warnings. Take as prescribed and immediately inform your doctor of any persistent or troublesome side effects.

Warning

You must be regularly monitored while on this drug, including tests for liver abnormalities. Make sure your doctor has your complete medical history, including a history of alcohol abuse, low blood pressure, diabetes, thyroid disease, muscle disease, or weakness.

Comments

Your total cholesterol level should be 200 or less, slightly higher if you're over age 65. Levels between 200 and 240 may be responsive to diet and exercise alone; if not, drug therapy may help. The total cholesterol-to-HDL ratio should not be higher than 4.5 to 1. Risk factors—smoking, hypertension, diabetes, and obesity—are also important in determining whether a cholesterol-lowering drug may be necessary. Low levels of "good" cholesterol and high levels of "bad" cholesterol (low-density, LDL, and triglycerides) are associated with an increased risk of heart disease, the number-one killer of women in the United States. Some research indicates that a high triglyceride level may present a greater risk for women than it does men.

Brand Name
Miacalcin Nasal*

Generic Name
calcitonin salmon

Type of Drug
Bone resorption inhibitor nasal spray. This drug helps to prevent bone loss, decrease the amount of calcium lost from bones, and increase bone density.

For
Treatment of osteoporosis in women who are more than 5 years past menopause.

Availability and Dosage
Nasal spray: 200 IU per metered spray. Follow package insert directions for use. Ask your pharmacist for a demonstration if you have questions.

Side Effects
More common include rhinitis, nasal congestion and nasal bleeding. Others include headache, diarrhea, loss of appetite, redness of facial skin and back pain.

Drug Interactions
No special warnings, although all drugs have the ability to interact with other drugs. Report any problems to your doctor or your pharmacist.

Food/Alcohol Interactions
Avoid alcohol, as it can stimulate bone loss. You may need to follow a diet low in calcium, but do not make any dietary changes without consulting your doctor.

Pregnancy/Nursing

Not recommended. It is unknown whether calcitonin passes into breast milk. Discuss with your doctor the potential benefits versus the risks.

Seniors

No special warnings. Take as prescribed and immediately inform your doctor of any persistent or troublesome side effects.

Warning

Periodic nasal examinations are important while you take this drug, to check for nasal ulcers or irritation. Tell your doctor if you have any allergic reactions to fish.

Comments

Osteoporosis is a progressive disease of the skeleton that leads to brittle bones and affects more than 20 million American women. After menopause, women should have their risk for osteroporosis assessed by their doctors and get bone density tests to determine bone loss. Risks are increased among women of Caucasian or Asian descent who are thin, had insufficient calcium intake, smoke, had or have an eating disorder, and who experienced early menopause (before age 50). Calcitonin salmon is also used to treat Paget's disease, a bone disorder.

Micro-K Extencaps

See K-Dur 20*

Brand Name
Migranal

Generic Name

dihydroergotamine mesylate

Type of Drug

Antimigraine nasal spray. This drug is used to treat active migraine attacks; it is not intended as a preventative.

For

Treatment of active migraine headache.

Availability and Dosage

Nasal spray: 0.5 mg per inhalation. Follow package directions or pharmacy instructions on how to use the nasal sprayer. Should be taken at the first sign of a migraine. Do not use this drug for tension headache or any other kind of headache except migraine. Do not take more of this medicine than is prescribed.

Side Effects

More common include light-headedness, drowsiness, dizziness, and constipation. Others include changes in taste, nausea, vomiting, and sore throat.

Drug Interactions

This drug may interact with erythromycin, antianginals, antihypertensives, insulin, diuretics, and beta-blockers. Do not take this drug within 24 hours of taking sumatriptan, naratriptan, or zolmitriptan. Always inform your doctors of every medication you are taking, including nonprescription medicines, vitamins, herbal remedies, and dietary supplements. *Do not take any over-the-counter medications unless approved by your doctor.*

Food/Alcohol Interactions

Avoid or limit alcohol. Avoid or limit caffeine. Your health care provider can supply you with a list of foods and beverages to avoid, including ripened cheeses, chocolate, fermented foods, bananas, nuts, monosodium glutamate, and citrus fruits.

Pregnancy/Nursing

Not recommended. This drug passes into breast milk with potentially serious side effects for the newborn. Bottle-feed your baby if you must take this drug.

Seniors

Older adults may experience increased side effects, including a sensitivity to cold.

Warning

This drug works by constricting blood vessels in the head and by depressing activity in parts of the brain. Serious side effects relating to insufficient blood supply include cold, bluish hands or feet and numbness or tingling in hands or feet. If you experience these symptoms or have an unusually fast or slow pulse rate, leg weakness, muscle pain, confusion, or chest pain, *seek emergency medical treatment.*

Comments

After using this drug, lie down in a dark, quiet room until symptoms subside. Migraine is a debilitating disease that affects 26 million Americans, most of them women. On an average day, an estimated 149,000 migraineurs require complete bed rest because of headache. This disease is often misunderstood by nonsufferers and often by physicians as well. Despite the range of treatments now available, a study by the National Headache Foundation in 1999 discovered that nearly half of migraine sufferers remained undiagnosed.

Brand Name
Mirapex

Generic Name

pramipexole

Type of Drug

Antiparkinsonian. This drug can be used without levodopa for early treatment of the disease and with levodopa to treat advanced cases.

For

Parkinson's disease.

Availability and Dosage

Tablets: 0.125 mg, 0.25 mg, 0.5 mg. 1.5 mg, 1 mg. Should be taken without food to minimize nausea. Do not take this medicine more often than is prescribed.

Side Effects

More common include nausea, dizziness, drowsiness, and insomnia. Others include constipation, weakness, dry mouth, increased sweating, leg pain, and hallucinations.

Drug Interactions

Pramipexole can interact with histamine H_2 blockers (cimetidine, ranitidine, famotidine, nizatidine), some diuretics, and calcium channel blockers. Always inform your doctors of every medication you are taking, including nonprescription medicines, vitamins, herbal remedies, and dietary supplements. *Do not take any over-the-counter medications unless approved by your doctor.*

Food/Alcohol Interactions

Avoid alcohol.

Pregnancy/Nursing

Not recommended. Bottle-feed your baby if you must take this drug.

Seniors

Older adults may experience more frequent or severe side effects if they have impaired kidney function. You may get dizzy; rise slowly from a sitting or reclining position. Your doctor may prescribe a low dose.

Warning

Pramipexole can cause extremely low blood pressure, which can cause dizziness, confusion, and fainting. This is known as postural hypotension and can occur when rising too quickly from a sitting or reclining position. Do not drive or operate machinery until you know how this drug will affect you.

Comments

Parkinson's disease is an illness that causes the depletion of dopamine-producing neurons in the brain that help the body to function normally. The loss of dopamine causes rigidity, tremors, slowed movement, a shuffling walk, and unsteadiness. This drug is believed to work by targeting dopamine receptors in the brain, binding to those receptors and stimulating them, thus enhancing motor-skill function.

Mircette

See Oral Contraceptives

misoprostol

See Cytotec

Modicon

See Oral Contraceptives

mometasone

See Elocon*

Brand Name
Monopril*

Generic Name
fosinopril

Type of Drug
Angiotensin-converting enzyme (ACE) inhibitor. ACE inhibitors are antihypertensives used to treat high blood pressure (hypertension). They work by blocking an enzyme in the body that is required to produce a substance that causes blood vessels to tighten. When this enzyme is blocked, blood vessels are relaxed, blood pressure is lowered, the workload of the heart and arteries is reduced, and blood and oxygen supplies are increased. ACE inhibitors do not cure hypertension; they control it for as long as the medication is used.

For
High blood pressure.

Availability and Dosage
Tablets: 10 mg, 20 mg, 40 mg. May be taken with or without food.

Side Effects
More common in women is a dry, hacking cough. Others include headache, dizziness, diarrhea, nausea, vomiting, chest pain, low blood pressure, palpitations, constipation, dry mouth, tingling in hands or feet, and blood cell count abnormalities.

Drug Interactions
Fosinopril may interact with lithium, allopurinol, some diuretics, antiemetics (antinausea), beta-blockers, and any other drugs that lower blood pressure. Do not take antacids within 2 hours of taking this drug. Always inform your doctors of every medication you are taking, including nonprescription medicines, vitamins, herbal remedies, and dietary supplements. *Do not take any over-the-counter medications unless approved by your doctor.*

Food/Alcohol Interactions
Avoid alcohol. Do not use salt substitutes.

Pregnancy/Nursing

Not recommended, especially during the second and third trimesters. Birth defects or fetal death may result. This drug passes into breast milk. Bottle-feed your baby if you must take this drug.

Seniors

Side effects may be more frequent in older adults. Your doctor may prescribe a low dose.

Warning

If you experience difficulty in breathing, arrhythmia, or any swelling of the face, lips, or throat, *seek emergency medical treatment*.

Comments

Hypertension can be aggravated by smoking, alcohol abuse, high salt intake, use of oral contraceptives, and obesity. Every year, nearly twice as many women as men die from heart disease and stroke as from all forms of cancer combined. Women are often misdiagnosed with regard to heart disease, because symptoms in women may differ from those in men—women often experience upper abdominal pain, nausea, and "burning" in the chest that is often mistaken for indigestion. The National Heart, Lung, and Blood Institute recommends that doctors evaluate their female patients' chest pain in conjunction with other symptoms and risk factors, including smoking, obesity, and high cholesterol.

Brand Name
Monurol

Generic Name

fosfomycin tromethamine

Type of Drug

Antibiotic.

For

Bladder infections; urinary-tract infections (UTIs).

Availability and Dosage

Sachet powder packet: Equivalent to 3 grams of fosfomycin. Empty the contents into 3 to 4 ounces of room-temperature water, stir to dissolve completely, and drink the entire dose immediately. The drug stays in your bladder for more than 3 days and begins to kill bacteria within hours.

Side Effects

More common include diarrhea, vaginitis, nausea, headache, dizziness, fatigue, and indigestion.

Drug Interactions

This medication may interact with gastrointestinal drugs. Always inform your doctors of every medication you are taking, including nonprescription medicines, vitamins, herbal remedies, and dietary supplements.

Food/Alcohol Interactions

Drink at least 8 glasses of water a day, preferably more. This will help flush bacteria out of the bladder and ease symptoms of burning and pain. Some health care practitioners recommend drinking cranberry juice to acidify the urine, but recently there has been some disagreement regarding that home remedy. Ask your doctor if cranberry juice, tea, or supplements are right for you.

Pregnancy/Nursing

No special warnings, although all drugs during pregnancy and breast-feeding should be avoided if possible. Before taking this drug, discuss with your doctor the benefits versus the potential risks.

Seniors

No special warnings. Take as prescribed and immediately inform your doctor of any persistent or troublesome side effects.

Warning

If your symptoms do not improve by the fourth day, contact your health care provider. This drug is not recommended for use by individuals age 18 or under, or by anyone who has kidney disease.

Comments

In controlled studies, almost 75% of women were cured of UTI after one dose of Monurol. According to the National Institutes of Health, half of all women by age 30 have had at least one urinary-tract infection (UTI). They are surpassed only by upper respiratory infections as the leading cause of absenteeism in working women. One of the leading causes of UTIs is a condition known as "honeymoon cystitis," in which vaginal bacteria is pushed into the urethral opening and moves into the bladder during sexual intercourse. To help avoid this, empty your bladder both shortly before and right after sex.

Brand Name
Motrin (also Advil, Medipren, Nuprin, Rufen)

Generic Name
ibuprofen*

Type of Drug
Nonsteroidal antiinflammatory drug (NSAID). Drugs in this group reduce pain, inflammation, and stiffness associated with a wide range of conditions affecting the bones, joints, and muscles. NSAIDs do not cure a disease; they are used for relief of symptoms. Your physician may routinely prescribe a series of different NSAIDs in order to find the one best suited for you.

For
Pain and inflammation; menstrual pain; headache; severe inflammation of arthritis, rheumatoid arthritis, and osteoarthritis.

Availability and Dosage
The prescription doses of these drugs usually start at 400 mg or more for inflammation associated with arthritis, rheumatoid arthritis, and osteoarthritis. Dosages will vary depending on the condition being treated. Take this medication with water, not coffee, tea, or carbonated beverages. Wait 30 minutes after taking ibuprofen before lying down, to reduce irritation of the esophagus.

Side Effects
More common include stomach upset or irritation, nausea, and constipation. Others include loss of appetite, drowsiness, and headache.

Drug Interactions
Ibuprofen can interact with other NSAIDs, including aspirin; do not take them at the same time. This drug may also interact with beta-blockers, anticoagulants (blood thinners), methotrexate, phenytoin, and lithium. Always inform your doctors of every

medication you are taking, including nonprescription medicines, vitamins, herbal remedies, and dietary supplements.

Food/Alcohol Interactions

Avoid alcohol, as it may increase the risk of stomach ulcers or gastric bleeding. Caffeine, cocoa, and carbonated drinks may aggravate stomach irritation.

Pregnancy/Nursing

Most NSAIDs are not recommended for pregnancy or for nursing mothers.

Seniors

Older patients may be more susceptible to stomach ulcers, gastrointestinal bleeding, and dizziness when rising from a sitting or reclining position.

Warning

If you experience vomiting of blood or "coffee grounds," heartburn, black, tarry stools, or stomach pain, contact your doctor immediately. These may be signs of a bleeding ulcer. Smoking may aggravate stomach irritation. If you are going to have surgery, you may need to discontinue this drug temporarily.

Comments

Ibuprofen is available without a prescription and is routinely used in self-medication. Follow package directions carefully and do not take more than 2400 mg in 24 hours. Women on higher doses of NSAIDs for the conditions described above should be monitored by their doctors for possible adverse side effects.

N.E.E.

See Oral Contraceptives

nabumetone

See Relafen*

Brand Name
Naprosyn (also Naprelan)

Generic Name

naproxen* (Naprelan is naproxen sodium)

Type of Drug

Nonsteroidal antiinflammatory drug (NSAID). Drugs in this group reduce pain, inflammation, and stiffness associated with a wide range of conditions affecting the bones, joints, and muscles. NSAIDs do not cure a disease; they are used for relief of symptoms.

For

Pain relief, including headache and menstrual cramps; pain and inflammation of rheumatoid arthritis and osteoarthritis.

Availability and Dosage

(Naprosyn) Tablets: 250 mg, 375 mg, 500 mg. Delayed-release tablets: 375, mg, 500 mg. Oral suspension: 125 mg per 5 ml. (Naprelan) Extended-release tablets: 375 mg, 500 mg, 750 mg.

Side Effects

More common include nausea, diarrhea, constipation, abdominal pain, dizziness, drowsiness, heartburn, vomiting, back pain, weakness, nasal congestion, sinusitis, and bronchitis. Others include urinary-tract infection (UTI), tingling sensation of the skin, and ringing in the ears.

Drug Interactions

NSAIDs have the potential to interact with many different drugs. Naproxen and naproxen sodium should not be taken together or with other NSAIDs including aspirin unless monitored by your physician. Interactions can also occur with anticoagulants (blood thinners), antihypertensives, anticonvulsants, beta-blockers, keto-conazole, steroids, elanapril, lisinopril, cyclosporine, methotrex-ate, diuretics (water pills), and lithium. Always inform your doctors of every medication you are taking, including nonprescription medicines, vitamins, herbal remedies, and dietary supplements.

Food/Alcohol Interactions

Avoid alcohol, as it can increase the risk of stomach irritation.

Pregnancy/Nursing

Not recommended. Bottle-feed your baby if you must take this drug.

Seniors

Older adults have a higher risk of side effects, especially ulcers and gastric bleeding. Your doctor may recommend a low dose.

Warning

NSAIDs can cause several potentially serious side effects, including gastrointestinal disorders such as gastric bleeding, ulceration, and perforation. They can have a highly toxic effect on the kidneys. If you have impaired kidney function, ulcers, anemia, asthma, or lupus, you should use this drug with caution. Symptoms of gastric bleeding include severe abdominal cramps, diarrhea or black, tarry stools, and vomiting of blood. *Seek emergency medical treatment immediately.*

Comments

Your physician may routinely prescribe a series of different NSAIDs in order to find the one best suited for you. Some, like naproxyn, are available only by prescription. Nonprescription versions of naproxen sodium (e.g., Aleve, store brands) are routinely used in self-medication for pain, headache, and menstrual cramps. Side effects and interactions remain the same. When using any nonprescription NSAID, follow package directions carefully and consult your doctor if problems arise. If you are going to have surgery, you may need to discontinue this drug temporarily. Women may have a higher risk of developing ulcers while taking NSAIDs, particularly if you smoke or drink alcohol, are over age 60, or use corticosteroid drugs.

naproxen*

See Naprosyn

naratriptan hydrochloride

See Amerge

Brand Name
Nardil

Generic Name

phenelzine sulfate

Type of Drug

Antidepressant; monoamine oxidase (MAO) inhibitor. By blocking the action of a brain enzyme that normally breaks down the
excitatory neurotransmitters in the brain, MAO inhibitors allow
the neurotransmitters to produce a greater stimulation of the
brain chemicals that help counteract depression.

For

Depression; anxiety; phobias.

Availability and Dosage

Tablets: 15 mg. May be taken with or without food. Dosages vary
individually and must be adjusted by your physician. Do not take
more of this medication than is prescribed. Do not abruptly stop
taking this medication without consulting your doctor. Your
dosage will need to be gradually decreased to avoid withdrawal
symptoms.

Side Effects

More common include blurred vision, dizziness, headache,
changes in appetite, weight gain, restlessness, and fatigue. Others include dry mouth, constipation, drowsiness, trembling, nausea, vomiting, insomnia, and fluid retention.

Drug Interactions

Phenelzine sulfate has an increased risk of potentially serious interactions with a wide variety of medications. This drug may interact with narcotics, other antidepressants, anesthetics,
antihistamines, sumatriptan, amphetamines, antiasthmatics, nefazodone, paroxetine, sertraline, venlafaxine, and fluoxetine. Always inform your doctors of every medication you are taking,
including nonprescription medicines, vitamins, herbal remedies,
and dietary supplements. *Do not take any over-the-counter medications unless approved by your doctor.*

Food/Alcohol Interactions

Avoid alcohol. Avoid or restrict caffeine in all forms: coffee, tea,
colas, and chocolate. MAO inhibitors carry a high risk of food in-

teractions. You will need to avoid foods high in tyramine, including aged cheeses (cheddar, Camembert, Stilton, and others), sauerkraut, chicken liver, chocolate, pickled herring, overripe avocados, fermented meats (salami, pepperoni), and yeast extracts. MAO inhibitor/food interactions can lead to dizziness, nausea, pounding headache, rapid heartbeat, and a dangerous rise in blood pressure. This is only a partial list. Your doctor or your pharmacist should supply you with a complete list of specific foods to avoid.

Pregnancy/Nursing

Not recommended. This drug may pass into breast milk. Bottle-feed your baby if you must take this drug.

Seniors

Older adults may be more susceptible to side effects. Your doctor may start you on a low dose.

Warning

Carry a medical ID card that states that you are taking an MAO inhibitor. With phenelzine, the most serious and potentially life-threatening reactions occur with drug/drug interactions and drug/food interactions. Phenelzine should not be taken within 14 days of taking any drugs or foods that have the possibility to interact with MAO inhibitors. If you have severe headaches, rapid heartbeat, heart arrhythmias, dizziness, or nausea, you may be experiencing a dangerously rapid rise in blood pressure that could lead to coma, stroke, or death. *Seek emergency medical treatment immediately.*

Comments

Regular monitoring by your doctor is essential while taking this or any other MAO inhibitor. If you are diabetic, this drug may affect your blood sugar level. Do not attempt to self-medicate with any over-the-counter products, including herbal remedies such as St. John's wort or products containing L-tryptophan. Many nonprescription remedies include ingredients known to interact adversely with MAO inhibitors, especially dextromethorphan, ephedrine, and pseudoephedrine.

Nasacort Aerosol

See Azmacort Aerosol*

Brand Name
Nasonex

Generic Name
mometasone furoate monohydrate

Type of Drug
Corticosteroid nasal spray.

For
Prevention of symptoms of seasonal allergies; allergic rhinitis.

Availability and Dosage
50 mcg per spray. Usual dosage is 2 sprays per nostril once daily, administered at the same time every day. Follow package directions carefully. Do not use more of this medicine than is prescribed.

Side Effects
More common include headache, viral infection, sore throat, blood-tinged mucus, and coughing. Others include upper respiratory-tract infection, increased menstrual cramping, muscle pain, sinusitis, chest pain, conjunctivitis, diarrhea, earache, flu-like symptoms, nausea, and rhinitis.

Drug Interactions
No special warnings, although all drugs have the ability to interact with any drugs. Report any problems to your doctor or your pharmacist. Always inform your doctors of every medication you are taking, including nonprescription medicines, vitamins, herbal remedies, and dietary supplements.

Food/Alcohol Interactions
No special warnings.

Pregnancy/Nursing
Not recommended. It is not known whether mometasone nasal spray passes into breast milk.

Seniors
No special warnings. Take as prescribed and immediately inform your doctor of any persistent or troublesome side effects.

Warning

Rare cases of nasal ulcers have been reported primarily in patients who use this drug for longer than 4 weeks. Long-term use of nasal corticosteroids may also cause cataracts.

Comments

Your physician should know if you have any of the following medical conditions before prescribing nasal mometasone: glaucoma, any recent nasal injury or nasal surgery, nasal sores, tuberculosis, herpes simplex infection of the eye, or any viral, bacterial, or fungal infections. If you think you have been exposed to chicken pox or measles while on this drug, notify your doctor at once.

Necon

See Oral Contraceptives

nefazodone

See Serzone*

Nelova

See Oral Contraceptives

Brand Name
Neurontin*

Generic Name

gabapentin

Type of Drug

Anticonvulsant. This type of drug is used to prevent seizures or to stop one in progress, and is the usual treatment for controlling epileptic seizures. This type of drug does not cure epilepsy. It works to control the symptoms for as long as you take it.

For

Epileptic seizures in adults.

Availability and Dosage

Tablets: 600 mg, 800 mg. Capsules: 100 mg, 300 mg, 400 mg. May be taken with or without food. It is important to take this medication exactly as prescribed, as the level of the drug in the body needs to be constant to be the most effective in preventing seizures. Do not abruptly stop taking this drug without consulting your doctor. The dosage may need to be gradually reduced.

Side Effects

More common include difficulty in walking or unsteadiness, vertigo, anxiety, vision changes, drowsiness, muscle aches, trembling, fatigue, and swelling of hands, feet, or lower legs. Others include dry skin, conjunctivitis, dry eyes, painful menstruation, slurred speech, indigestion, abnormal dreams, changes in sex drive, diarrhea, confusion, and insomnia.

Drug Interactions

Gabapentin may interact with cimetidine. Antacids have been shown to decrease absorption of this drug. Do not take any prescription or over-the-counter antacids within 2 hours of taking gabapentin. Always inform your doctors of every medication you are taking, including nonprescription medicines, vitamins, herbal remedies, and dietary supplements.

Food/Alcohol Interactions

Avoid alcohol.

Pregnancy/Nursing

Not recommended. It is not known whether gabapentin passes into breast milk.

Seniors

Older adults sometimes eliminate a drug more slowly, resulting in higher blood levels of a drug than might occur in a younger person. Your doctor may start you on a low dose.

Warning

When used in conjunction with other antiepileptic drugs, gabapentin can cause an adverse reaction known as nystagmus, the uncontrolled, continuous movement of the eyes either back and forth or in a rolling motion. If you experience this, notify your doctor at once.

Comments

If you suffer from a seizure disorder, you should wear a medical identification tag and carry an ID card that lists all the medications you are taking.

nifedipine

See *Procardia XL**

nitrofurantoin

See *Macrobid**

nitroglycerin

See *Nitrostat**

Brand Name
Nitrostat* (also Nitro-Dur)

Generic Name

nitroglycerin

Type of Drug

Antianginal. Nitroglycerin is a vasodilator, a drug that relaxes the muscular wall of the blood vessel and opens the blood vessel.

For

Acute sudden-onset anginal pain; coronary artery disease.

Availability and Dosage

Nitrostat is a sublingual (under the tongue) tablet. Nitroglycerin dosages range from 0.1 mg/hour to 0.6 mg/hour in various forms: sublingual tablets and aerosol sprays, extended-release capsules and tablets, (Nitro-Dur) transdermal patches and ointment. Follow directions carefully when using any form of this medicine. Consult your doctor or your pharmacist if you have questions about how to take this drug. Do not abruptly stop taking this medication, as doing so may result in an angina attack.

Side Effects

More common include dizziness, headache, flushing of the skin, rapid pulse, nausea, and restlessness. Others include shortness of breath, fatigue, and fainting.

Drug Interactions

Nitroglycerin should be used with caution when taking any drugs for hypertension (high blood pressure) or heart disease. Always inform your doctors of every medication you are taking, including nonprescription medicines, vitamins, herbal remedies, and dietary supplements. *Do not take any over-the-counter medications unless approved by your doctor.*

Food/Alcohol Interactions

Do not eat, drink, or smoke at the same time as you take a sublingual (under the tongue) form of nitroglycerin. Avoid alcohol while taking this medication, as low blood pressure and increased dizziness may result.

Pregnancy/Nursing

Not recommended. It is not known whether nitroglycerin passes into breast milk.

Seniors

Older adults may be more susceptible to side effects, especially dizziness or light-headedness when rising too quickly from a sitting or reclining position.

Warning

If your symptoms do not improve after taking nitroglycerin, *seek emergency medical treatment immediately.* Do not take nitroglycerin with sildenafil (Viagra). Although Viagra has not been approved for use by women, some doctors are prescribing it anyway and some women are borrowing their male partners' prescriptions. The combination of Viagra and nitroglycerin has caused death.

Comments

Nitroglycerin has been in continual use since the late 1800s, making it one of the oldest drugs still used to treat heart disease. It belongs to a group of drugs called nitrates, which treat angina in three ways: by relieving an ongoing attack, by preventing an anticipated attack, and by reducing the risk of recurring attacks. Make sure your doctor has your complete medical history, including a history of glaucoma, kidney or liver disease, thyroid disease, stroke, or anemia. Regular and careful monitoring by your physician is essential while you are taking this medication.

nizatidine

See Axid*

Brand Name
Nizoral

Generic Name

ketoconazole

Type of Drug

Antifungal. This type of drug is now widely available over-the-counter in a variety of topical creams, ointments, and gels, but prescription antifungals are still necessary in some cases.

For

Various fungal infections including thrush and candidiasis; ringworm; athlete's foot; seborrheic dermatitis.

Availability and Dosage

Tablets: 200 mg. Topical cream: 2% strength. Topical shampoo: 2%. Oral forms should be taken with food. Follow instructions carefully for the form of ketoconazole used.

Side Effects

More common include nausea, vomiting, abdominal pain, and upset stomach. Others include headache, fatigue, drowsiness, and increased sensitivity of your eyes to light.

Drug Interactions

Ketaconazole has the potential to interact with a wide variety of medications, including anticonvulsants, antacids, antiulcers, terfenadine, corticosteroids, histamine (H_2) blockers (including ranitidine and cimetidine), anticoagulants (blood thinners), and cisapride. Always inform your doctors of every medication you are taking, including nonprescription medicines, vitamins, herbal remedies, and dietary supplements. *Do not take any over-the-counter medications unless approved by your doctor.*

Food/Alcohol Interactions

Avoid alcohol. The combination of ketoconazole and alcohol can increase dizziness and the risk of liver damage.

Pregnancy/Nursing

Not recommended. Ketoconazole passes into breast milk.

Seniors

No special warnings. Take as prescribed and immediately inform your doctor of any persistent or troublesome side effects.

Warning

Oral forms of this drug may cause severe damage to the liver. Your doctor may want to perform regular blood tests to monitor liver function. If you experience dark urine, jaundice, extreme fatigue, fever, diarrhea, or vomiting, notify your doctor at once.

Comments

Nonprescription versions of ketoconazole are available in topical creams and shampoos. Follow package directions carefully and consult your doctor if you have any problems.

Brand Name
Nolvadex

Generic Name

tamoxifen citrate

Type of Drug

Anticancer (antineoplastic); antiestrogen. More than half of breast cancers are promoted by the female hormone estrogen. This drug prevents estrogen from linking to cells that recognize the hormone, thereby slowing its growth.

For

To reduce the recurrence of breast cancer in patients who have had surgery and/or radiation therapy to treat early breast cancer; to reduce the risk of breast cancer in high-risk women; to treat women with breast cancer who are at risk of developing cancer in the opposite breast.

Availability and Dosage

Tablets: 10 mg, 20 mg. Dosage is individualized depending on the patient. Do not change your dosage without your doctor's approval. For women who have early breast cancer, tamoxifen is usually taken for 5 years.

Side Effects

More common include hot flashes, vaginal discharge or bleeding, and menstrual irregularities. Others include hair loss, skin rash, weight gain, nausea, and headache. This drug is used for only 5 years; after that, it causes so many side effects that it must be discontinued.

Drug Interactions

Tamoxifen may interact with anticoagulants (blood thinners). Always inform your doctors of every medication you are taking, including nonprescription medicines, vitamins, herbal remedies, and dietary supplements. *Do not take any over-the-counter medications unless approved by your doctor*.

Food/Alcohol Interactions

No special warnings.

Pregnancy/Nursing

Not recommended while taking this drug or for two months after the drug is stopped. If you become pregnant while on this drug, stop taking it immediately.

Seniors

Adverse effects have been found to be more common in women over age 50.

Warning

Rare but serious side effects are associated with tamoxifen, including blood clots, uterine cancer, cataracts or other eye damage, and excessive calcium in the blood (hypercalcemia). If you experience sudden shortness of breath, chest pain, coughing up blood, lower-leg swelling or pain, any unusual vaginal discharge or bleeding, menstrual irregularities, pain or pressure in the pelvic area, or changes in vision, notify your doctor immediately.

Comments

Tamoxifen has been used for more than 20 years to treat breast cancer, a disease that kills 44,000 women each year. In 1998, it became the first drug to be approved to reduce the risk of breast cancer in healthy women who are at high risk for breast cancer but have never had the disease. A risk-assessment test given by your doctor can estimate your chances of developing breast cancer; a score of 1.7 or above is considered high risk. A study by the National Cancer Institute found that healthy, high-risk women who took tamoxifen daily reduced their risk of breast cancer by 44%. A 5-year study of 13,000 women, conducted by Allegheny University of Health Sciences, indicated that tamoxifen reduced the cancer rate by almost 50% in healthy, high-risk women.

However, a Duke University Medical School study in 1999 found that tamoxifen may lose its effectiveness over time, and may allow estrogen-related cancers to reappear. You and your doctor should discuss the benefits versus the potential risks of tamoxifen before beginning treatment.

Norcet

See Vicodin

Nordette

See Oral Contraceptives

Norethin

See Oral Contraceptives

norethindrone and ethinyl estradiol

See Oral Contraceptives

norethindrone acetate and ethinyl acetate

See Oral Contraceptives

norethindrone and mestranol

See Oral Contraceptives

norgestimate and ethinyl estradiol

See Oral Contraceptives

norgestrel and ethinyl estradiol

See Oral contraceptives

Norinyl

See Oral Contraceptives

Brand Name
Norvasc*

Generic Name

amlodipine

Type of Drug

Calcium channel blocker. These types of drugs are used for the prevention of chest pain, or angina. They are also used to correct certain heart arrhythmias (irregular heartbeats) and to lower blood pressure by blocking or slowing the flow of blood into the two chambers of the heart. Amlodipine increases the supply of blood and oxygen to the heart and reduces its workload. This type of drug does not cure heart disease; it helps to control the symptoms for as long as it is taken.

For

High blood pressure; angina pectoris.

Availability and Dosage

Tablets: 2.5 mg, 5 mg, 10 mg. May be taken with or without food. Do not abruptly stop taking this drug. Your dosage may have to be gradually reduced.

Side Effects

More common include skin flushing, headache, dizziness, nausea, and anxiety. Others include heart arrhythmias, pounding heartbeat, swelling of ankles or feet, fatigue, drowsiness, weakness, and muscle cramps.

Drug Interactions

Caution should be used when combining amlodipine with other heart drugs, including beta-blockers, antihypertensives, and other calcium channel blockers. Always inform your doctors of every medication you are taking, including nonprescription medicines, vitamins, herbal remedies, and dietary supplements. *Do not take any over-the-counter medications unless approved by your doctor.*

Food/Alcohol Interactions

Avoid alcohol, as it may increase dizziness and rapid heartbeats. Avoid grapefruit juice.

Pregnancy/Nursing

Not recommended.

Seniors

Elderly people may be more susceptible to side effects from this medication, particularly if they have liver disease. Your doctor may start you on a low dose.

Warning

Make sure your doctor has your complete medical history, including a history of congestive heart failure, low blood pressure (hypotension), or liver disease.

Comments

People who have hypertension should be regularly monitored to keep track of their blood pressure and heart rate. Treatment often includes lifestyle changes such as weight control and appropriate exercise. Hypertension is often referred to as "the silent killer" because it has no symptoms, yet forces the heart to work harder. If hypertension remains untreated, it can result in heart failure, kidney disease, or stroke. Heart disease is the leading cause of death for women in the United States, claiming more than 500,000 lives each year.

Brand Name
Norvir

Generic Name

ritonavir

Type of Drug

Antiviral; protease inhibitor.

For

HIV infection.

Availability and Dosage

Capsules: 100 mg. Oral solution: 80 mg per ml. Drug management therapy for patients who have HIV infection or AIDS is a complex process involving a combination of drugs in what is now commonly referred to as an "AIDS cocktail." There is no one "cocktail"—these combinations, including protease inhibitors and nucleoside analogs, are providing increased life expectancy and dramatic improvement in symptoms for some patients. Patients play a critical role in the management of this disease by taking medications for HIV and AIDS exactly as prescribed, in the proper dosages and at the proper times. Ritonavir may be taken with or without food.

Side Effects

More common include abdominal pain, diarrhea, and fatigue. Others include loss of appetite, mouth ulcers, anxiety, dizziness, depression, vomiting, headache, heartburn, stomach pain, drowsiness, skin problems, and muscle pain.

Drug Interactions

This drug has the potential to interact with a wide variety of medications, including anticancer drugs, acetaminophen, aspirin and other NSAIDs, anticonvulsants, some antifungals, antidiabetics, some antidepressants, heart drugs, antianxiety drugs, cisapride, cholesterol-lowering drugs, anticoagulants (blood thinners), and indomethacin. Always inform your doctors of every medication you are taking, including nonprescription medicines, vitamins, herbal remedies, and dietary supplements. *Do not take any over-the-counter medications unless approved by your doctor.*

Food/Alcohol Interactions

Avoid alcohol if you have decreased liver function.

Pregnancy/Nursing

A guide published by the American Medical Association in 1995 recommends that all pregnant women be tested for HIV. Bottle-feeding is recommended to reduce any possible risk of infection from an HIV-positive mother. Before taking this drug, discuss with your doctor the benefits versus the potential risks.

Seniors

No special warnings. Take as prescribed and immediately inform your doctor of any persistent or troublesome side effects.

Warning

Ritonavir does not reduce the risk of transmission of HIV, so precautions against infection must still be practiced. Regular and careful monitoring by your physician is required while on this or any drugs to treat this disease.

Comments

Although overall deaths from AIDS are on the decline, the disease is increasing faster among women than among men, and it still affects minorities disproportionately. Women who have HIV often have difficulty accessing proper health care, and the prohibitive cost of the drugs involved ($16,000 or more a year) often exclude those who need them. Given the rise in heterosexually transmitted HIV, more prevention efforts—namely, insisting that partners use latex condoms—are being aimed at women. Although there is presently no cure for this disease, new drug trials and research continue. See the Women's Resource Directory at the back of this book for the names of organizations that have the latest information on treatments.

ofloxacin

See Floxin

Brand Name
Ogen

Generic Name

estropipate

Type of Drug

Estrogen. Estrogens are used to maintain normal female functions when the ovaries are not producing enough, such as after either natural or surgical menopause. Estrogens can relieve menopausal symptoms, treat hormonal imbalances, and slow down the onset of osteoporosis.

For

Relief of menopausal symptoms including hot flashes, mood changes, night sweats, and vaginal dryness.

Availability and Dosage

Tablets: 0.75 mg, 1.5 mg, 3 mg, 6 mg. Vaginal cream: 1.5 mg. Individual doses vary greatly. Follow your doctor's instructions for taking any form of estrogen. Tablets may be taken with or without food.

Side Effects

More common include changes in appetite, stomach upset or bloating, mood changes, fatigue, and changes in sex drive. Others include swelling or bleeding of the gums, diarrhea, headaches, skin rash, eye lesions, dizziness, migraine headaches, and vaginal yeast infections. Side effects with the vaginal cream include uterine bleeding, vaginal discharge, and breast tenderness.

Drug Interactions

Estropipate has the potential to interact with a wide variety of medications, including androgens (male hormones), thyroid drugs, cimetidine, cortisone and other steroids, oral contraceptives, anticonvulsants, raloxifene, tamoxifen, anticoagulants (blood thinners), some antibiotics, and methotrexate. Always inform your doctors of every medication you are taking, including nonprescription medicines, vitamins, herbal remedies, and dietary supplements.

Food/Alcohol Interactions

No special alcohol warnings. Avoid grapefruit juice while taking this medication.

Pregnancy/Nursing

Not recommended. Can cause birth defects. If you think you are pregnant, stop taking the drug and contact your health care practitioner. This drug passes into breast milk; bottle-feeding your baby is recommended.

Seniors

No special warnings. Take as prescribed and immediately inform your doctor of any persistent or troublesome side effects.

Warning

Estrogens have been linked to an increased risk of endometrial cancer and breast cancer when taken for extended periods of time. Risks usually increase with dosage. Taking a progestin drug concurrently with estrogen can reduce the chance of certain types of cancers. If you experience recurrent vaginal bleeding, breast pain or enlargement, or swelling of the legs and feet, notify your doctor immediately.

Comments

It is important to be regularly monitored by your doctor while on any form of estrogen, including a Pap test and pelvic exam every

6 to 12 months, along with regular mammograms. Make sure that your doctor knows if you have a history of breast, cervical, endometrial, or uterine cancer, migraine, fibroids, edema (fluid retention), or blood clots.

omeprazole

See Prilosec*

Oral Contraceptives

• Brand Names

Desogen*, Mircette, Ortho-Cept*

Generic Name

desogestrel and ethinyl estradiol

• Brand Names

Demulen 1/35, Demulen 1/50, Zovia 1/35E, Zovia 1/50E

Generic Name

ethynodial diacetate and ethinyl estradiol

• Brand Names

Alesse-21, Alesse-28*, Levlen, Levlite, Levora 0.15/30, Nordette, Tri-Levlen*, Triphasil*, Trivora

Generic Name

levonorgestrel and ethinyl estradiol

• Brand Names

Estrostep, Estrostep FE, Loestrin 1.5/30, Loestrin 1/20, Loestrin Fe 1.5/30*, Loestrin Fe 1/20*

Generic Name

norethindrone acetate and ethinyl estradiol

• Brand Names

Brevicon, Genora 0.5/35, Genora 1/35, Intercon 0.5/35, Jenest-28, Modicon, N.E.E. 1/35, N.E.E. 1/50, Necon 0.5/35, Necon 1/35*, Necon 10/11, Nelova 1/35, Nelova 10/11, Norethin 1/35, Norinyl 1+35, Ortho-Novum 1/35, Ortho-Novum 10/11 28, Ortho-Novum 7–7–7 28*, Ovcon-35, Ovcon-50, Tri-Norinyl 28

Generic Name

norethindrone and ethinyl estradiol

• Brand Names

Genora 1/50, Intercon 1/50, Necon 1/50, Nelova 1/50M, Norethin 1/50M, Norinyl 1+50, Ortho-Novum 1/50

Generic Name

norethindrone and mestranol

• Brand Names

Ortho-Cyclen*, Ortho Tri-Cyclen*

Generic Name

norgestimate and ethinyl estradiol

• Brand Names:

Lo-Ovral 28*, Ovral

Generic Name

norgestrel and ethinyl estradiol

Type of Drug

Hormonal oral contraceptive.

For

Birth control and other uses as directed by your doctor, including regulation of erratic menstrual cycles, alleviation of painful, heavy periods, and reduction of the symptoms of perimenopause. Ortho Tri-Cyclen is also prescribed for acne.

Availability and Dosage

Dosages and administration depend on the type and number of pills (21 or 28). Estradiol (estrogen) is the common denominator in almost all oral contraceptives; the amount of progestin varies. "Mini-pills" contain only progestin. Follow package insert instructions. Take these drugs exactly as prescribed and follow instructions exactly for what to do when you miss a dose. Any interruption in taking the pill (especially the mini-pill) may result in pregnancy. May be taken with or without food. Should be taken at the same time every day. Use a backup form of birth control for the first month (some doctors recommend two) you take this drug.

Side Effects

Side effects vary according to the type of drug, but the more common include nausea, bleeding between menstrual periods, changes in mood, and depression. Others include weight gain, dry eyes, headache, breast tenderness, increased sun sensitivity, and decrease in sex drive. Your doctor may change your brand of oral contraceptive depending on the number and severity of side effects, your age, hormonal changes, and other factors as determined by regular physical and gynecological examinations. Always keep your doctor informed of any side effects.

Drug Interactions

Unplanned pregnancies have occurred due to interactions between some prescription drugs and oral contraceptives, mainly by reducing the pill's effectiveness. These include some antibiotics (including amoxicillin, ampicilllin, cephalexin, erythromycin, penicillin, sulfa drugs, and tetracycline drugs), carbamazepine, phenytoin, and some antimigraines. Oral contraceptives can also affect how other drugs work, including acetaminophen, aspirin, anticoagulants (blood thinners), some benzodiazepines, and corticosteroids.

Food/Alcohol Interactions

No special warnings.

Pregnancy/Nursing

Not recommended. These drugs can cause birth defects. *If you become pregnant while on the pill, stop taking it immediately.* Some oral contraceptives (usually the progestin-only or the mini-pill) are safe during nursing; others are not recommended. Consult your obstetrician if you wish to take any of these drugs while breast-feeding. Progestin-only pills are not recommended for women who have had gestational diabetes: Studies have shown that the risk of of developing Type II (non-insulin–dependent) diabetes nearly tripled.

Seniors

Not usually prescribed.

Warning

Women are strongly cautioned not to smoke while taking oral contraceptives, as it significantly raises the risk of blood clots, heart attack, and stroke. Make sure your doctor knows of any history of diabetes, hypertension, high cholesterol, stroke, liver disease, breast cancer, or a family history of breast cancer. Obese women have a significantly increased risk of side effects.

Comments

"The pill," as the entire group of oral contraceptives is commonly known, has undergone significant changes since its introduction in 1960, along with the attendant controversies over its safety and side effects. Older pills contained higher doses of estrogens and progestins; today's lower-dose versions are generally considered safer. Although the pill has been found to help prevent ovarian and endometrial cancer, there are still questions surrounding whether it increases the risk of breast or cervical cancer. Almost 11 million women use the pill, which has an effectiveness rating of more than 99%. According to the FDA, more studies have been done on the pill than on any other medicine in history. Some oral contraceptives can be used as "emergency" contraception as instructed by your doctor, or you may be prescribed one of the new "morning after" pill kits (see Plan B and Preven).

Orasone

*See Deltasone**

orlistat

See Xenical

Ortho-Cept*

See Oral Contraceptives

Ortho-Novum

See Oral Contraceptives

Ortho-Cyclen*

See Oral Contraceptives

Ortho Tri-Cyclen*

See Oral Contraceptives

Brand Name
Orudis (also Oruvail)

Generic Name

ketoprofen

Type of Drug

Nonsteroidal antiinflammatory analgesic (NSAID). Drugs in this group reduce pain, inflammation, and stiffness associated with a wide range of conditions that affect the bones, joints, and muscles. NSAIDs do not cure a disease; they are used for relief of symptoms. Your physician may routinely prescribe a series of different NSAIDs in order to find the one best suited for you.

For

Pain relief; relief of pain and inflammation of rheumatoid arthritis and osteoarthritis.

Availability and Dosage

(Orudis) Capsules: 25 mg, 50 mg, 75 mg. (Oruvail) Extended-release capsules: 100 mg, 150 mg, 200 mg. Take with food or immediately after meals with a full glass of water. To minimize adverse effects on your esophagus and stomach, do not take this drug right before lying down. When using this drug to relieve menstrual pain, take at the first sign of pain for best results.

Side Effects

More common include nausea, vomiting, heartburn, dizziness, drowsiness, and headache. Others include ringing in the ears, tingling or numbness in the hands and feet, gum or dental problems, and diarrhea or constipation. Side effects are more likely with large doses or prolonged use.

Drug Interactions

Do not take ketoprofen with other NSAIDs (such as ibuprofen and aspirin) unless instructed by your doctor. Ketoprofen can also interact with steroids, anticoagulants (blood thinners), some antibiotics, anticonvulsants, beta-blockers, antihypertensives, digoxin, lithium, oral antidiabetics, and methotrexate. Always inform your doctors of every medication you are taking, including nonprescription medicines, vitamins, herbal remedies, and dietary supplements.

Food/Alcohol Interactions

Avoid alcohol, as it may increase the risk of stomach ulcers or gastric bleeding. Smoking may also aggravate stomach irritation.

Pregnancy/Nursing

Most NSAIDs are not recommended for pregnancy or for nursing mothers.

Seniors

Older adults may be more susceptible to the side effects of this drug, particularly stomach ulcers, gastrointestinal bleeding, and dizziness when rising from a sitting or reclining position.

Warning

NSAIDs can cause several potentially serious side effects, including gastrointestinal disorders, dizziness, and gastric bleeding. If you have impaired kidney function, ulcers, anemia, asthma, or lupus, you should use this drug with caution. Women may have a higher risk of developing ulcers while taking NSAIDs, particularly if they smoke or drink alcohol, are over age 60, or use corticosteroid drugs. Symptoms of gastric bleeding include severe abdominal cramps, diarrhea, black, tarry stools, and vomiting of blood. *Seek emergency medical treatment.*

Comments

Orudis KT is the nonprescription version of this drug. Many NSAIDs are now available without a prescription and are routinely used in self-medication. Side effects and interactions remain the same. When using any nonprescription NSAID, follow package directions carefully and do not exceed the recommended dose. If you are going to have surgery, you may need to discontinue this drug temporarily.

Oruvail

*See **Orudis***

Ovcon

*See **Oral Contraceptives***

Ovral

*See **Oral Contraceptives***

oxaprozin

See Daypro*

Panacet

See Vicodin

Brand Name
Parnate

Generic Name

tranylcypromine sulfate

Type of Drug

Antidepressant; monoamine oxidase (MAO) inhibitor. By blocking the action of a brain enzyme that normally breaks down the excitatory neurotransmitters in the brain, MAO inhibitors allow the neurotransmitters to produce a greater stimulation of the brain chemicals that help counteract depression.

For

Depression.

Availability and Dosage

Tablets: 10 mg. May be taken with or without food. Dosages vary individually and must be adjusted by your physician. Do not take more of this medication than is prescribed. Do not abruptly stop taking this medication without consulting your doctor. Your dosage will need to be gradually decreased to avoid withdrawal symptoms.

Side Effects

More common include blurred vision, dizziness, headache, changes in appetite, restlessness, and fatigue. Others include dry mouth, constipation, drowsiness, nausea, vomiting, insomnia, and fluid retention.

Drug Interactions

Tranylcypromine sulfate has an increased risk of potentially serious interactions with a wide variety of medications. This drug may interact with narcotics, other antidepressants, anesthetics, antihistamines, sumatriptan, amphetamines, antiasthmatics, nefazodone, paroxetine, sertraline, venlafaxine, and fluoxetine. Always inform your doctors of every medication you are taking, including nonprescription medicines, vitamins, herbal remedies, and dietary supplements. *Do not take any over-the-counter medications unless approved by your doctor.*

Food/Alcohol Interactions

Avoid alcohol. Avoid or limit caffeine. MAO inhibitors carry a high risk of food interactions. You will need to avoid foods high in tyramine, including aged cheeses (cheddar, Camembert, Stilton, and others), sauerkraut, chicken liver, chocolate, pickled herring, overripe avocados, fermented meats (salami, pepperoni), and yeast extracts. MAO inhibitor/food interactions can lead to dizziness, nausea, pounding headache, rapid heartbeat, and a dangerous rise in blood pressure. This is only a partial list. Your doctor or your pharmacist should supply you with a complete list of specific foods to avoid.

Pregnancy/Nursing

Not recommended. This drug may pass into breast milk. Bottle-feed your baby if you must take this drug.

Seniors

Older adults may be more susceptible to side effects. Your doctor may start you on a low dose.

Warning

Carry a medical ID card that states that you are taking an MAO inhibitor. With tranylcypromine, the most serious and potentially life-threatening reactions occur with drug/drug interactions and drug/food interactions. Tranylcypromine should not be taken within 14 days of taking any drugs or foods that have the possibility to interact with MAO inhibitors. If you have severe headaches, rapid heartbeat, heart arrhythmias, dizziness, or nausea, you may be experiencing a dangerously rapid rise in blood pressure that could lead to coma, stroke, or death. *Seek emergency medical treatment immediately.*

Comments

Regular monitoring by your doctor is essential while taking this or any other MAO inhibitor. If you are diabetic, this drug may affect your blood sugar level. Do not attempt to self-medicate with any over-the-counter products, including herbal remedies such as St. John's wort and products containing L-tryptophan. Many nonprescription remedies include ingredients known to interact adversely with MAO inhibitors, especially dextromethorphan, ephedrine, and pseudoephedrine.

paroxetene

*See Paxil**

Brand Name
Paxil*

Generic Name

paroxetine

Type of Drug

Selective serotonin reuptake inhibitor (SSRI) antidepressant. This drug belongs to a newer class of antidepressants that work by raising the brain's level of serotonin, a chemical associated with mood and mental alertness. It can also help to relieve the repetitive rituals and anxiety associated with obsessive-compulsive disorder.

For

Depression; panic disorder; obsessive-compulsive disorder (OCD); social anxiety disorder.

Availability and Dosage

Tablets: 20 mg, 30 mg. May be taken with or without food. Do not take more of this medicine than is prescribed.

Side Effects

More common include weakness, abdominal pain, and nausea. Others include loss of appetite, constipation, drowsiness, dizziness, insomnia, tremor, and palpitations.

Drug Interactions

The most serious interactions occur with monoamine oxidase (MAO) inhibitor antidepressants (selegiline, phenelzine, tranylcypromine). These drugs and paroxetene should never be taken together or within 2 weeks of each other. Interactions may occur with anticoagulants (blood thinners), cimetidine, phenytoin, digoxin, and tryptophan. Always inform your doctors of every medication you are taking, including nonprescription medicines, vitamins, herbal remedies, and dietary supplements.

Food/Alcohol Interactions

Avoid alcohol. Avoid or limit caffeine, as it may increase central-nervous-system stimulant effects of this drug.

Pregnancy/Nursing

Not recommended. Paroxetine passes into breast milk. Bottle-feed your baby if you must take this drug.

Seniors

No special warnings unless you have impaired kidney or liver function. Your doctor may prescribe a low dose.

Warning

Make sure that your doctor has your complete medical history, including a history of liver or kidney disease or seizures. Do not take this drug with over-the-counter remedies containing trypto-phan or St. John's wort.

Comments

Paxil was the first drug approved for the treatment of social anx-iety disorder, in which fears of scrutiny in social or performance situations go beyond a simple case of nerves. Symptoms include sweating, trembling, blushing, shaky voice, pounding heart, and tense muscles. It is estimated that more than 10 million Ameri-cans have this condition.

penicillin VK

See **Veetids***

Brand Name
Pepcid*

Generic Name

famotidine

Type of Drug

Histamine H_2 blocker.

For

Decreasing stomach acid; stomach and duodenal ulcers; gas-troesophageal reflux disease (GERD).

Availability and Dosage

Tablets: 20 mg, 40 mg. Orally disintegrating tablets: 20 mg, 40 mg. Oral suspension: 40 mg per 5 ml. May be taken with or without food. Dosages will vary depending on the condition being treated. Do not take more of this medicine than is prescribed.

Side Effects

More common include headache, dry mouth, and constipation. Others include nausea, stomach pain, joint pains, and dizziness.

Drug Interactions

No special warnings, although all drugs have the ability to interact with other drugs. Report any problems to your doctor or your pharmacist. Always inform your doctors of every medication you are taking, including nonprescription medicines, vitamins, herbal remedies, and dietary supplements.

Food/Alcohol Interactions

No special warnings.

Pregnancy/Nursing

Not recommended. Famotidine passes into breast milk. Bottle-feed your baby if you must take this drug.

Seniors

Side effects may be more frequent and severe in older patients if they have impaired kidney function. Your doctor may prescribe a low dose.

Warning

Smoking may aggravate ulcers and may interfere with the effectiveness of famotidine.

Comments

Each year approximately 500,000 new cases of ulcers are diagnosed in the United States, half of them women. According to the Centers for Disease Control and Prevention (CDC), women generally develop first-onset symptoms at age 35, and the risk of ulcer disease rises with age. The majority of peptic ulcers are caused by the bacterium *H. pylori*, and antibiotics are often used in conjunction with antiulcer drugs. Nonprescription H_2 blockers are among most popular over-the-counter medications. The nonprescription form of famotidine is Pepcid AC, used for heartburn, indigestion, and upset stomach. Follow package directions carefully. Do not take more often than needed, and consult your doctor if symptoms worsen.

Brand Name

Percocet (also Endocet*, Roxicet*, Roxilox, Tylox)

Generic Name

acetaminophen and oxycodone hydrochloride

Type of Drug

Narcotic analgesic.

For

Pain relief.

Availability and Dosage

Tablets: 325 acetaminophen with 5 mg oxycodone; 500 mg acetaminophen with 5 mg oxycodone. Should be taken with food. Do not take more of this medicine than is prescribed.

Side Effects

More common include drowsiness, dizziness, nausea, and loss of appetite. Others include constipation, difficulty in urinating, dry mouth, light-headedness, euphoria, and sweating.

Drug Interactions

This drug can interact with other central nervous system (CNS) depressants, narcotic painkillers, monoamine oxidase (MAO) inhibitor antidepressants, antihistamines, and tranquilizers. Always inform your doctors of every medication you are taking, including nonprescription medicines, vitamins, herbal remedies, and dietary supplements. *Do not take any over-the-counter medications unless approved by your doctor.*

Food/Alcohol Interactions

Avoid alcohol, as it can increase the sedative effect of this drug.

Pregnancy/Nursing

Not recommended. Narcotics used during pregnancy can result in addiction in the newborn. This drug may pass into breast milk. Bottle-feed your baby if you must take this drug.

Seniors

Side effects involving central-nervous-system depression may be more frequent and severe in older patients. Your doctor may prescribe a low dose.

Warnings

This drug has a high incidence of physical and psychological dependence. Tell your doctor if you have a history of alcohol or substance abuse, depression, or suicidal thoughts. Do not drive or operate machinery until you know how this drug will affect you. Do not take over-the-counter products containing acetaminophen, as overdose may result.

Comments

This drug was the first oxycodone/acetaminophen product. It has been prescribed for relief of more than 500 types of pain.

Brand Name
Periactin

Generic Name

cyproheptadine

Type of Drug

Antihistamine. These drugs counteract the effect of histamine, a chemical released in the body that can cause itching and swelling.

For

Relief of symptoms of seasonal allergy; skin rash, itching, or hives caused by allergies; anorexia.

Availability and Dosage

Tablets: 4 mg. Oral syrup: 2 mg per 5 ml. May be taken with or without food.

Side Effects

More common include drowsiness and dizziness, which may diminish as your body adjusts to the drug. Others include impaired coordination, restlessness, tremor, insomnia, weakness, euphoria, and fainting.

Drug Interactions

Cyproheptadine can interact with other antihistamines, monoamine oxidase (MAO) inhibitor antidepressants, other central nervous system (CNS) depressants, tranquilizers, antianxiety drugs, and benzodiazepines. Always inform your doctors of every medication you are taking, including nonprescription medicines, vitamins, herbal remedies, and dietary supplements. *Do not take any over-the-counter medications unless approved by your doctor.*

Food/Alcohol Interactions

Avoid alcohol, as it can increase the sedative effect of this drug.

Pregnancy/Nursing

Not recommended, especially during the last trimester. Bottle-feed your baby if you must take this drug.

Seniors

Side effects involving sedation, dizziness, and hypotension (low blood pressure) are more likely in older patients. Your doctor may prescribe a low dose.

Warning

Do not take any over-the-counter antihistamines, sleep aids, or cough or cold medications while taking this drug. Do not drive or operate machinery until you know how this drug will affect you.

Comments

Cyproheptadine is used for a wide variety of conditions, including dermatitis, eczema, and migraine headaches. It is also prescribed for anorexia because it can increase appetite, which may lead to weight gain. There are dozens of over-the-counter antihistamines available, and many people self-medicate, using them for everything from hay fever to hives. OTC antihistamines can interact with many different drugs, including those for heart disease, hypertension, diabetes, thyroid disease, and glaucoma. Always check with your doctor or your pharmacist before taking an over-the-counter antihistamine if you are taking any prescription drug.

phenazopyridine hydrochloride

See Pyridium

phenelzine sulfate

*See **Nardil***

Brand Name
Phenergan Suppository*

Generic Name
promethazine

Type of Drug
Antihistamine; antiemetic (antinausea).

For
Relief of allergy symptoms; motion sickness; nausea; vomiting.

Availability and Dosage
Rectal suppository: 12.5 mg, 25 mg, 50 mg. Tablets: 12.5 mg, 25 mg, 50 mg. Oral syrup: 6.25 mg per 5 ml, 25 mg per 5 ml. Cream: 2%. Oral form may be taken with food. Follow package instructions for insertion of the suppository form.

Side Effects
More common include drowsiness and dry mouth. Others include weakness, dizziness, fainting, impaired coordination, hand tremor, and blurred vision.

Drug Interactions
Promethazine can interact with central nervous system (CNS) depressants, narcotic painkillers, levodopa, methyldopa, tricyclic antidepressants, and thyroid drugs. Do not take any monoamine oxidase (MAO) inhibitor antidepressant within 2 weeks of taking promethazine. Always inform your doctors of every medication you are taking, including nonprescription medicines, vitamins, herbal remedies, and dietary supplements. *Do not take any over-the-counter medications unless approved by your doctor.*

Food/Alcohol Interactions
Avoid alcohol.

Pregnancy/Nursing
Not recommended, especially during the last trimester. Bottle-feed your baby if you must take this drug.

Seniors

Side effects may be more frequent and severe in older patients, including drowsiness, dizziness, and low blood pressure. Your doctor may prescribe a low dose.

Warning

Do not use over-the-counter medications for coughs, colds, sinus, or appetite suppression while taking this drug.

Comments

Promethazine is an ingredient used in numerous medications for relief of allergy symptoms. It is also used for nausea and vomiting caused by use of other drugs.

phentermine

See Fastin

phenytoin

See Dilantin*

pioglitazone

See Actos

Brand Name
Plan B

Generic Name

levonorgestrel

Type of Drug

Progestin; postcoital contraceptive. It is not known exactly how this drug works. It is believed to delay ovulation or prevent fertilization, depending on what phase of the monthly cycle a woman is in when she takes this drug. Emergency contraception prevents pregnancy from occurring. It will not terminate an existing pregnancy.

For

Emergency contraception (the "morning after" pill).

Availability and Dosage

Two tablets of levonorgestrel: 0.75 mg. The first tablet should be taken within 72 hours of unprotected intercourse, the second tablet 12 hours after the first. The sooner this drug is taken after unprotected sex, the more effective it will be.

Side Effects

More common include nausea and vomiting. Ask your health care provider if an antinausea medication can be prescribed. Other side effects include lower abdominal pain, fatigue, headache, dizziness, breast tenderness, and changes in menstrual bleeding.

Drug Interactions

No studies have been conducted on drug interactions. Always inform your doctors of every medication you are taking, including nonprescription medicines, vitamins, herbal remedies, and dietary supplements.

Food/Alcohol Interactions

No special warnings.

Pregnancy/Nursing

Do not use this drug if you think you might be pregnant. It will not terminate an existing pregnancy. Although there is no evidence to suggest that using emergency contraception while pregnant causes birth defects, you should avoid taking all drugs while pregnant.

Seniors

Not usually prescribed.

Warning

Emergency contraception may not be right for women who have a history of breast cancer, stroke, blood clots, hypertension, migraine headaches, diabetes, or heart, kidney, or liver disease. Make sure your health care provider has your complete medical history. Do not use emergency contraception as a substitute for ongoing contraceptive methods; doing so may increase your risk of a tubal pregnancy. Although it is highly effective (an 89% reduction in risk of pregnancy for a single act of unprotected sex), other methods of birth control have a higher effective rate without the unpleasant side effects of nausea and vomiting. This drug provides no protection against sexually transmitted diseases.

Comments

This drug is available by prescription through Planned Parenthood clinics and other health care providers. Ask your doctor or your health care professional if he or she can provide it. For more information, see Contraception in the Women's Resource Directory at the back of this book.

Brand Name
Plaquenil

Generic Name

hydroxychloroquine

Type of Drug

Antimalarial; antiinflammatory. This is a disease-modifying antirheumatic drug (DMARD), similar to nonsteroidal antiinflammatory drugs (NSAIDs) but stronger and slower acting.

For

Relief of symptoms of rheumatoid arthritis: swelling, joint pain, stiffness; symptoms of systemic lupus erythematosus; treatment of malaria.

Availability and Dosage

Tablets: 200 mg. Should be taken with food to minimize upset stomach. Dosages will vary depending on the condition being treated.

Side Effects

More common include diarrhea, loss of appetite, and nausea. Others include headache, dizziness, and skin rash. These may subside as your body adjusts to the medication. Side effects can occur at any time, including months after the course of treatment has finished.

Drug Interactions

Hydroxychloroquine can interact with digoxin and antacids. Do not take this drug within 2 hours of taking an antacid. Always inform your doctors of every medication you are taking, including nonprescription medicines, vitamins, herbal remedies, and dietary supplements. *Do not take any over-the-counter medications unless approved by your doctor.*

Food/Alcohol Interactions

Avoid alcohol.

Pregnancy/Nursing

Not recommended, but discuss with your doctor the benefits versus the potential risks. You must not breast-feed your baby, however, as toxic doses are excreted in breast milk. Bottle-feed your baby if you must take this drug.

Seniors

Older adults may experience increased side effects. Take as prescribed and notify your doctor of any persistent or troublesome side effects.

Warning

You must be regularly examined by an ophthalmologist while taking this drug; retinal damage has occurred with long-term use. If you experience vision changes including blurred vision, flashes or streaks of light, night blindness, or problems in focusing, contact your doctor. Make sure your doctor has your complete medical history, including a history of anemia, blood disorders, seizures, eye disorders, or liver, stomach, or intestinal disease. If you have psoriasis, your symptoms may worsen while taking this drug.

Comments

You may need to take hydroxychloroquine for several months before you notice any improvement in your symptoms. Regular monitoring is required to check your eyesight and hearing, as well as blood tests for anemia or liver dysfunction.

Brand Name
Plendil*

Generic Name

felodipine

Type of Drug

Calcium channel blocker. These drugs are used for the prevention of angina, or chest pain. They are also used to correct certain heart arrhythmias (irregular heartbeats) and to lower blood pressure by blocking or slowing the flow of blood into the two chambers of the heart. This type of drug does not cure hypertension; it helps to control it for as long as it is taken. Felodipine is sometimes prescribed when diuretics or beta-blockers were ineffective or caused intolerable side effects.

For

Mild to moderate hypertension.

Availability and Dosage

Extended-release tablets: 2.5 mg, 5 mg, 10 mg. Tablets must be swallowed whole; do not break or crush. May be taken with or without food.

Side Effects

More common include headache, dizziness, muscle weakness, swelling of the ankles, and constipation. Others include cough, palpitations, upset stomach, abdominal pain, back pain, sore throat, and rash.

Drug Interactions

Felodipine can interact with other heart drugs, including antihypertensives and beta-blockers, cimetidine, ranitidine, anticoagulants (blood thinners), some anticonvulsants, carbamazepine, and erythromycin. Always inform your doctors of every medication you are taking, including nonprescription medicines, vitamins, herbal remedies, and dietary supplements. *Do not take any over-the-counter medications unless approved by your doctor.*

Food/Alcohol Interactions

Avoid alcohol. Do not take felodipine with grapefruit juice, as it can significantly raise blood levels of the drug. Your doctor may recommend dietary changes to help treat hypertension.

Pregnancy/Nursing

Not recommended. The effects of the drug on nursing infants is unknown; bottle-feed your baby if you must take this drug.

Seniors

Older patients (65 and older, in the drug studies) and those who have liver impairment may have elevated blood levels of this drug, due to the length of time it takes to be cleared from the body. Your doctor may prescribe a low dose.

Warning

Make sure your doctor has your complete medical history, including a history of liver disease, low blood pressure, edema, and heart attack.

Comments

You should have your blood pressure checked regularly and know where it falls under the following four stages: Stage 1 (mild hypertension) ranges from 140/90 to 159/99. Stage 2 (moderate hypertension) ranges from 160/100 to 179/109. Stage 3 (severe hypertension) ranges from 180/110 to 209/119. Stage 4 (very severe) is 210/120 and higher.

podofilox

See Condylox

Polymox

See Amoxil*

potassium chloride*

See K-Dur 20*

pramipexole

See Mirapex

Brand Name
Pravachol*

Generic Name

pravastatin

Type of Drug

Cholesterol-lowering. These drugs are usually prescribed after dietary and lifestyle changes have failed to lower cholesterol, but they do not take the place of those changes. You still need to incorporate lifestyle modifications, if indicated, including quitting smoking, reducing saturated fats in your diet, and getting adequate aerobic exercise as recommended by your physician.

For

High cholesterol.

Availability and Dosage

Tablets: 10 mg, 20 mg, 40 mg. May be taken with or without food.

Side Effects

More common include nausea, vomiting, and diarrhea. Others include fatigue, heartburn, constipation, abdominal pain, muscle pain, headache, and dizziness.

Drug Interactions

Pravastatin can interact with other cholesterol-lowering drugs, diltiazem, gemfibrozil, erythromycin, ketoconazole, itraconazole, niacin, cimetidine, anticoagulants (blood thinners), and digoxin. Always inform your doctors of every medication you are taking, including nonprescription medicines, vitamins, herbal remedies, and dietary supplements. *Do not take any over-the-counter medications unless approved by your doctor.*

Food/Alcohol Interactions

Avoid or limit alcohol. Avoid grapefruit juice. Foods high in fiber may interfere with absorption. Pravastatin should be used as part of a complete cholesterol-management program that includes a healthy diet and appropriate exercise.

Pregnancy/Nursing

A woman must never become pregnant while taking this drug.

Seniors

Side effects may be more frequent and severe in older patients. Your doctor may prescribe a low dose.

Warning

You must be regularly and carefully monitored by your physician while taking this drug. Make sure your doctor has your complete medical history, including a history of heavy alcohol use, liver disease, musculoskeletal problems, and tumors.

Comments

This drug has proven effective in preventing a first heart attack, and women are more likely to die from a first heart attack than men are. However, the prevention study included only men and it is unclear how that data applies to women. This type of drug (statin) can raise HDL (the "good" cholesterol), reduce triglycerides, and reduce overall cholesterol. Your total cholesterol level should be 200 or less, slightly higher if you're over age 65. Levels between 200 and 240 may be responsive to diet and exercise alone; if not, drug therapy may help. Artery-clogging LDL cholesterol should be between 100 and 130.

pravastatin

See Pravachol*

prazepam

See Centrax

prednisone*

See Deltasone*

Brand Name
Premarin*

Generic Name

conjugated estrogens

Type of Drug

Estrogen. Estrogens are used to maintain normal female functions when the ovaries are not producing enough, such as after menopause. Estrogens can relieve menopausal symptoms, treat hormonal imbalances, and reduce the risk or slow the onset of osteroporosis.

For

Relief of menopausal symptoms including hot flashes, mood changes, night sweats, vaginal dryness; prevention of osteoporosis.

Availability and Dosage

Tablets: 0.3 mg, 0.625 mg, 0.9 mg, 1.25 mg, 2.5 mg. Should be taken with food.

Side Effects

More common include blood clots, nausea, vomiting, and breast tenderness. Others include breakthrough bleeding or spotting, vaginal yeast infections, fluid retention, headache, migraines, dizziness, skin rash, hair loss, changes in weight, and changes in sex drive.

Drug Interactions

Estrogens can interact with anticoagulants (blood thinners), carbamazepine, phenytoin, calcium, and tricyclic antidepressants. Always inform your doctors of every medication you are taking, including nonprescription medicines, vitamins, herbal remedies, and dietary supplements. *Do not take any over-the-counter medications unless approved by your doctor.*

Food/Alcohol Interactions

Do not drink grapefruit juice while taking this drug.

Pregnancy/Nursing

A woman must never become pregnant while taking this drug. If you think you are pregnant, stop taking it immediately and consult your gynecologist. Bottle-feed your baby if you must take this drug.

Seniors

No special warnings, unless you smoke, which can increase adverse side effects. Take as prescribed and immediately inform your doctor of any persistent or troublesome side effects.

Warning

Estrogens increase the risk of uterine cancer. To reduce that risk, your doctor may prescribe a progestin to be used concurrently with estrogens. If you experience vaginal bleeding after menopause, contact your doctor immediately. There is also an increased risk of blood clots, gallbladder disease, and hypercalcemia (excess calcium in the blood). If you develop chest pain, pain in your calves, shortness of breath, severe headache, dizziness, fainting, or loss of vision, you could be experiencing a blood clot. *Seek emergency medical treatment.* Smoking increases your risk of serious medical conditions.

Comments

Women should start discussing menopause with their doctors between age 40 and age 49, when perimenopause and the symptoms of menopause start to occur. This can help you decide on a course of traditional and alternative treatments as well as prepare you for the physical and psychological changes of that time of life. A 1998 survey of women by the North American Menopause Society found that more than half of all American women between age 50 and 65 who had reached menopause said they were happiest and most fulfilled now, as compared to when they were in their twenties, thirties, or forties. The negative consequences of growing older are often more visible in a youth-oriented society, but many women find menopause to be a time of personal growth, as they focus on their relationships, hobbies, or other interests.

Brand Name
Prempro* (also Premphase)

Generic Name

conjugated estrogens and medroxyprogesterone

Type of Drug

Estrogen/progestin. This combination of female sex hormones reduces the risk of endometrial cancer, which increases when estrogen is used alone. Hormone-replacement therapy (HRT) is also used to help prevent osteoporosis (see Premarin, above).

For

Relief of menopausal symptoms including hot flashes, mood changes, night sweats, vaginal dryness; prevention of osteoporosis.

Availability and Dosage

Tablets: 0.625 mg, 2.5 mg. One tablet is taken for 28 days and one is added for days 15 through 28. May be taken with or without food.

Side Effects

More common include nausea, breast tenderness, headache, and abdominal pain. Others include fibroid-tumor enlargement, vaginal yeast infections, breakthrough bleeding or spotting, fluid retention, headache, migraines, dizziness, changes in weight, and changes in sex drive.

Drug Interactions

This combination drug can interact with anticoagulants (blood thinners), carbamazepine, phenytoin, antidiabetics, thyroid drugs, corticosteroids, calcium, and tricyclic antidepressants. Always inform your doctors of every medication you are taking, including nonprescription medicines, vitamins, herbal remedies, and dietary supplements. *Do not take any over-the-counter medications unless approved by your doctor.*

Food/Alcohol Interactions

Do not drink grapefruit juice while on this drug.

Pregnancy/Nursing

A woman must never become pregnant while taking this drug. If you think you are pregnant, stop taking it immediately and consult your gynecologist. Bottle-feed your baby if you must take this drug.

Seniors

No special warnings, unless you smoke, which can increase adverse side effects. Take as prescribed and immediately inform your doctor of any persistent or troublesome side effects.

Warning

If you have diabetes, taking this drug may worsen your condition. This combination drug is not for women who have blood-clotting disorder, cancer, liver or gallbladder disease, heart attack, or unusual vaginal bleeding. Smoking increases your risk of developing a serious medical condition.

Comments

The loss of estrogen during menopause can lead to osteoporosis, a bone-thinning disorder that often results in fractures of the wrist, spine, and hip. Talk to your doctor about a bone-density test, a quick and effective way to determine whether hormone-replacement therapy might help or to check if your current HRT is beneficial. Excessive alcohol, protein, and caffeine intake over time can contribute to bone loss.

Brand Name
Prevacid*

Generic Name

lansoprazole

Type of Drug

Antiulcer.

For

Duodenal ulcers; gastroesophageal reflux disease (GERD).

Availability and Dosage

Delayed-release capsules: 15 mg, 30 mg. Should be taken on an empty stomach, 1 hour before or 2 hours after meals. Dosages will vary depending on the condition being treated.

Side Effects

More common include dizziness, headache, and diarrhea. Others include abdominal pain, changes in appetite, and nausea.

Drug Interactions

Lansoprazole can interact with digoxin, ketoconazole, and medications containing iron. Always inform your doctors of every medication you are taking, including nonprescription medicines, vitamins, herbal remedies, and dietary supplements.

Food/Alcohol Interactions

Do not take lansoprazole with food as it will interfere with absorption of the drug. If you are being treated for GERD, avoid or restrict foods and beverages that may worsen your condition: alcohol, coffee, chocolate, and fried foods.

Pregnancy/Nursing

Not recommended. Bottle-feed your baby if you must take this drug.

Seniors

No special warnings, except in cases where dosages exceed 30 mg a day. Your doctor may prescribe a low dose. Take as prescribed and immediately inform your doctor of any persistent or troublesome side effects.

Warning

Make sure your doctor has your complete medical history, including a history of liver or kidney disease. If you have an ulcer, notify your doctor immediately if any of the following occurs: diarrhea, black, tarry stools, vomiting of "coffee grounds," fever, chills, or worsening stomach pain. These may be signs of a bleeding ulcer.

Comments

Gastroesophageal reflux disease (GERD) occurs when stomach contents flow back into the esophagus, irritating the sensitive lining and causing heartburn. Erosive esophagitis, a severe form of GERD, can result in sores or erosions in the esophagus.

Brand Name
Preven

Generic Name

levonorgestrel and ethinyl estradiol

Type of Drug

Progestin/estrogen; postcoital contraceptive. These drugs are combination oral contraceptive (COC) pills designed to prevent pregnancy from occurring by interfering with ovulation, fertilization, and implantation. They will not terminate an existing pregnancy.

For

Emergency contraception (the "morning after" pill).

Availability and Dosage

Preven Emergency Contraceptive Kit contains four tablets (0.25 levonorgestrel and 0.05 mg ethinyl estradiol), a urine pregnancy test, and a detailed patient information book. Follow instructions exactly for timing of doses. For maximum effectiveness, take these pills as soon as possible, within 72 hours of unprotected intercourse.

Side Effects

More common are nausea and vomiting. Others include menstrual irregularities, breast tenderness, headache, abdominal pain, and dizziness.

Drug Interactions

No studies have been conducted on drug interactions, but interactions can occur between estradiol (estrogen) and other drugs. Always inform your doctors of every medication you are taking, including nonprescription medicines, vitamins, herbal remedies, and dietary supplements.

Food/Alcohol Interactions

No special warnings.

Pregnancy/Nursing

Do not use these drugs if you think you might be pregnant.

Seniors

Not usually prescribed.

Warning

Emergency contraception should not be used by women with a history of heart disease, blood clots, hypertension, diabetes, breast cancer, or liver disease. Smokers over age 35 run a significantly higher risk of serious conditions when using combination oral contraceptives. Do not use emergency contraception as a substitute for ongoing contraceptive methods, as doing so may increase your risk of a tubal pregnancy. Although it is highly effective (about 2% of women might become pregnant after a single act of unprotected intercourse), other methods of birth control are more effective without the unpleasant side effects of nausea and vomiting. This drug provides no protection against sexually transmitted diseases.

Comments

Emergency contraception has long been called "the best-kept secret in women's health." Many doctors have been prescribing specific doses of oral contraceptives for the purpose of preventing a possible pregnancy, keeping the issue of reproductive rights between a woman and her health care professional. In the future, it's possible that a woman may be able to receive emergency contraception directly from her pharmacist.

Brand Name
Prilosec*

Generic Name
omeprazole

Type of Drug
Antiulcer. This drug is often prescribed in combination with clarithromycin (an antibiotic) to treat ulcers caused by the bacteria *H. pylori*.

For
Short-term treatment of active duodenal ulcers; gastric ulcers; gastroesophageal reflux disease (GERD).

Availability and Dosage
Delayed-release capsules: 10 mg, 20 mg, 40 mg. Dosages will vary depending on condition being treated. Should be taken on an empty stomach, 1 hour before or 2 hours after meals, usually in the morning. Do not take more of this medicine than is prescribed. Do not stop taking this medicine even if your symptoms improve.

Side Effects
More common include headache, diarrhea, and abdominal pain. Others include nausea, dizziness, vomiting, rash, constipation, cough, and back pain.

Drug Interactions
Omeprazole may interact with diazepam, ketoconazole, phenytoin, anticoagulants (blood thinners), and medications containing iron. Always inform your doctors of every medication you are taking, including nonprescription medicines, vitamins, herbal remedies, and dietary supplements. *Do not take any over-the-counter medications unless approved by your doctor.*

Food/Alcohol Interactions
Because the effectiveness of this drug lasts 24 hours, it is usually prescribed for use on an empty stomach before breakfast. Avoid or restrict alcohol, caffeine, and citrus foods and beverages, as they can aggravate ulcers.

Pregnancy/Nursing
Not recommended. Bottle-feed your baby if you must take this drug.

Seniors

Side effects may be more frequent or severe if you have impaired kidney or liver function. Your doctor may prescribe a low dose.

Warning

Omeprazole causes serious side effects in only 1% or fewer users. If you develop chest pain, dark yellow or brownish urine, sore throat, fever, shortness of breath, or skin rash, you may be experiencing an allergic reaction. *Seek emergency medical treatment.*

Comments

Once thought to be a "man's" disease, ulcers now affect women equally—half of the 500,000 new cases diagnosed every year are women. In the early 1980s, it was discovered that most ulcers are caused by the *H. pylori* bacteria, although most doctors were slow to combine antibiotic therapy with traditional antiulcer drugs. Doctors now routinely use a combination of clarithromycin with omeprazole to treat ulcers caused by *H. pylori*, and studies have shown that a month of combination therapy healed almost 90% of patients' ulcers, and 52% of them were still ulcer-free 6 months later.

Prinivil*

*See Zestril**

Brand Name
Procardia XL* (also Adalat CC*)

Generic Name

nifedipine

Type of Drug

Calcium channel blocker. These drugs are used for the prevention of angina, or chest pain. They are also used to correct certain heart arrhythmias (irregular heartbeats) and to lower blood pressure by blocking or slowing the flow of blood into the two chambers of the heart. This type of drug does not cure heart disease; it helps to control the symptoms for as long as it is taken.

For

Angina pectoris; high blood pressure, including pregnancy-related high blood pressure; migraine headache.

Availability and Dosage

Extended-release tablets: 30 mg, 60 mg, 90 mg. May be taken with or without food. Should be taken at regular intervals. Do not break or crush tablets. Do not take more of this medicine than is prescribed. Do not abruptly stop taking this drug without consulting your doctor.

Side Effects

More common include edema, headache, fatigue, dizziness, constipation, and nausea. Others include palpitations, rash, insomnia, nervousness, dry mouth, leg cramps, skin flushing, weakness, and heartburn.

Drug Interactions

Nifedipine may interact with beta-blockers, digoxin, anticoagulants (blood thinners), cimetidine, antiinflammatory drugs, oral contraceptives, antihypertensives, aspirin, phenytoin, ranitidine, diuretics, and antiarrhythmia drugs. Always inform your doctors of every medication you are taking, including nonprescription medicines, vitamins, herbal remedies, and dietary supplements. *Do not take any over-the-counter medications unless approved by your doctor.*

Food/Alcohol Interactions

Avoid alcohol. Do not drink grapefruit juice while taking this drug. If you have hypertension, your doctor may recommend dietary and exercise guidelines.

Pregnancy/Nursing

Not recommended. Bottle-feed your baby if you must take this drug.

Seniors

Side effects may be more frequent and severe in older patients, including hypotension (low blood pressure). Your doctor may prescribe a low dose.

Warning

If your doctor prescribes nifedipine, make sure that you are receiving the extended-release version of this drug (Procardia XL). In studies, older versions of nifedipine (Procardia) were linked to a 60% increased risk of heart attack.

Comments

People who have hypertension should be regularly monitored to keep track of their blood pressure and heart rate. Treatment often includes lifestyle changes such as weight control and appropriate exercise. If hypertension remains untreated, it can result in heart failure, kidney disease, or stroke. Heart disease is the leading cause of death for women in the United States, claiming more than 500,000 lives each year.

promethazine

See Phenergan Suppository*

Propacet 100

See Darvocet-N 100

propoxyphene napsylate and acetaminophen

See Darvocet-N 100

propranolol

See Inderal

Brand Name
Propulsid*

Generic Name

cisapride

Type of Drug

Gastrointestinal stimulant. This drug speeds up the rate at which food moves through the stomach, reducing irritation.

For

Gastroesophageal reflux disease (GERD); heartburn.

Availability and Dosage

Tablets: 10 mg, 20 mg. Should be taken on an empty stomach, fifteen minutes before meals, and at bedtime with a beverage. Do not take more of this medicine than is prescribed.

Side Effects

More common include diarrhea and abdominal pain. Others include nausea, headache, rash, low blood pressure, back pain, vertigo, and dizziness.

Drug Interactions

Cisapride may interact with cimetidine, antidiabetics, antifungals, ranitidine, tetracycline, anticoagulants (blood thinners), indinavir, diazepam, levodopa, and lithium. Always inform your doctors of every medication you are taking, including nonprescription medicines, vitamins, herbal remedies, and dietary supplements. *Do not take any over-the-counter medications unless approved by your doctor.*

Food/Alcohol Interactions

Avoid alcohol, caffeine, carbonated drinks, chocolate, and fried or fatty foods, as they can aggravate heartburn.

Pregnancy/Nursing

Not recommended. Bottle-feed your baby if you must take this drug.

Seniors

Side effects may be more frequent and severe if you have kidney or liver impairment. Your doctor may prescribe a low dose.

Warning

As of July 14, 2000, Propulsid was discontinued due to 341 reports of serious cardiac arrhythmias and 80 deaths from July 1993 to December 1999. In 85 percent of these cases, the events occurred when Propulsid was used in patients with known risk factors. The drug is currently available only through an investigational limited access program. If all other standard treatments have failed, your physician can determine if you are eligible for enrollment in this program, which includes extensive diagnostic screening and close monitoring by a gastroenterologist.

Comments

Gastroesophageal reflux disease (GERD) occurs when stomach contents flow back into the esophagus, irritating the sensitive lining and causing heartburn. Erosive esophagitis, a severe form of GERD, can result in sores or erosions in the esophagus. Cisapride is used specifically for nighttime heartburn caused by GERD.

Protostat

See Flagyl

Brand Name
Proventil (also Ventolin)

Generic Name
albuterol*

Type of Drug
Bronchodilator. This drug relaxes bronchial muscles to alleviate wheezing caused by asthma.

For
Asthma; bronchial spasms.

Availability and Dosage
Tablets: 2 mg, 4 mg. Extended-release tablets: 4 mg. Tablets should be taken on an empty stomach, 1 hour before or 2 hours after meals. Inhalation aerosol: Each canister provides 200 inhalations. Follow instructions for use and ask your pharmacist for a demonstration.

Side Effects
More common include nausea, vomiting, nervousness, rapid heartbeat, and rhinitis. Others include back pain, allergic reaction, fever, and tremor.

Drug Interactions
Albuterol can interact with beta-blockers, diuretics, and digoxin. Albuterol should not be used within 2 weeks of taking monoamine oxidase (MAO) inhibitor antidepressants or tricyclic antidepressants. Always inform your doctors of every medication you are taking, including nonprescription medicines, vitamins, herbal remedies, and dietary supplements. *Do not take any over-the-counter medications unless approved by your doctor.*

Food/Alcohol Interactions
No special warnings.

Pregnancy/Nursing
Not recommended. Bottle-feed your baby if you must take this drug.

Seniors
Side effects may be more frequent and severe, including heart arrhythmias and angina.

Warning

Do not take more of this medicine or use your inhaler more often than is prescribed, as your condition may worsen. You should be regularly monitored while on this drug. Do not drive or operate machinery until you know how this drug will affect you. Make sure your doctor has your complete medical history, including a history of heart arrhythmia, hypertension, stroke, glaucoma, seizure, or diabetes.

Comments

Proventil Inhalation Aerosol does not contain ozone-depleting chlorofluorocarbons (CFCs), unlike most of the metered-dose inhalers (MDIs) in the United States. MDIs are being reformulated to eliminate use of CFCs, but they will not be removed from the market until there is a suitable replacement.

Brand Name
Provera* (also Cycrin*)

Generic Name

medroxyprogesterone acetate

Type of Drug

Progestin. This drug is a synthetic steroid that mimics the effects of progesterone, a naturally occurring hormone essential to the female reproductive system.

For

Irregular menstrual periods; correction of a hormonal imbalance that may cause abnormal uterine bleeding; endometriosis; premenstrual syndrome (PMS).

Availability and Dosage

Tablets: 2.5 mg, 5 mg, 10 mg. Vaginal or rectal suppositories are used to treat premenstrual syndrome (PMS). Oral tablets may be taken with food to minimize stomach upset.

Side Effects

More common include changes in menstrual flow, breakthrough bleeding or spotting, changes in weight, and fluid retention. Others include increased sweating, hot flashes, changes in mood, changes in sex drive, headache, stomach pain, and growth of facial hair.

Drug Interactions

This drug may interact with other medications depending on the form and dosage. Always inform your doctors of every medication you are taking, including nonprescription medicines, vitamins, herbal remedies, and dietary supplements. *Do not take any over-the-counter medications unless approved by your doctor.*

Food/Alcohol Interactions

No special warnings.

Pregnancy/Nursing

A woman must never become pregnant while taking this drug. If you think you are pregnant, stop taking it and notify your doctor immediately. This drug may occasionally be used to prevent premature labor or spontaneous abortion, but only under the supervision of a physician. This drug may pass into breast milk and increase the flow. Discuss with your doctor whether you should bottle-feed your baby while taking this drug.

Seniors

Adverse side effects may be more likely if you have liver impairment. Take as prescribed and notify your doctor immediately of any persistent or troublesome side effects.

Warning

Make sure your doctor has your complete medical history, including a history of blood clots, stroke, breast cancer, asthma, migraine, seizures, diabetes, unexplained vaginal bleeding, high cholesterol, or heart or kidney disease. This drug can adversely affect fertility even after treatment is stopped; discuss with your doctor how long it may take to get pregnant. If you experience numbness or pain in an arm or leg, chest pain, severe headache, problems with vision or speech, swelling, shortness of breath, or loss of coordination, *seek emergency medical treatment.*

Comments

An injectable form of medroxyprogesterone is used as a contraceptive (see Depo-Provera).

Brand Name
Prozac*

Generic Name

fluoxetine

Type of Drug

SSRI (selective serotonin reuptake inhibitor) antidepressant. These drugs comprise a newer class of antidepressants that work by raising the brain's level of serotonin, a chemical associated with mood and mental alertness. Fluoxetine is used extensively for depression, anxiety, and other emotional problems.

For

Depression; bulimia; obsessive-compulsive disorder (OCD).

Availability and Dosage

Capsules: 10 mg, 20 mg. Liquid: 20 mg per 5 ml. May be taken with or without food. Do not take more of this medicine than is prescribed.

Side Effects

More common include anxiety, insomnia, and nervousness. Others include rash, tremor, dizziness or light-headedness, weakness, abnormal dreams, fatigue, increased sweating, nausea, changes in appetite, diarrhea, bronchitis, rhinitis, weight loss, muscle or joint pain, back pain, painful menstrual cramps, sexual dysfunction, chills, and vision changes.

Drug Interactions

Fluoxetine has the potential to interact with a wide variety of medications, including tricyclic antidepressants, lithium, buspirone, cimetidine, carbamazepine, metoprolol, benzodiazepines, phenytoin, and anticoagulants (blood thinners). The most serious and potentially fatal interactions can occur with monoamine oxidase (MAO) inhibitor antidepressants. You should not start taking any MAO inhibitor for at least 5 weeks after the end of fluoxetine treatment, nor should you start taking fluoxetine within 2 weeks of stopping an MAO inhibitor. Do not take tryptophan, St. John's wort, or any prescription or nonprescription products containing dextromethorphan (found in cough and cold remedies). Always inform your doctors of every medication you are taking, including nonprescription medicines, vitamins, herbal remedies, and dietary supplements. *Do not take any over-the-counter medications unless approved by your doctor.*

Food/Alcohol Interactions

Avoid alcohol.

Pregnancy/Nursing

No studies have been conducted on fluoxetine and pregnancy. Discuss with your doctor the benefits versus the potential risks.

Fluoxetine passes into breast milk. Bottle-feed your baby if you must take this drug.

Seniors

No special warnings, unless you have impaired liver or kidney function. Your doctor may prescribe a low dose. Older adults are also more likely to be taking multiple medications that may interact with fluoxetine.

Warning

Fluoxetine is accumulative and can remain in the body for a long period of time. Drug interactions can occur even after you have stopped taking it. Some women find their sexual desire decreased while on fluoxetine and have difficulty reaching orgasm.

Comments

Nearly 23 million prescriptions for Prozac were filled in 1998. Although the drug has proven effective in treating depression, bulimia, obsessive-compulsive disorder, and premenstrual syndrome (PMS), and has fewer side effects than some of the older medications, there is some controversy as to whether doctors are prescribing this drug without thorough physical and psychological evaluations and follow-up. Women are 10 times more likely than men to suffer from moderate depression and are more likely to seek treatment. Any drugs prescribed for mental disorders should be part of an overall treatment plan that includes behavioral therapy, lifestyle changes, and regular monitoring by a physician or other health care professional.

Brand Name
Pyridium

Generic Name

phenazopyridine hydrochloride

Type of Drug

Urinary-tract analgesic. This drug is used to relieve the pain and burning associated with urinary-tract infections (UTIs). It is not an antibiotic and will not treat or cure the infection.

For

Pain relief of urinary-tract infections (UTIs).

Availability and Dosage

Tablets: 95 mg, 100 mg, 200 mg. Sustained-release tablets: 200 mg. Should be taken with food.

Side Effects

More common include headache, dizziness, and indigestion. Others include stomach cramps, rash, vomiting, and blue or purplish skin color (report this immediately to your health care provider).

Drug Interactions

No special warnings, although all drugs have the ability to interact with other drugs. Report any problems to your doctor or your pharmacist.

Food/Alcohol Interactions

Drink plenty of water while on this medication.

Pregnancy/Nursing

Not recommended, but discuss with your doctor the benefits versus the potential risks. It is not known whether phenazopyridine passes into breast milk. Bottle-feed your baby while taking this drug.

Seniors

No special warnings. Take as prescribed and immediately inform your doctor of any persistent or troublesome side effects.

Warning

There are several nonprescription versions of urinary-tract analgesics. They contain the same active ingredient as the prescription medication. They are useful for immediate pain relief in conjunction with your drug therapy, but do not use them in place of the proper prescription medications to treat urinary-tract infections. You will be relieving the pain of a UTI without eliminating the underlying infection, which may result in kidney infection. Certain medical tests may be affected by this drug; tell your doctor you are using it if any urine-sugar tests or urine-ketone tests are run.

Comments

Phenazopyridine is used to provide symptomatic relief of UTIs and is not intended for long-term use. This medication (and its nonprescription versions) may turn your urine bright orange or red. This is harmless and will occur only as long as you take this drug. It may stain your clothing. It may also stain soft contact lenses, sometimes permanently. Do not wear contact lenses while on this medication.

quinapril

See Accupril*

ramipril

See Altace*

ranitidine

See Zantac*

Brand Name
Relafen*

Generic Name

nabumetone

Type of Drug

Nonsteroidal antiinflammatory drug (NSAID). Drugs in this group reduce pain, inflammation, and stiffness associated with a wide range of conditions affecting the bones, joints, and muscles. NSAIDs do not cure a disease; they are used for relief of symptoms.

For

Relief of symptoms of osteoarthritis and rheumatoid arthritis.

Availability and Dosage

Tablets: 500 mg, 750 mg. May be taken with food to reduce stomach upset. To minimize potentially damaging effects on your esophagus and stomach, do not take this drug right before lying down.

Side Effects

More common include nausea, heartburn, diarrhea, constipation, drowsiness, bloating, and dizziness. Others include fluid retention, ringing in the ears, blurred vision, mouth ulcers, and numbness or tingling in the hands or feet.

Drug Interactions

NSAIDs have the potential to interact with many different drugs. Nabumetone should not be taken with other NSAIDs, including aspirin, unless monitored by your physician. Interactions can also occur with anticoagulants (blood thinners), antihypertensives, anticonvulsants, ketoconazole, steroids, captopril, cyclosporine, methotrexate, diuretics (water pills), and lithium. Always inform your doctors of every medication you are taking, including nonprescription medicines, vitamins, herbal remedies, and dietary supplements.

Food/Alcohol Interactions

Avoid alcohol, as it can increase the risk of stomach irritation.

Pregnancy/Nursing

Not recommended. Bottle-feed your baby if you must take this drug.

Seniors

Older adults have a higher risk of side effects, especially ulcers and gastric bleeding. Your doctor may recommend a low dose.

Warning

NSAIDs can cause several potentially serious side effects, including gastrointestinal disorders, dizziness, and gastric bleeding. They can have a highly toxic effect on the kidneys. If you have impaired kidney function, ulcers, anemia, asthma, or lupus, you should use this drug with caution. Symptoms of gastric bleeding include severe abdominal cramps, diarrhea or black, tarry stools, and vomiting of blood. *Seek emergency medical treatment immediately.*

Comments

Nabumetone has a lower risk of stomach irritation than other NSAIDs. Your physician may routinely prescribe a series of different NSAIDs in order to find the one best suited for you. Some, like nabumetone, are available only by prescription, but many NSAIDs can be obtained over-the-counter and are routinely used in self-medication. Side effects and interactions remain the same with nonprescription NSAIDs. When using any nonprescription NSAID, follow package directions carefully and consult your doctor if problems arise. If you are going to have surgery, you may need to discontinue this drug temporarily. Women may have a higher risk of developing ulcers while taking NSAIDs, particularly if they smoke, drink alcohol, are over age 60, or use corticosteroid drugs.

Brand Name

Restoril

Generic Name

temazepam*

Type of Drug

Benzodiazepine sedative. Benzodiazepines are central nervous system (CNS) depressants, and work on the part of the brain that controls emotion by slowing nervous-system transmissions. They are often used to relieve the symptoms of anxiety but do not address the underlying cause.

For

Short-term treatment of insomnia.

Availability and Dosage

Capsules, 7.5 mg, 15 mg, 30 mg. Should be taken only at bedtime. May be taken with or without food. Do not take more of this medicine than is prescribed. Do not abruptly stop taking this medication; doing so may cause adverse reactions including seizures and confusion.

Side Effects

More common include drowsiness and headache. Others include fatigue, nervousness, lethargy, dizziness, dry mouth, excess saliva, rapid heartbeat, and nausea.

Drug Interactions

Benzodiazepines have the potential to interact with other central nervous system (CNS) depressants, resulting in increased sedation. Temazepam can interact with antianxiety drugs, antihistamines, some antidepressants, narcotic pain relievers, antipsychotics, and drugs used for insomnia. Other interactions can occur with cimetidine and oral contraceptives, resulting in the possibility of increased toxic effects of temazepam. Always inform your doctors of every medication you are taking, including nonprescription medicines, vitamins, herbal remedies, and dietary supplements. *Do not take any over-the-counter medications unless approved by your doctor.*

Food/Alcohol Interactions

Avoid alcohol; it may increase the sedative effect.

Pregnancy/Nursing

A pregnant woman must never take this drug. Temazepam affects fetal development. If you suspect you are pregnant, notify your doctor immediately. Bottle-feed your baby if you must take this drug.

Seniors

Older adults may experience an increase in side effects, especially oversedation. Your doctor may prescribe a low dose.

Warning

This drug is usually prescribed for 7 to 10 days. Your doctor will not likely give you a prescription for more than a 1-month supply. Temazepam has a high risk of physical and psychological dependency. Temazepam should be administered with caution in severely depressed patients or those with suicidal tendencies. Be sure to notify your doctor if you have a history of depression, suicidal thoughts, sleep apnea, convulsions, or hallucinations.

Comments

Benzodiazepines are often the drug of choice to treat anxiety. In larger doses, they are used for insomnia. This drug may lose its effectiveness over time. If you must take this drug on a regular basis, careful monitoring by your doctor is essential. When it is time to stop taking this drug, the dosage will have to be gradually reduced to avoid withdrawal symptoms.

Brand Name
Retin-A*

Generic Name

tretinoin

Type of Drug

Topical antiacne.

For

Acne.

Availability and Dosage

Topical cream: 0.025%, 0.05%, 0.1%. Topical gel: 0.025%, 0.01%, 0.1%. Topical solution: 0.05%. Usual dosage is once daily, usually at night. You may feel a slight warmth or tingling when applied.

Side Effects

More common include peeling, mild stinging or redness, and skin irritation. Others include rash, blistering, and changes in skin color. Your doctor may adjust the dosage to minimize side effects.

Drug Interactions

Do not use this drug in combination with any prescription or non-prescription medication without consulting your doctor, including treatments containing resorcinol, sulfa, benzoyl peroxide, or salicylic acids. Do not use exfoliating agents or abrasive cleansers. Do not use cosmetic skin lotions containing alpha hydroxy or beta hydroxy acids, alcohol, astringents, or medicated cosmetics.

Food/Alcohol Interactions

No special warnings.

Pregnancy/Nursing

Not recommended.

Seniors

No special warnings. Take as prescribed and immediately inform your doctor of any persistent or troublesome side effects.

Warning

Do not apply more of this drug than is prescribed; using more does not make the drug more effective, and you may experience excess peeling of the skin. Avoid direct sunlight. Do not use tanning lamps or tanning beds while on this medication. If you experience severe peeling or redness, or have an allergic reaction (excessively red, blistery skin), notify your doctor. Topical tretinoin is flammable. Use caution around candles, lighted matches, or other open flames.

Comments

Acne is the most common skin disease treated by physicians, with adolescent boys being the primary group affected. But women represent the fastest-growing segment of acne patients, with up to 50% of adult women suffering from some form of the disease, sometimes due to hormonal fluctuations and stress. Chocolate does not cause acne, although in some individuals it may aggravate it. When using topical tretinoin, it may take up to 3 months to see significant improvement in your condition, and your acne may get worse during the first days or weeks of treatment.

Brand Name
Retrovir

Generic Name
zidovudine (AZT)

Type of Drug
Antiviral. AZT was approved in 1987, one of the first drugs to be used against HIV infection.

For
HIV.

Availability and Dosage
Drug management therapy for patients who have HIV infection or AIDS is a complex process involving a combination of drugs in what is now commonly referred to as an "AIDS cocktail." There is no one "cocktail"—these combinations, including protease inhibitors and nucleoside analogs, are providing increased life expectancy and dramatic improvement in symptoms for some patients. For example, zidovudine is used in one of the newer drugs (brand name Combivir), in combination with lamivudine in a single tablet. Patients play a critical role in the management of these diseases by taking medications for HIV and AIDS exactly as prescribed, in the proper dosages at the proper times.

Side Effects
More common include anemia, nausea, vomiting, shortness of breath, fatigue, and skin pallor. Others include insomnia, restlessness, muscle aches, sore throat, chills, mouth sores, chest pains, bleeding gums, hoarseness, nosebleeds, changes in urinary habits, and dizziness.

Drug Interactions
This drug has the potential to interact with a wide variety of medications, including anticancer drugs, acetaminophen, aspirin, anticonvulsants, some antifungals, and indomethacin. Always inform your doctors of every medication you are taking, including nonprescription medicines, vitamins, herbal remedies, and dietary supplements. *Do not take any over-the-counter medications unless approved by your doctor.*

Food/Alcohol Interactions
No special warnings.

Pregnancy/Nursing

A guide published by the American Medical Association in 1995 recommends that all pregnant women be tested for HIV. A newborn's risk of infection can be greatly reduced if the mother receives zidovudine treatment during pregnancy and the baby continues to receive the treatment for the first 6 weeks. Bottle-feeding is recommended to reduce any possible risk of infection from an HIV-positive mother.

Seniors

Reduced kidney function may be a factor among older adults. Your doctor will determine the proper dosage of this drug.

Warning

This drug is not for use in people who have bone marrow disease. Zidovudine does not reduce the risk of transmission of HIV, so precautions against infection must still be practiced. Regular and careful monitoring by a physician is required while on this or any other drugs used to treat HIV.

Comments

Although overall deaths from AIDS are on the decline, the disease is increasing faster among women than men and still affects minorities disproportionately. Women who have HIV often have difficulty in accessing proper health care, and the prohibitive cost of the drugs involved ($16,000 or more a year) often excludes those who need them. Given the rise in heterosexually transmitted HIV, more prevention efforts—namely, insisting that a partner use latex condoms—are being aimed at women. Although there is presently no cure for this disease, new drug trials and research continue. See the Women's Resource Directory at the back of this book for the names of organizations that have the latest information on treatments.

Brand Name
Rheumatrex

Generic Name

methotrexate

Type of Drug

Anticancer; antipsoriatic; antirheumatic. Methotrexate belongs to a group of medicines called disease-modifying antirheumatic drugs (DMARDs), which act to suppress inflammation.

For

Certain types of cancer (uterine, lymphoma, leukemia); rheumatoid arthritis; psoriasis.

Availability and Dosage

Tablets: 2.5 mg. Also available by injection. Dosages will vary depending on the condition being treated. Follow your doctor's instructions carefully, as an overdose can produce serious side effects. Generally, dosages are higher for cancer therapy and lower for rheumatoid arthritis. Should be taken on an empty stomach, 1 hour before or 2 hours after meals.

Side Effects

More common include nausea, vomiting, loss of appetite, headaches, and dizziness. Others include mood swings, weight loss, acne, skin pallor, rash, and itching.

Drug Interactions

This drug has the potential to interact with a wide variety of medications, including tetracycline antibiotics, sulfa drugs, aspirin, some anticonvulsants, and folic acid. Always inform your doctors of every medication you are taking, including nonprescription medicines, vitamins, herbal remedies, and dietary supplements. *Do not take any over-the-counter medications unless approved by your doctor.*

Food/Alcohol Interactions

Avoid alcohol.

Pregnancy/Nursing

A woman must never become pregnant while taking this drug. Methotrexate can cause miscarriage and birth defects. If you must take this drug after delivery, bottle-feeding your baby is recommended.

Seniors

The risk of side effects is increased in older adults, particularly if they have decreased kidney or liver function.

Warning

Potentially life-threatening interactions have occurred between methotrexate and certain NSAIDs (ketoprofen and naproxen). If you experience difficulty in breathing, bloody vomit, seizures, swollen feet, dark urine, extreme fatigue, jaundice, painful or difficult urination, cough, or fever, *seek emergency treatment immediately.*

Comments

Methotrexate is usually prescribed for rheumatoid arthritis when other therapies, such as antimalarials and gold salts, have not produced favorable results. Because methotrexate is generally well tolerated, it is frequently used as a second-line therapy. Recent studies have indicated that methotrexate, when used in combination with sulfasalazine and prednisolone, controlled symptoms of rheumatoid arthritis in more than 70% of patients. Careful monitoring by your doctor and regular laboratory tests are essential while you take this drug.

Brand Name
Rhinocort*

Generic Name
budesonide

Type of Drug
Nasal corticosteroid.

For
Relief of symptoms of hay fever and allergic rhinitis; prevention of nasal polyp regrowth after surgery.

Availability and Dosage
Inhalation aerosol: 0.032 mg per inhalation. Follow directions for proper administration.

Side Effects
More common include nosebleeds, irritation of nasal passages, sore throat, and hoarseness. Others include eye pain, vision impairment, stomach pain, and indigestion.

Drug Interactions
Tell your doctor if you are taking other inhalation corticosteroids, other steroids, or any medications that suppress immune-system function.

Food/Alcohol Interactions
No special warnings.

Pregnancy/Nursing
Not recommended. This drug may pass into breast milk.

Seniors

No special warnings. Take as prescribed and immediately inform your doctor of any persistent or troublesome side effects.

Warning

This drug is not to be used to stop an acute asthma attack. In rare instances, inhaled steroids can result in yeast infections of the mouth. Gargling with plain water after each use may reduce this risk.

Comments

If symptoms persist or get worse during treatment, call your health care practitioner.

Brand Name
Ridaura

Generic Name

auranofin

Type of Drug

Antiarthritic; gold compound. This drug is an oral form of gold, which can reduce painful joint inflammation associated with arthritis and rheumatoid arthritis. It is usually prescribed in cases where other therapies have not been effective.

For

Rheumatoid arthritis: to reduce joint pain, swelling, and tenderness. This drug is not to be used for osteoarthritis.

Availability and Dosage

Capsules: 3 mg. Also available in injection form.

Side Effects

More common include hives, itching, loss of appetite, diarrhea, indigestion, nausea, stomach pain, and cramps. Others are hoarseness, coughing, vision impairment, hair loss, painful or difficult urination, weakness, fatigue, and fluid retention in the face, feet, or legs.

Drug Interactions

Although auranofin is sometimes prescribed concurrently with aspirin and other nonsteroidal antiinflammatory drugs (NSAIDs), interactions can occur. Auranofin can also interact with carbamazepine, anticancer drugs, some anticonvulsants, and zidovudine (AZT). Always inform your doctors of every medication you are taking, including nonprescription medicines, vitamins, herbal remedies, and dietary supplements.

Food/Alcohol Interactions

Avoid alcohol.

Pregnancy/Nursing

Not recommended.

Seniors

There is an increased risk of side effects in older adults. Your doctor may adjust your dosage accordingly.

Warning

Careful monitoring by your doctor or rheumatologist along with periodic laboratory tests are essential while taking this drug in order to check for gold toxicity or adverse effects such as anemia or a low white-blood-cell count.

Comments

You may take this drug for up to 6 months before you see any benefits. Do not stop taking this medicine without consulting your doctor. The long-term effectiveness of this drug is unpredictable. After a gold injection, you may experience a worsening of your symptoms. Injections must be given under a health care professional's supervision.

Brand Name
Risperdal*

Generic Name

risperidone

Type of Drug

Antipsychotic.

For

Symptoms of psychosis. This drug may also be prescribed for Alzheimer's patients who develop psychotic symptoms such as aggression, delusions, and hallucinations in addition to memory loss and confusion. In a study of 625 patients in 40 U.S. nursing homes, low doses of risperidone helped calm approximately one-third of the patients.

Availability and Dosage

Tablets: 1 mg, 2 mg, 3 mg, 4 mg. Oral solution: 1 mg per ml. May be taken with or without food. Should be taken at regular intervals. Do not abruptly stop taking this medication; your doctor will have to gradually decrease your dose.

Side Effects

More common include drowsiness, agitation, anxiety, vision changes, decreased sex drive, loss of balance, menstrual changes, memory problems, difficulty in concentrating, and increased sensitivity to sunlight. Others include headache, stomach pain, constipation, fatigue, and weight gain.

Drug Interactions

Risperdal can interact with levodopa, beta-blockers, carbamazepine, central nervous system (CNS) depressants, cimetidine, tricyclic antidepressants, and other drugs used for mental problems. Always inform your doctors of every medication you are taking, including nonprescription medicines, vitamins, herbal remedies, and dietary supplements. *Do not take any over-the-counter medications unless approved by your doctor.*

Food/Alcohol Interactions

Avoid alcohol, as it can increase drowsiness or dizziness.

Pregnancy/Nursing

Not recommended. This drug may pass into breast milk.

Seniors

The risk of side effects is increased in older adults. Older women may be more at risk for side effects involving uncontrolled movements of the face, tongue, and jaw. Your doctor may prescribe a low dose.

Warning

If you experience convulsions, difficulty in breathing, rapid, weak, or irregular heartbeat, wormlike movements of the tongue, urinary incontinence, or severe muscle stiffness, seek emergency medical treatment. Risperdal should be used with caution by people who have heart disease; this drug can cause potentially life-threatening abnormal heart rhythms.

Comments

It is possible that your judgment could become impaired while taking this drug. Do not drive, operate machinery, or perform any tasks requiring mental alertness until you know how this drug affects you.

risperidone

See Risperdal*

ritonavir

See Norvir

rofecoxib

See Vioxx

rosiglitazone

See Avandia

Roxicet*

See Percocet

Roxilox

See Percocet

Rufen

See Motrin

salmeterol xinafoate

See Serevent*

Brand Name
Sandimmune (also Neoral, SangCya)

Generic Name
cyclosporine

Type of Drug
Immunosuppressive agent.

For

Prevention of organ rejection after a heart, kidney, or liver transplant. It may also be used for rheumatoid arthritis, psoriasis, and other conditions as prescribed by your doctor.

Availability and Dosage

Sandimmune and Neoral capsules: 25 mg, 50 mg, 100 mg. Sandimmune, Neoral, and SangCya oral solution: 100 mg per ml. This drug should be taken at the same time each day. Capsules may be taken with or without food. Follow directions carefully for oral solution; it should be mixed in a glass container (not plastic or paper) with the beverage recommended on the instructions provided by your pharmacist—usually milk or orange juice for Sandimmune; orange juice or apple juice for Neoral and SangCya. Do not take this medication with grapefruit juice.

Side Effects

More common include headache, swelling or bleeding of gums, unusual growth of gum tissue, high blood pressure, increased hair growth, and loss of appetite. Others include tremors, nausea, vomiting, leg cramps, hiccups, and a lowered resistance to infection.

Drug Interactions

Cyclosporine has the potential to interact with a variety of drugs. It must be used with caution in combination with other kidney-toxic drugs. Cyclosporine may also interact with cimetidine, diltiazem, erythromycin, estrogens, ketoconazole, some cholesterol-lowering drugs, antibiotics and other antibacterials, prednisone, cortisone, antihypertensives, diuretics (water pills), and warfarin. Always inform your doctors of every medication you are taking, including nonprescription medicines, vitamins, herbal remedies, and dietary supplements. *Do not take any over-the-counter medications unless approved by your doctor.*

Food/Alcohol Interactions

Do not take any form of this drug with grapefruit juice. Do not mix the oral solution of this drug with any liquids other than the ones usually recommended (above) or by your pharmacist.

Pregnancy/Nursing

A pregnant woman must never take this drug. Cyclosporine has been proven to cause birth defects. If you suspect you are pregnant, notify your doctor immediately. Bottle-feed your baby if you must take this drug.

Seniors

Kidney function is often reduced in older adults and may be more susceptible to the kidney-toxic effects of this drug. Careful monitoring of kidney function is essential.

Warning

You should never switch brands of cyclosporine unless directed by your doctor. They are not interchangeable. The two brands of capsules (Sandimmune, Neoral) and the three brands of oral solution (Sandimmune, Neoral, and SangCya) are each absorbed differently. Prolonged use of these drugs may impair kidney function. You must have regular lab work performed during treatment. Do not have any vaccinations while on this drug.

Comments

Cyclosporine suppresses the body's immune system function, thereby suppressing the body's natural reaction to rejecting an organ transplant. This drug is also used to treat rheumatoid arthritis, an autoimmune disorder that affects a greater number of women than men.

Sanorex

See Mazanor

selegiline

See Eldepryl

Septra

See Bactrim

Septra DS

See Bactrim

Brand Name
Serevent*

Generic Name

salmeterol xinafoate

Type of Drug

Bronchodilator (inhalation).

For

Symptoms of chronic asthma and bronchial spasms. Not for acute asthma attacks.

Availability and Dosage

Inhalation aerosol: 21 mcg. Usual dose is twice a day, 12 hours apart. Do not take this medicine more often than is prescribed. Follow the instructions for using the inhaler, and consult your pharmacist if you need a demonstration.

Side Effects

More common include headache, tremor, and cough. Others include sinus irritation, stomach pain, respiratory infection, and dry mouth.

Drug Interactions

This drug may interact with some antihypertensives, including beta-blockers. Interactions may also occur with monoamine oxidase (MAO) inihibitor antidepressants, thyroid drugs, tricyclic antidepressants, and prescription and nonprescription antihistamines. Always inform your doctors of every medication you are taking, including nonprescription medicines, vitamins, herbal remedies, and dietary supplements.

Food/Alcohol Interactions

No special warnings.

Pregnancy/Nursing

Not recommended, but women who have asthma must continue treatment in some form. Discuss with your doctor the benefits versus the potential risks. The effects of this drug on newborns is unknown. Bottle-feed your baby if you must take this drug.

Seniors

No special warnings. Take as prescribed and immediately inform your doctor of any persistent or troublesome side effects.

Warning

Do not use this drug to stop an acute asthma attack; it will not work in time. If you experience difficulty in breathing, wheezing, rapid heartbeat, or chest pain, call your doctor or seek medical treatment immediately. Use this drug cautiously if you have a history of diabetes, heart disease, hypertension, arrhythmia, or thyroid disease. Ask your doctor how long you will need to be on this drug; there is some evidence of an increased risk of ovarian tumors.

Comments

More than 1% of pregnant women have asthma, a condition in which the airways and the bronchi (breathing tubes) in the lungs are constricted. You must get emergency treatment if you have an asthma attack that does not respond to treatment. Oxygen deprivation to the fetus may result. Asthma can also be triggered by exercise; salmeterol is also prescribed for use in those cases.

sertraline

*See Zoloft**

Brand Name

Serzone*

Generic Name

nefazodone

Type of Drug

Antidepressant. This drug is not chemically related to any other antidepressant. It is often prescribed for patients unable to tolerate other types of antidepressants.

For

Depression.

Availability and Dosage

Tablets: 50 mg, 100 mg, 150 mg, 200 mg, 250 mg. Take on an empty stomach, 1 hour before or 2 hours after meals. Take at regular intervals. Do not take more of this medicine than is prescribed.

Side Effects

More common include dry mouth, constipation, fatigue, dizziness, and headache. Others include nausea, skin flushing, heartburn, cough, insomnia, and tremor.

Drug Interactions

Nefazodone may interact with alprazolam, digoxin, calcium channel blockers, cholesterol-lowering drugs, and erythromycin. Do not take this drug within 2 weeks of taking a monoamine oxidase

(MAO) inhibitor antidepressant. Always inform your doctors of every medication you are taking, including nonprescription medicines, vitamins, herbal remedies, and dietary supplements. *Do not take any over-the-counter medications unless approved by your doctor.*

Food/Alcohol Interactions

Avoid alcohol. It is important to take this drug on an empty stomach, as food will interfere with its absorption and effectiveness.

Pregnancy/Nursing

Not recommended. It is unknown whether this drug passes into breast milk. Discuss with your doctor the benefits versus the potential risks.

Seniors

This drug is eliminated more slowly in older women. Your doctor may prescribe a low dose.

Warning

You must be regularly monitored by a physician while taking this drug. Make sure your doctor has your complete medical history, including a history of liver disease, seizure, heart disease, or suicidal thoughts. Women with mitral valve prolapse (MVP) syndrome may have a lower blood volume (hypovolemia) and be at increase risk for hypotension (low blood pressure).

Comments

It may take several weeks to notice significant benefits from this drug. In drug studies, nefazodone was found to significantly improve the symptoms of severe premenstrual syndrome (PMS). Unlike some other antidepressants, nefazodone does not cause weight gain or decreased libido.

sibutramine hydrochloride monohydrate

See Meridia

sildenafil citrate

See Viagra*

simvastatin

See Zocor*

Brand Name
Sinemet (also Sinemet CR)

Generic Name

carbidopa and levodopa

Type of Drug

Antiparkinsonian. This drug is used alone or with tolcapone (Tasmar) to help relieve the symptoms of Parkinson's disease—head and limb trembling, muscular stiffness, and inability to control movement.

For

Parkinson's disease.

Availability and Dosage

This combination drug of carbidopa and levodopa comes in various strengths—$10/100$, $25/100$, and $25/250$ (carbidopa is the first number and levodopa the second). Dosages are specific to individual needs and must be determined by your doctor. Sinemet may be taken with or without food. Sinemet CR (sustained-release) should be taken on an empty stomach, 1 hour before or 2 hours after meals.

Side Effects

More common include involuntary muscle movements, nausea, stomach pain, and confusion. Others include difficulty in sleeping, skin flushing, fatigue, shakiness, dizziness when rising from a sitting or reclining position, loss of appetite, headache, dry mouth, anxiety, depression, and heart palpitations. Dark urine is a harmless side effect.

Drug Interactions

This drug may interact with antihypertensives, oral antidiabetics, some antidepressants, phenytoin, and diuretics. Do not take this drug within 2 weeks of taking a monoamine oxidase (MAO) inhibitor antidepressant. Use caution when taking vitamin B_6 (pyridoxine). Always inform your doctors of every medication you are taking, including nonprescription medicines, vitamins, herbal remedies, and dietary supplements. *Do not take any over-the-counter medications unless approved by your doctor.*

Food/Alcohol Interactions

Avoid alcohol. A diet high in protein can interfere with absorption and effectiveness of levodopa. Your doctor or other health care professional may give you a list of foods to restrict.

Pregnancy/Nursing

Not recommended. Bottle-feed your baby if you must take this drug.

Seniors

Adverse side effects may be increased in older people, especially those who have heart disease. Your doctor may prescribe a low dose.

Warning

Make sure your doctor has your complete medical history, including a history of heart disease, arrhythmia, glaucoma, or any mental disorders.

Comments

You must be carefully and regularly monitored by your doctor while taking this drug. Parkinson's disease is a degenerative, progressive neurological disorder marked by four main symptoms: tremors, rigidity or stiffness in limbs, slowed movement, and balance disorder. Its average age of onset is 55, and more men than women are affected.

Brand Name
Soma

Generic Name

carisoprodol*

Type of Drug

Muscle relaxant. This drug is used to relieve symptoms of sprains and muscle spasms and may be used with other medications or treatments.

For

Painful muscle conditions.

Availability and Dosage

Soma compound tablets: 325 mg aspirin and 200 mg cariso-prodol. Soma compound with codeine tablets: 325 mg aspirin, 200 mg carisoprodol, and 16 mg codeine. May be taken with or without food.

Side Effects

More common include drowsiness, dry mouth, and dizziness. Others include headache, mouth ulcers, constipation, restlessness, skin redness, heartburn, sleep disturbances, nausea, vomiting, and unsteadiness.

Drug Interactions

No special warnings, although all drugs have the ability to interact with other drugs. Always inform your doctors of every medication you are taking, including nonprescription medicines, vitamins, herbal remedies, and dietary supplements.

Food/Alcohol Interactions

Avoid alcohol, as it may increase drowsiness.

Pregnancy/Nursing

Before taking this drug, discuss with your doctor the benefits versus the potential risks. Bottle-feed your baby if you must take this drug.

Seniors

Older adults may experience more adverse side effects. Your doctor may prescribe a low dose.

Warning

Although there are no known drug interactions, caution should be used when taking this drug with other medications known to cause drowsiness, including antihistamines, sedatives, tranquilizers, anticonvulsants, and painkillers. Ask your pharmacist's advice regarding over-the-counter drugs that may cause drowsiness: sleep aids, antihistamines, analgesics, and motion-sickness medications.

Comments

If you are taking the form of this drug that contains codeine, follow dosage instructions exactly and report any adverse side effects to your physician. Drowsiness may be intensified, along with the potential for more adverse reactions and drug interactions. Consult your pharmacist or your physician before taking any over-the-counter medication (see Warning).

sotalol HCl

*See **Betapace***

spironolactone

*See **Aldactone***

Brand Name

Sporanox

Generic Name

itraconazole

Type of Drug

Antifungal.

For

Relief of fungal infections.

Availability and Dosage

Capsules: 100 mg. Oral solution: 10 mg per ml. Should be taken with food.

Side Effects

More common include nausea and vomiting. Others include elevated liver enzymes, diarrhea, rash, fluid retention, headache, and hypertension.

Drug Interactions

This drug can interact with cisapride, triazolam, lovastatin, simvastatin, oral antidiabetics, antiviral drugs, cimetidine, famotidine, ranitidine, and phenytoin. Always inform your doctors of every medication you are taking, including nonprescription medicines, vitamins, herbal remedies, and dietary supplements.

Food/Alcohol Interactions

No special warnings.

Pregnancy/Nursing

Not recommended. Bottle-feed your baby if you must take this drug.

Seniors

No special warnings. Take as prescribed and immediately inform your doctor of any persistent or troublesome side effects.

Warning

In rare cases, hepatitis and other liver damage can result from this drug. If you experience extreme fatigue, flu-like symptoms, jaundice, dark urine, or pale stools, call your doctor immediately. Make sure your doctor knows if you have a history of liver impairment or disease.

Comments

This drug was originally approved to treat internal fungus infections of the esophagus, brain, lungs, and other organs. It is now also used to treat fungal infections of the nails. It can take up to 3 months before there is visible improvement. Nail fungus (onychomycosis) is characterized by cracked, yellowed, or rotting nails, usually on the big toe but also on the fingernails. You should not use acrylic nails or any "press-on" type of artificial nails if you have this fungus. Itraconazole is not a cure; symptoms may recur when you stop treatment.

sulfisoxazole

See **Gantrisin**

sumatriptan

See **Imitrex***

Brand Name
Sumycin*

Generic Name
tetracycline HCL

Type of Drug

Antibiotic. These drugs are among the most commonly prescribed, resulting in such widespread use that the bacteria they were developed to kill have become resistant to them. These "resistant" forms are then passed from person to person, further causing the spread of infections that become even more difficult to treat. Your doctor will prescribe the correct antibiotic depending on the type of infection. Antibiotics are useless against viral infections such as colds and flu.

For

Various bacterial infections.

Availability and Dosage

Tablets: 250 mg, 500 mg. Capsules: 250 mg, 500 mg. Oral suspension: 125 mg per 5 ml. Should be taken with 8 ounces of water on an empty stomach, 1 hour before or 2 hours after meals. It is essential to take the complete course of antibiotics prescribed. If you fail to do so, increased drug resistance by any leftover bacteria is likely to occur.

Side Effects

More common include nausea, diarrhea, upset stomach, and rash. Others include increased sun sensitivity, genital or rectal itching, sore tongue, dizziness, and stomach cramps.

Drug Interactions

Tetracycline can interact with oral contraceptives, other antibiotics, digoxin, anticoagulants (blood thinners), and antacids. Separate your dose of tetracycline by 2 hours from any over-the-counter medications or from vitamins that contain calcium, magnesium, zinc, or iron. Always inform your doctors of every medication you are taking, including nonprescription medicines, vitamins, herbal remedies, and dietary supplements. *Do not take any over-the-counter medications unless approved by your doctor.*

Food/Alcohol Interactions

Avoid or limit alcohol. Avoid dairy products.

Pregnancy/Nursing

Not recommended, especially during the second and third trimesters. Bottle-feed your baby if you must take this drug.

Seniors

No special warnings. Take as prescribed and immediately inform your doctor of any persistent or troublesome side effects. Tell your doctor if you have impaired kidney function.

Warning

Women who take a combination of birth control pills and tetracycline have become pregnant. Use an additional method of birth control while taking this drug. Avoid direct sunlight. Do not use tanning beds or tanning lamps. Check the drug's expiration date and do not use it beyond that time.

Comments

If you are taking tetracycline for a sexually transmitted disease (STD), your male partner should wear a condom and may also need to be treated for an STD.

Brand Name
Symmetrel

Generic Name

amantadine

Type of Drug

Antiparkinsonian.

For

Parkinson's disease; fatigue associated with multiple sclerosis; involuntary muscle movements.

Availability and Dosage

Capsules: 100 mg. May be taken with or without food. Do not abruptly stop taking this medication without consulting your doctor, as your symptoms of Parkinson's disease may worsen. Your dose may have to be gradually decreased.

Side Effects

More common include dizziness or light-headedness, nausea, and nervousness. Others include headache, loss of appetite, skin blotches, difficulty in sleeping, constipation, dry mouth and nightmares.

Drug Interactions

Amantadine may interact with some diuretics, appetite suppressants, antiasthmatics, some antihistamines, levodopa, some antidepressants, and triamterene. Always inform your doctors of every medication you are taking, including nonprescription medicines, vitamins, herbal remedies, and dietary supplements. *Do not take any over-the-counter medications unless approved by your doctor.*

Food/Alcohol Interactions

Avoid alcohol. Avoid or limit caffeine.

Pregnancy/Nursing

Not recommended. Bottle-feed your baby if you must take this drug.

Seniors

Side effects may be more pronounced in older adults, primarily because of a decrease in kidney function. Your doctor may prescribe a low dose.

Warning

Do not take any over-the-counter antihistamines, appetite suppressants, sinus or cold medications, water pills, or drugs containing caffeine. Make sure your doctor has your complete medical history, including a history of seizures, eczema, heart disease, circulatory problems, mental or emotional disorders, or kidney disease.

Comments

This drug is also an antiviral used to treat some types of flu viruses. If you are taking this drug for flu and your symptoms do not improve or become worse, call your doctor. Parkinson's disease is a degenerative, progressive neurological disorder marked by four main symptoms: tremors, rigidity or stiffness in limbs, slowed movement, and balance disorder. Its average age of onset is 55, and more men than women are affected. You may see improvement in symptoms shortly after starting this drug, but in some cases it can take up to 2 weeks to see the maximum benefit.

Brand Name
Synarel

Generic Name

nafarelin acetate

Type of Drug

Gonadotropin-releasing hormone (GnRH) nasal spray. This drug reduces estrogen production by the ovaries, thereby shrinking the uterine lining (endometrium). It is also used in conjunction with treatments for infertility, when infertility is caused by uterine tissue growing outside the uterus (endometriosis).

For

Endometriosis; menstrual cramps; abnormal menstrual bleeding; infertility.

Availability and Dosage

Nasal spray: 2 mg per ml. Frequency is determined based on the condition being treated.

Side Effects

More common include vaginal dryness, acne, and hot flashes. Others include headache, changes in weight, breast pain, and changes in mood.

Drug Interactions

This drug may interact with nasal decongestants, corticosteroids, and some anticonvulsants. Always inform your doctors of every medication you are taking, including nonprescription medicines, vitamins, herbal remedies, and dietary supplements. *Do not take any over-the-counter medications unless approved by your doctor.*

Food/Alcohol Interactions

Avoid alcohol. Avoid or limit caffeine.

Pregnancy/Nursing

Not recommended during pregnancy. If you are taking this drug for infertility, consult your doctor immediately if you think you might be pregnant. Bottle-feed your baby if you must take this drug (for endometriosis or other menstrual disorders).

Seniors

Not usually applicable.

Warning

Untreated endometriosis can lead to infertility. Regular pelvic exams are important, plus vaginal ultrasound or laparoscopy if endometriosis is suspected based on your symptoms (severe menstrual pain, pelvic pain, pain during sexual intercourse, or inability to get pregnant). If your gynecologist dismisses or minimizes severe menstrual symptoms without a complete examination including diagnostic tests, get a second opinion. If you experience vaginal bleeding between periods while taking this drug, notify your doctor.

Comments

Endometriosis can be painful and debilitating, or it may have few symptoms. More than 15% of women between age 15 and 44 have some degree of it. Uterine tissue can travel outside the pelvic cavity (e.g., to the lungs and brain) and still respond to the hormonal changes as if it were inside the uterus. Up to 50% of women who explore fertility treatments have some form of endometriosis. Another gonadotropic-releasing hormone (GnRH) used for endometriosis is Lupron. It is available in injection form and administered by your doctor. Like Synarel, it causes a chemical menopause.

Brand Name
Synthroid* (also Levoxyl*, Levoxine, Levothroid, Synthrox)

Generic Name

levothyroxine

Type of Drug

Thyroid hormone.

For

Treatment of thyroid disorders, including insufficient thyroid hormone production or enlarged thyroid due to goiter.

Availability and Dosage

Tablets: 0.025 mg, 0.05 mg, 0.075 mg, 0.1 mg, 0.112 mg, 0.125 mg, 0.15 mg, 0.175 mg, 0.2 mg, 0.3 mg. This drug should be taken on an empty stomach at the same time every day, usually in the morning before eating.

Side Effects

Side effects are rare and can be controlled by dosage adjustments. They include menstrual changes, headache, weight gain, constipation, nervousness, and tremor.

Drug Interactions

Levothyroxine may interact with oral contraceptives, estrogen, oral antidiabetics, digoxin, insulin, anticoagulants (blood thinners), aspirin, tricyclic antidepressants, appetite suppressants, and beta-blockers. Always inform your doctors of every medication you are taking, including nonprescription medicines, vitamins, herbal remedies, and dietary supplements. *Do not take any over-the-counter medications unless approved by your doctor.*

Food/Alcohol Interactions

No special warnings.

Pregnancy/Nursing

No special warnings, although all drugs during pregnancy and breast-feeding should be avoided if possible. Before taking this drug, discuss with your doctor the benefits versus the potential risks. Your dosage may need to be adjusted during pregnancy.

Seniors

Side effects, although generally rare, may be more pronounced in older adults. Your doctor may prescribe a low dose.

Warning

Do not change brands of levothyroxine without consulting your doctor or your pharmacist. With the ability to order prescription drugs over the Internet, this is especially important to remember. Different brands of levothyroxine may not produce the same results, and proper dosage is essential. You may be taking this medication for the rest of your life; do not stop taking it without your doctor's approval. Regular monitoring by your physician is required while on thyroid replacements.

Comments

Levothyroxine was introduced in 1953 and is used to replace thyroxine, the hormone produced by the thyroid gland, when there is a deficiency or absence (due to thyroid surgery or radiation treatment). Before taking any nonprescription medications for colds, coughs, allergies, asthma, sinus, or weight loss (OTC appetite suppressants), check with your doctor or your pharmacist.

Synthrox

See Synthroid*

T-Stat

See Ery-Tab*

tacrine hydrochloride

See Cognex

Brand Name

Tagamet

Generic Name

cimetidine*

Type of Drug

Histamine H_2 blocker. Histamine is a chemical that produces a variety of effects, including increased secretion of stomach acid. Antihistamines traditionally used for allergies do not block the effect of histamine on stomach acid.

For

Stomach ulcers and duodenal ulcers; gastroesophageal reflux disease (GERD).

Availability and Dosage

Tablets: 200 mg, 300 mg, 400 mg, 800 mg. Oral liquid: 300 mg per 5 ml, with 2.8% alcohol. Dosages will vary depending on the condition being treated. Take tablets with water, not juice or soda.

Side Effects

More common include headache, fatigue, diarrhea, nausea, vomiting, and abdominal pain. Others include breast swelling, hair loss (temporary), and skin rash.

Drug Interactions

This drug has the potential to interact with a wide variety of medications, including aspirin, antiinflammatories, beta-blockers, calcium channel blockers, carbamazepine, anticoagulants (blood thinners), metoprolol, itraconazole, ketoconazole, oral contraceptives, some antidepressants, nifedipine, oral antidiabetics, benzodiazepines, narcotic pain relievers, tetracycline antibiotics, and digoxin. Always inform your doctors of every medication you are taking, including nonprescription medicines, vitamins, herbal remedies, and dietary supplements. *Do not take any over-the-counter medications unless approved by your doctor.*

Food/Alcohol Interactions

Avoid alcohol. Avoid caffeinated foods and beverages. Acidic foods and beverages may irritate the stomach.

Pregnancy/Nursing

Not recommended. Bottle-feed your baby if you must take this drug.

Seniors

Older adults may experience increased side effects, especially if they have liver or kidney impairment. Your doctor may prescribe a low dose.

Warning

If stomach pain worsens while using this drug, call your doctor at once. If you experience black, tarry stools, confusion, hallucinations, or vomiting of "coffee ground" material, *seek emergency medical treatment*.

Comments

Ulcer disease—once considered a condition that affected mostly men—now counts an equal number of women among its sufferers. Each year approximately 500,000 new cases of ulcers are diagnosed in the United States, half of them women. According to the Centers for Disease Control and Prevention (CDC), women generally develop first-onset symptoms at age 35, and the risk of ulcer disease rises with age. The majority of peptic ulcers are caused by the bacterium *H. pylori*, and antibiotics are often used in conjunction with antiulcer drugs. Nonprescription H_2 blockers are among the most popular over-the-counter medications. The nonprescription form of cimetidine is Tagamet HB, which is used for heartburn, indigestion, and upset stomach. Follow package directions carefully, do not take more often than needed, and consult your doctor if symptoms worsen.

tamoxifen citrate

*See **Nolvadex***

Brand Name
Tasmar

Generic Name

tolcapone

Type of Drug

Antiparkinsonian. This drug is used with carbidopa/levodopa (Sinemet) to help relieve the symptoms of Parkinson's disease—head and limb trembling, muscular stiffness, and inability to control movement.

For

Parkinson's disease.

Availability and Dosage

Tablets: 100 mg, 200 mg. May be taken with or without food. Your doctor may need to adjust your dose of carbidopa/levodopa (Sinemet) to minimize side effects. Do not stop taking this drug without consulting your doctor.

Side Effects

More common include nausea, dizziness or fainting when rising quickly from a sitting or reclining position, and diarrhea. Others include heartburn, constipation, drowsiness, dry mouth, fatigue, headache, abdominal pain, involuntary muscle movements, and dark yellow or brown urine (bright yellow is a harmless side effect of this drug).

Drug Interactions

Tolcapone has the potential to interact with monoamine oxidase (MAO) inhibitor antidepressants, antihypertensives, methyldopa, anticoagulants (blood thinners), and drugs for insomnia. Always inform your doctors of every medication you are taking, including nonprescription medicines, vitamins, herbal remedies, and dietary supplements. *Do not take any over-the-counter medications unless approved by your doctor.*

Food/Alcohol Interactions

Limit alcohol.

Pregnancy/Nursing

No special warnings, although all drugs during pregnancy and breast-feeding should be avoided if possible. Before taking this drug, discuss with your doctor the benefits versus the potential risks.

Seniors

Older adults may be more susceptible to side effects, including hallucinations and postural low blood pressure (dizziness or fainting when standing up too quickly).

Warning

In rare instances, this drug can cause severe liver damage. Liver problems may manifest as light-colored stools, dark urine, weakness, or jaundice. If you experience any of these, notify your doctor immediately. Make sure your doctor has your complete medical history, including a history of low blood pressure, fainting, anorexia, hallucinations, or kidney or liver disease. Do not drive, operate machinery, or perform tasks requiring mental alertness until you know how this drug affects you.

Comments

You must be carefully and regularly monitored by your doctor while taking tolcapone. Periodic tests for liver function will be necessary. This drug is the first in a new class of antiparkinsonian agents called COMT (catechol-O-methyltransferase) inhibitors. Parkinson's disease is a degenerative, progressive neurological disorder marked by four main symptoms: tremors, rigidity or stiffness in limbs, slowed movement, and balance disorder. Its average age of onset is 55, and more men than women are affected.

Brand Name
Tegretol

Generic Name

carbamazepine

Type of Drug

Anticonvulsant. This drug is used to prevent seizures or to stop one in progress.

For

Seizure disorders; certain emotional disorders including manic depression; migraine headache.

Availability and Dosage

Tablets: 200 mg. Extended-release tablets: 100 mg, 200 mg, 400 mg. Chewable tablets: 100 mg. Oral suspension: 100 mg per 5 ml. Dosages vary widely depending on the condition being treated. Do not change the dose that your doctor prescribes. Do not abruptly stop taking this medication, as doing so may induce seizures.

Side Effects

More common include drowsiness, unsteadiness, nausea, vomiting, stomach pain, and diarrhea. Others include dry mouth, nervousness, changes in mood, constipation, headache, increased sun sensitivity, mouth pain, tingling or numbness in the feet and hands, blurred vision, swelling, and rash.

Drug Interactions

Carbamazepine has the potential to interact with a wide variety of medications, including other anticonvulsants, anticoagulants (blood thinners), cimetidine, lithium, corticosteroids, erythromycin, verapamil, estrogens, oral contraceptives, fluvoxamine, antifungals, monoamine oxidase (MAO) inhibitor antidepressants, central nervous system (CNS) depressants, risperidone, tricyclic antidepressants, and flu vaccines. Always inform your doctors of every medication you are taking, including nonprescription medicines, vitamins, herbal remedies, and dietary supplements. *Do not take any over-the-counter medications unless approved by your doctor.*

Food/Alcohol Interactions

Avoid alcohol.

Pregnancy/Nursing

Not recommended, but seizures during pregnancy also pose risks to the fetus. You and your doctor will have to weigh the benefits against the potential risks. This drug passes into breast milk. Bottle-feed your baby if you must take this drug.

Seniors

Increased side effects have been noted in older adults, including heart arrhythmias, slow heartbeat, restlessness, and confusion.

Warning

Carbamazepine is a very potent drug, and its levels in the bloodstream must be carefully and regularly monitored by proper monitoring and tests. Make sure your doctor has your complete medical history, including a history of glaucoma, lupus, or diabetes.

Comments

Unplanned pregnancies have occurred in women who are taking this drug in combination with oral contraceptives containing estrogen. Use an additional method of birth control while on this drug.

temazepam*

See **Restoril**

Brand Name
Tenormin

Generic Name

atenolol

Type of Drug

Beta-blocker. These drugs block the response of the heart and blood vessels, lower pulse rate, and reduce the force of the heartbeat, thereby reducing the workload of the heart. They are sometimes prescribed after a heart attack to help prevent future attacks.

For

High blood pressure; angina pectoris; irregular heartbeat; anxiety.

Availability and Dosage

Tablets: 25 mg, 50 mg, 100 mg. May be taken with or without food. Do not abruptly stop taking this drug, as doing so could result in adverse reactions.

Side Effects

More common include muscle aches. Others include dizziness, anxiety, changes in sex drive, sleep disturbance, nightmares, fatigue, weakness, rash, diarrhea, headache, nausea, swelling of the legs or ankles, slow heartbeat, fainting, and tremors.

Drug Interactions

Atenolol may interact with oral antidiabetics, antihypertensives, other heart medications, diuretics (water pills), aspirin, estrogens, thyroid drugs, monoamine oxidase (MAO) inhibitors, phenytoin, and some antiasthmatics. Do not take this drug within 2 hours of taking an antacid. Always inform your doctors of every medication you are taking, including nonprescription medicines, vitamins, herbal remedies, and dietary supplements. *Do not take any over-the-counter medications unless approved by your doctor.*

Food/Alcohol Interactions

Avoid alcohol, as it may cause dizziness and drowsiness.

Pregnancy/Nursing

Not recommended. If this drug must be taken, discuss with your doctor the benefits versus the potential risks. Bottle-feed your baby if you must take this drug.

Seniors

Adverse reactions are more common in older adults, including an increased sensitivity to cold, chest pains, and changes in heart rate. Your doctor may prescribe a low dose.

Warning

Make sure your doctor has your complete medical history, including a history of diabetes, bradycardia (slow heartbeat), emphysema, depression, psoriasis, thyroid disease, asthma, or heart, kidney, or liver disease. Your blood pressure and heart rate should be regularly monitored while you take this drug. This medication may reduce exercise-related chest pain and cause you to become overly active. You and your doctor should determine a safe level of activity.

Comments

If you are being treated for hypertension, it is essential to learn as much as possible about the causes and risks of this disease. In 2000, the National Council on the Aging (NCOA) surveyed 1500 Americans over age 50—a group at great risk for complications from uncontrolled high blood pressure—and found that they are largely unaware about what their blood pressure goals should be. Interestingly, the sample did not indicate gender, but included 900 whites, 300 African-American, and 300 Hispanic respondents. Half of the respondents in the survey were unaware that kidney failure can result from hypertension, and nearly half incorrectly believe that the main cause of high blood pressure is stress. One-third were unaware that they have high blood pressure, and only 27% know the importance of the systolic (top) number as an indicator of high blood pressure. Recent recommendations indicate that blood pressure should be under 140/90.

Brand Name
Tenuate

Generic Name
diethylpropion

Type of Drug
Nonamphetamine appetite suppressant. This drug is used in conjunction with a weight-management program that involves a healthy diet plan and appropriate exercise.

For
Short-term weight reduction.

Availability and Dosage
Tablets: 25 mg. Extended-release tablets: 75 mg. Should be taken on an empty stomach, 1 hour before meals. Do not take more of this medicine than is prescribed. Do not use longer than 8 to 12 weeks unless directed by your doctor.

Side Effects
More common include dry mouth, light-headedness, rapid heartbeat, sleeplessness, stomach upset, and constipation. Others include sore throat, fever, and irritability.

Drug Interactions
Diethylpropion may interact with antihypertensives, monoamine oxidase (MAO) inhibitor antidepressants, antiasthmatics, other appetite suppressants, amantadine, and decongestants. Always inform your doctors of every medication you are taking, including nonprescription medicines, vitamins, herbal remedies, and dietary supplements. *Do not take any over-the-counter medications unless approved by your doctor.*

Food/Alcohol Interactions
Avoid alcohol. Avoid caffeinated foods and beverages.

Pregnancy/Nursing
Not recommended. If you must take this drug, bottle-feed your baby. If you are trying to become pregnant you should not take this drug. If you suspect you are pregnant, stop taking this drug and notify your doctor immediately.

Seniors

Not usually prescribed. If you must take this drug, make sure your doctor knows if you have a history of hypertension, glaucoma, or heart, kidney, or thyroid disease.

Warning

A rare but potentially fatal reaction called primary pulmonary hypertension is more likely in patients who take appetite-suppressant drugs for more than 3 months. If you experience difficulty in breathing, swelling in the lower legs or ankles, chest pain, or fainting, *seek emergency medical treatment*. Do not take any nonprescription drugs for allergies, colds, or coughs as they may contain ingredients that will intensify a stimulant effect and cause a rapid rise in heart rate. Make sure your doctor has your complete medical history before you take this drug, including a history of alcohol or substance abuse.

Comments

Studies indicate that most patients regain the weight they lost during appetite suppression drug therapy, not because of the drug, but because they did not change their basic eating and exercise habits. This type of drug therapy is not appropriate for individuals who are only slightly overweight.

Brand Name
Terazol 3 (also Terazol 7)

Generic Name

terconazole

Type of Drug

Antifungal.

For

Candidiases, specifically vaginal yeast infections.

Availability and Dosage

Vaginal suppositories or vaginal cream 0.8% (Terazol 3). Vaginal cream 0.4% (Terazol 7). Follow package directions for correct application or insertion of this medication. Use this drug consistently for the full course of treatment, even during your menstrual period.

Side Effects

Headache, body pain, genital pain, stinging, irritation, and menstrual pain.

Drug Interactions

No special warnings, although all drugs have the ability to interact with other drugs. Report any problems to your doctor or your pharmacist.

Food/Alcohol Interactions

No special warnings.

Pregnancy/Nursing

The vaginal cream form should not be used during the first trimester. Bottle-feed your baby if you must take this drug.

Seniors

No special warnings. Take as prescribed and immediately inform your doctor of any persistent or troublesome side effects.

Warning

Do not use tampons while taking this drug, as they may absorb the medication. To avoid reinfection, your male partner should use a nonlatex condom during intercourse and should consult a doctor if penile itching, burning, or irritation results. The suppository form of this drug may cause erosion of latex condoms or diaphragms. Use another method of birth control to ensure proper protection. Do not use feminine hygiene sprays or douches.

Comments

Wear sanitary napkins or pantiliners to prevent your clothing from being stained. Cotton underwear is recommended; synthetic fabrics do not "breathe" and can delay improvement in your symptoms because moisture encourages yeast growth. Nonprescription medications are available for treatment of yeast infections. However, do not self-medicate unless you have been first diagnosed by a doctor to determine the type of infection. Oral antifungals may be necessary in some cases of candidiasis.

terazosin

*See Hytrin**

terconazole

See Terazol 3

timolol

See Timoptic XE*

Brand Name
Timoptic XE*

Generic Name

timolol

Type of Drug

Ophthalmic beta-blocker. This drug lowers pressure in the eyes and is used to treat some types of glaucoma, a condition that causes damage to the optic nerve and can lead to blindness.

For

Reduction of internal eye pressure in glaucoma.

Availability and Dosage

Eyedrops: 0.25%, 0.5%. Ophthalmic solution-gel: 0.25%, 0.5% Usual dosage is 1 drop once or twice daily. Follow directions for administration, and do not rub eyes afterward. Do not touch the tip of the eyedropper to any surface. Remove contact lenses, including the soft ones, before application.

Side Effects

More common include eye irritation or stinging during application and temporary blurred vision after application. Others include dry eyes, increased sensitivity to light, redness, watering, and inflammation.

Drug Interactions

Interactions may occur with other ophthalmic beta-blockers, oral antidiabetics, antihypertensives, some heart medications, and some antidepressants. Always inform your doctors of every medication you are taking, including nonprescription medicines, vitamins, herbal remedies, and dietary supplements. *Do not take any over-the-counter medications unless approved by your doctor.*

Food/Alcohol Interactions

Avoid alcohol, as it may increase drowsiness.

Pregnancy/Nursing

No special warnings, although all drugs during pregnancy should be avoided if possible. Before taking this drug, discuss with your doctor the benefits versus the potential risks. This drug passes into breast milk. Bottle-feed your baby if you must take this drug.

Seniors

There may be an increased risk of side effects. Take exactly as prescribed and notify your doctor at once of any persistent or troublesome side effects.

Warning

Make sure your doctor has your complete medical history, including a history of low blood sugar, diabetes, emphysema, thyroid disease, asthma, or heart disease. If you experience a slow heartbeat (50 beats per minute or less), call your doctor immediately.

Comments

Do not use these drops while you are wearing contact lenses; wait at least 15 minutes after application before inserting lenses. Your eyes may become especially sensitive to light and glare while using this drug.

tizanidine

See Zanaflex

Brand Name
Tobradex*

Generic Name

tobramycin/dexamethasone

Type of Drug

Antibiotic/corticosteroid combination (ophthalmic).

For

Prevention or treatment of eye infections. Tobramycin treats the infection while dexamethasone suppresses inflammation.

Availability and Dosage

Ophthalmic suspension: 0.1%, 0.3%. Ophthalmic ointment: 0.1%, 0.3%. Follow directions carefully for administering. Do not touch the dropper tip to any surface. Do not rub your eyes after application.

Side Effects

More common include stinging or burning of eyes after application. These should be temporary, but notify your doctor if irritation continues.

Drug Interactions

This drug may interact with other eye medications. Always inform your doctors of every medication you are taking, including nonprescription medicines, vitamins, herbal remedies, and dietary supplements.

Food/Alcohol Interactions

Avoid or limit alcohol.

Pregnancy/Nursing

No special warnings, although all drugs during pregnancy and breast-feeding should be avoided if possible. Before taking this drug, discuss with your doctor the benefits versus the potential risks.

Seniors

No special warnings. Take as prescribed and immediately inform your doctor of any persistent or troublesome side effects.

Warning

This drug may cause temporary blurred vision or other vision disturbances. Do not drive or operate machinery until you know how this medication will affect you. Make sure your doctor knows if you have a history of herpes simplex, conjunctivitis, untreated eye infections, or allergies to antibiotics or steroids.

Comments

You will need to be regularly monitored by a physician and/or an ophthamologist while on this medication. Long-term use can lead to fungal infections of the cornea; glaucoma; optic nerve damage; and other defects in vision.

Brand Name
Tofranil

Generic Name

imipramine hydrochloride

Type of Drug

Tricyclic antidepressant. These drugs increase the levels of nor-epinephrine and serotonin in the brain, may have a mild sedative effect, and generally work to correct a chemical imbalance believed to be the basis for certain types of depression. Your physician will prescribe one of several tricyclics based on your particular symptoms.

For

Depression.

Availability and Dosage

Tablets: 10 mg, 25 mg, 50 mg. Capsules: 75 mg, 100 mg, 125 mg, 150 mg. May be taken with or without food. Taking at bedtime may minimize side effects. Do not take more of this medicine than is prescribed. Do not abruptly stop taking this medication without consulting your doctor.

Side Effects

More common include drowsiness, headache, dry mouth, fatigue, weight gain, dizziness, and nausea. Others include sweating, blurred vision, diarrhea, anxiety, changes in sex drive, breast enlargement, rash, palpitations, and abnormal breast-milk production.

Drug Interactions

The most serious interactions may occur with monoamine oxidase (MAO) inhibitors. Do not take any MAO inhibitor drug within 2 weeks of taking imipramine. Other interactions can occur with sedatives, thyroid drugs, oral contraceptives, narcotic painkillers, carbamazepine, cimetidine, appetite suppressants, amphetamines, methyldopa, promethazine, and any central nervous system (CNS) depressants including diazepam and alprazolam. Always inform your doctors of every medication you are taking, including nonprescription medicines, vitamins, herbal remedies, and dietary supplements. *Do not take any over-the-counter medications unless approved by your doctor.*

Food/Alcohol Interactions

Avoid alcohol.

Pregnancy/Nursing

Not recommended, especially during the first trimester.

Seniors

Older patients may be more susceptible to side effects, including dizziness when standing up quickly and heart arrhythmias. Your doctor may prescribe a low dose.

Warning

Make sure your doctor has your complete medical history, including a history of alcohol or substance abuse, bipolar disorder (manic depression), suicidal thoughts, hypertension, glaucoma, Parkinson's disease, or heart, liver, or kidney disease. Do not take any over-the-counter medications for allergies, colds, or coughs without checking with your doctor. These may contain ingredients that could intensify side effects.

Comments

Tricyclic antidepressants may cause a decrease in sexual drive for women. Drugs in this group generally take 2 to 4 weeks before any improvement is shown, although some symptoms such as insomnia may improve earlier. Tricyclics were much more commonly prescribed before the development of newer antidepressants such as fluoxetine (Prozac). They are often used for other conditions, including migraine, nerve pain, and incontinence in older women.

tolcapone

See Tasmar

Toprol XL*

See Lopressor

tramadol HCl

See Ultram*

tranylcypromine sulfate

See Parnate

Brand Name
Tranxene

Generic Name

clorazepate dipotassium

Type of Drug

Benzodiazepine tranquilizer, antianxiety. Benzodiazepines are central nervous system (CNS) depressants and work on the part of the brain that controls emotion by slowing central-nervous-system transmissions. They are often the drug of choice to relieve the symptoms of anxiety but do not address the underlying cause.

For

Anxiety disorders; anxiety-related insomnia; irritable bowel syndrome (IBS); treatment of alcohol withdrawal.

Availability and Dosage

Tablets: 3.75 mg, 7.5 mg, 15 mg, 22.5 mg. Should be taken on an empty stomach, but may be taken with food to avoid stomach upset. Do not take more of this medicine than is prescribed. Clorazepate has a high risk of physical or psychological dependence. Do not abruptly stop taking this medication without consulting your doctor.

Side Effects

More common include drowsiness, dizziness, and unsteadiness. Others include headache, forgetfulness, confusion, depression, nightmares, constipation, and dry mouth.

Drug Interactions

Clorazepate can interact with other central nervous system (CNS) depressants, tranquilizers, some antidepressants, digoxin, antihistamines, oral contraceptives, levodopa, erythromycin, narcotic painkillers, and cimetidine. Do not take antacids within 1 hour of taking this drug. Always inform your doctors of every medication you are taking, including nonprescription medicines, vitamins, herbal remedies, and dietary supplements. *Do not take any over-the-counter medications unless approved by your doctor.*

Food/Alcohol Interactions

Avoid alcohol, as it may increase the sedative effect of this drug. Avoid grapefruit juice while taking this drug.

Pregnancy/Nursing

Not recommended, especially during the first trimester. Bottle-feed your baby if you must take this drug.

Seniors

Older adults may be more susceptible to side effects, especially if they have impaired kidney function. Your doctor may prescribe a low dose.

Warning

Make sure your doctor has your complete medical history, including a history of alcohol or substance abuse, glaucoma, depression, suicidal thoughts, or kidney, liver, or lung disease. Do not use over-the-counter medicines for allergies, colds, or coughs without consulting your doctor. They may contain ingredients that can interact with clorazepate. You must be regularly monitored while on this drug.

Comments

You will need to be regularly monitored by your physician while on this medication, especially if you are taking it for a prolonged period of time. Women are often prescribed antianxiety agents while the underlying cause remains untreated. If you suspect that your symptoms are being prematurely ascribed to anxiety without a complete medical checkup, get a second opinion.

trazodone*

See Desyrel

tretinoin

See Retin-A*

Tri-Levlen

See Oral Contraceptives

Tri-Norinyl

See Oral Contraceptives

triamcinolone acetonide

See Azmacort Aerosol*

triamterine and hydrochlorothiazide (HCTZ)

*See Dyazide**

triazolam

See Halcion

trimethoprim and sulfamethoxazole

See Bactrim

Trimox*

*See Amoxil**

Triphasil*

See Oral Contraceptives

Brand Name
Tylenol with Codeine

Generic Name

acetaminophen and codeine phosphate*

Type of Drug

Narcotic/analgesic combination.

For

Relief of moderate to severe pain.

Availability and Dosage

Tablets: 300 mg acetaminophen with 7.5 mg, 15 mg, 30 mg, or 60 mg codeine; 325 mg acetaminophen with 30 mg or 60 mg codeine; 650 mg acetaminophen with 30 mg codeine. Caplets: 325 mg acetaminophen with 15 mg, 30 mg, or 60 mg codeine. Oral solution: 120 mg acetaminophen and 12 mg codeine per 5 ml, with 7% alcohol. May be taken with or without food. Do not take more of this medicine than is prescribed. Codeine has a high risk of physical and psychological dependence.

Side Effects

More common include drowsiness, dizziness, and constipation. Others include nausea, dry mouth, and itching.

Drug Interactions

This combination can interact with other narcotics, tranquilizers, anticoagulants (blood thinners), cimetidine, some anticonvulsants, some antihistamines, oral antidiabetics, some antidepressants, and muscle relaxants. Always inform your doctors of every medication you are taking, including nonprescription medicines, vitamins, herbal remedies, and dietary supplements. *Do not take any over-the-counter medications unless approved by your doctor.*

Food/Alcohol Interactions

Avoid alcohol, as it can increase the sedative effect and can also cause liver damage. Tell your doctor if you routinely drink more than 3 alcoholic beverages a day.

Pregnancy/Nursing

Not recommended. Bottle-feed your baby if you must take this drug.

Seniors

Older adults should use this drug with caution, due to increased susceptibility to side effects. Your doctor may prescribe a low dose.

Warning

Potentially life-threatening interactions can occur when this drug is taken with monoamine oxidase (MAO) inhibitor antidepressants. Do not take this drug within 14 days of taking an MAO inhibitor. Make sure your doctor has your complete medical history, including a history of alcohol or substance abuse, seizures, constipation, gallbladder disease, asthma, any blood disorder, or heart, kidney, liver, or lung disease. Do not drive or operate machinery until you know how this drug will affect you. If you experience anxiety, difficulty in breathing, palpitations, weakness, or jaundice, contact your doctor immediately.

Comments

Do not take over-the-counter products containing acetaminophen while you are taking this medication. Always check ingredient labels. There are numerous versions of acetaminophen (Tylenol) that can be used safely when self-medicating for mild to moderate pain, including pain from osteoarthritis. (Narcotics are controlled substances and are not available over-the-counter.) Availability ranges from regular-strength (325 mg) to extra-strength (500 mg) in tablet, capsule, caplet, and gelcap forms. Follow package directions carefully and notify your doctor if pain or symptoms persist. A 5-year Johns Hopkins study of more than 500 women indicates that OTC acetaminophen (Tylenol) may reduce the risk of ovarian cancer, although researchers have not yet discovered how the drug works in these cases.

Tylox

See Percocet

Brand Name
Ultram*

Generic Name
tramadol hydrochloride

Type of Drug
Analgesic.

For
Relief of mild to moderate pain.

Availability and Dosage
Tablets: 50 mg. May be taken with or without food. Do not increase your dosage without your doctor's approval.

Side Effects
More common include dizziness, nausea, constipation, drowsiness, dry mouth, and loss of appetite. Others include anxiety, heart arrhythmia, mood changes, changes in frequency of urination, and menopausal symptoms.

Drug Interactions
Interactions may occur with anticonvulsants, diazepam, monoamine oxidase (MAO) inhibitors, and some antidepressants and psychiatric drugs. Always inform your doctors of every medication you are taking, including nonprescription medicines, vitamins, herbal remedies, and dietary supplements.

Food/Alcohol Interactions

Avoid alcohol.

Pregnancy/Nursing

Not recommended. Bottle-feed your baby if you must take this drug.

Seniors

Adults age 75 and older may be more sensitive to this medication. Your doctor may start you on a low dose. Take as prescribed and immediately inform your doctor of any persistent or troublesome side effects.

Warning

This drug has been known to cause seizures in certain patients, particularly when used in combination with other drugs. Tell your doctor if you have a history of seizures, head injury, or lung, kidney, or liver disease. The most serious side effects are difficulty in breathing, chest pains, disorientation, and hallucinations. *Seek emergency medical treatment immediately.*

Comments

Tramadol is used for a wide range of pain relief, including postsurgical pain of hysterectomy or C-sections, chronic pain, and lower-back pain. Use caution when driving or operating machinery until you know how this drug will affect your mental alertness. Tramadol has a high incidence of drug dependency. Tell your doctor of any history of alcohol or drug abuse.

Brand Name
Urispas

Generic Name

flavoxate hydrochloride

Type of Drug

Antispasmodic.

For

Urinary tract spasms; relief of painful and frequent urination; pubic area pain.

Availability and Dosage

Tablets: 100 mg. This drug is more effective when taken 30 minutes before meals, but may be taken with food if stomach upset occurs.

Side Effects

More common include dry mouth, nausea, drowsiness, dizziness, nervousness, and blurred vision. Others include difficulty in concentrating, abdominal pain, heart arrhythmia, and constipation. Some side effects may subside as your body adjusts to the medication.

Drug Interactions

This drug may interact with blood-pressure–lowering medications and certain antidepressants. Always inform your doctors of every medication you are taking, including nonprescription medicines, vitamins, herbal remedies, and dietary supplements.

Food/Alcohol Interactions

No special warnings.

Pregnancy/Nursing

No special warnings, although all drugs during pregnancy and breast-feeding should be avoided if possible. Before taking this drug, discuss with your doctor the benefits versus the potential risks. This drug may pass into breast milk. You may want to bottle-feed your baby while on this medication.

Seniors

This drug has a higher risk of side effects, especially mental confusion, in older adults. Notify your doctor immediately of any persistent or severe side effects.

Warning

Flavoxate can cause drowsiness or blurred vision. Use caution when driving, operating machinery, or performing any tasks that require mental alertness until you know how this drug affects you. Also avoid strenuous activity, as flavoxate reduces the ability to sweat and can increase your risk of heatstroke. If you develop a rash, rapid pulse, or fever, notify your doctor immediately.

Comments

Flavoxate works by relaxing urinary-tract muscles, preventing or reducing painful spasms. Tell your doctor if you have a history of stomach or intestinal problems, or urinary-track blockage, or if you have glaucoma.

ursodiol USP

See Actigall

valacyclovir, HCl

See **Valtrex**

Brand Name

Valium

Generic Name

diazepam*

Type of Drug

Benzodiazepine tranquilizer; central nervous system (CNS) depressant. These drugs work on the part of the brain that controls emotion by slowing the nervous-system transmissions. They are often the drugs of choice to relieve the symptoms of anxiety but do not address the underlying cause. A large class of drugs, benzodiazepines are also used as sedatives and muscle relaxants.

For

Anxiety disorders; panic attacks; muscle spasms; tremors; insomnia.

Availability and Dosage

Tablets: 2 mg, 5 mg, 10 mg. Sustained-release capsules: 15 mg. May be taken with or without food. Do not take more of this medicine than is prescribed. Do not abruptly stop taking this drug without consulting your doctor.

Side Effects

More common include drowsiness, fatigue, dizziness or light-headedness, and slurred speech. Others include headache, blurred vision, changes in sex drive, nausea, forgetfulness, confusion, changes in urinary habits, and loss of coordination.

Drug Interactions

Diazepam has the ability to interact with a wide variety of drugs, including anticonvulsants, antihistamines, tricyclic antidepressants, monoamine oxidase (MAO) inhibitor antidepressants, selective serotonin reuptake inhibitor (SSRI) antidepressants, fluoxetine, digoxin, narcotic pain relievers, cimetidine, levodopa, oral contraceptives, tranquilizers, other benzodiazepines, and any drug that acts as a CNS depressant. Always inform your doctors of every medication you are taking, including nonprescription medicines, vitamins, herbal remedies, and dietary supplements. *Do not take any over-the-counter medications unless approved by your doctor.*

Food/Alcohol Interactions

Avoid alchohol, as it can increase the sedative effect.

Pregnancy/Nursing

Not recommended. Diazepam passes into breast milk. Bottle-feed your baby if you must take this drug.

Seniors

Elderly patients have an increased risk of adverse effects, particularly oversedation. Your doctor will usually prescribe the lowest possible effective dose of this drug. Take exactly as prescribed and notify your doctor of any persistent or troublesome side effects.

Warning

Benzodiazepines have a high risk of physical and psychological dependence. While taking this drug, you will need to be monitored by a physician who should reassess your treatment on a regular basis. Make sure your doctor knows your complete medical history, especially a history of alcohol or other substance abuse, depression, psychosis, suicidal thoughts, sleep apnea, stroke, or kidney or liver disease. This drug can impair your ability to drive, operate machinery, or perform tasks requiring mental alertness. Do not drive until you know how this medication will affect you.

Comments

Women of all ages are often prescribed drugs to control symptoms of anxiety and panic disorder without receiving counseling or addressing the underlying cause, but older women appear to be more vulnerable. One study involving 13,000 women age 60 and older taking psychoactive drugs during a 6-month period found that half of the prescriptions for sleeping pills and tranquilizers either 1) should not have been given at all or 2) should have been prescribed for shorter periods of time. In 1999, Columbia University's National Center on Addiction and Substance Abuse in New York reported that of the more than 25 million American women over age 60, an estimated 2.8 million abuse diazepam and other psychiatric drugs.

valsartan

See Diovan*

Brand Name
Valtrex

Generic Name

valacyclovir HCL

Type of Drug

Antiviral.

For

Treatment of symptoms of herpes zoster (shingles) and treatment or suppression of genital herpes.

Availability and Dosage

Caplets: 500 mg. May be taken with or without food. Dosages for herpes zoster (shingles) are different from those for herpes simplex (genital herpes). Take the full course of treatment prescribed even if you begin to feel better. Drink plenty of water while on this medication.

Side Effects

More common include nausea, headache, vomiting, and diarrhea. Others include constipation, dizziness, abdominal pain, anorexia, rash, agitation, and confusion.

Drug Interactions

Valacyclovir may interact with prescription and over-the-counter antacids. This drug may also interact with zidovudine (AZT) and cause extreme drowsiness. Always inform your doctors of every medication you are taking, including nonprescription medicines, vitamins, herbal remedies, and dietary supplements.

Food/Alcohol Interactions

No special warnings.

Pregnancy/Nursing

No special warnings, although all drugs during pregnancy and breast-feeding should be avoided if possible. Before taking this drug, discuss with your doctor the benefits versus the potential risks.

Seniors

Older adults who have reduced kidney function may be started on a low dose of this drug.

Warning

This drug does not cure herpes, nor does it prevent the spread of infection. Genital herpes is spread by sexual contact, especially when there are sores or blisters on the vulva, the vaginal or anal area, or when a pelvic exam has discovered sores on the cervix. But herpes can also be transmitted even when there are no sores visible. Viral particles may be shedding on the skin that may not be easily detected. The use of condoms by your partner is recommended at all times. Genital herpes can be transmitted to a newborn and increase his or her risk of brain damage and blindness. If you know or suspect you have herpes, make sure that you tell your ob/gyn. This drug should be used with extreme caution in patients who have kidney disease, are infected with HIV, or are taking immunosuppressant drugs such as those used after an organ transplant.

Comments

There is no known cure for genital herpes, although patients now have better treatment options for this viral disease. Valacyclovir has been shown to work as well as acyclovir and in a shorter period of time. It is important that women who have genital herpes have annual Pap smears; some evidence suggests that the disease increases a woman's risk of cervical cancer.

Brand Name

Vancenase AQ Nasal Spray (also Vancenase AQ DS*, Beconase AQ, Vanceril Inhaler)

Generic Name

beclomethasone

Type of Drug

Corticosteroid nasal spray; corticosteroid inhalation aerosol. These drugs work by reducing nasal-passage inflammation. In allergic rhinitis it decreases the allergic response to allergens. In asthmatic patients, it reduces inflammation of the lining of the airways.

For

Nasal inflammation; relief of hay fever symptoms; prevention of nasal polyps after surgical removal; bronchial asthma (not to be used for acute asthma).

Availability and Dosage

(Vancenase AQ) Nasal Spray: 0.042 mg per spray. (Vancenase AQ DS) Nasal Spray: 0.084 mg per spray. (Beconase AQ): 0.042 mg per spray. (Vanceril): 0.042 mg per inhalation. (Vanceril Double Strength): 0.08 mg per inhalation. Dosages will vary depending on the condition being treated. Nasal inhaler: 1 or 2 inhalations in each nostril, 1 or 2 times a day. Oral inhalation: 2 inhalations, 3 or 4 times a day. People who have severe asthma may be directed to use the inhalation form more frequently. All forms of this drug include specific instructions for use and administration; if you have questions, consult your doctor or your pharmacist. Do not take more of this medicine than is prescribed.

Side Effects

More common (nasal spray) include nosebleed, nasal irritation or burning, sore throat, and headache. More common (inhalation aerosol) include white patches in mouth or throat, sore throat, and hoarseness.

Drug Interactions

Few interactions have been reported with this medication. Inform your doctor if you are taking oral corticosteroids (including other inhalation forms of corticosteroid) or any drugs that suppress the immune system.

Food/Alcohol Interactions

No special warnings.

Pregnancy/Nursing

No special warnings, although all drugs during pregnancy and breast-feeding should be avoided if possible. Before taking this drug, discuss with your doctor the benefits versus the potential risks. Beclomethasone passes into breast milk. Bottle-feed your baby if you must take this drug.

Seniors

No special warnings. Take as prescribed and immediately inform your doctor of any persistent or troublesome side effects.

Warning

Some inhaled corticosteroids can result in yeast infections of the mouth or throat. To reduce this risk, gargle with plain water after each use. Make sure your doctor knows if you have a history of tuberculosis, diabetes, glaucoma, any infection of the nose, sinuses, throat, or lungs, herpes infections, or kidney or liver disease.

Comments

It may take up to 3 weeks before you receive the maximum benefits of this medication, but it usually starts to work within 1 week. Beclomethasone is prescribed to reduce the frequency and severity of asthma attacks, but it will not relieve symptoms once an attack has begun.

Vanceril Inhaler

See Vancenase AQ

Brand Name

Vasotec*

Generic Name

enalapril maleate

Type of Drug

Angiotensin-converting enzyme (ACE) inhibitors. ACE inhibitors are antihypertensives used to treat high blood pressure (hypertension). They work by blocking an enzyme in the body that is required to produce a substance that causes blood vessels to tighten. When this enzyme is blocked, blood vessels are relaxed, blood pressure is lowered, the workload of the heart and arteries is reduced, and blood and oxygen supplies are increased. ACE inhibitors do not cure hypertension; they control it for as long as the medication is taken. Controlling high blood pressure may reduce the risk of heart attack, stroke, and kidney failure.

For

High blood pressure; congestive heart failure; diabetic kidney disease.

Availability and Dosage

Tablets: 2.5 mg, 5 mg, 10 mg, 20 mg. Should be taken on an empty stomach, 1 hour before or 2 hours after meals. Do not abruptly stop taking this drug, as doing so can cause serious reactions. Your doctor will need to gradually decrease your dose.

Side Effects

A side effect that appears to occur more frequently in women is a dry, hacking cough. More common include fatigue, dizziness, nausea, and headache. Some side effects may diminish as your body adjusts to the drug. Others include chest pain, diarrhea, bronchitis, rash, tingling in the hands, feet, or around the mouth, and vivid dreams. A serious side effect, called angioedema, occurs in about 1 in 200 people who take enalapril. Severe swelling of the tongue and lips occurs, which is treated with steroids and antihistamines. This condition is life-threatening.

Drug interaction

ACE inhibitors have the potential to interact with many types of drugs including potassium-sparing diuretics, potassium supplements, beta-blockers, antihypertensives, lithium, anticoagulants (blood thinners), some tranquilizers, allopurinol, digoxin, and antiinflammatories including nonsteroidal antiinflammatory drugs (NSAIDs). Always inform your doctors of every medication you are taking, including nonprescription medicines, vitamins, herbal remedies, and dietary supplements. *Do not take any over-the-counter medications unless approved by your doctor.*

Food/Alcohol Interactions

Avoid alcohol. Do not use salt substitutes. Your doctor may advise you to restrict foods high in potassium, such as bananas, citrus fruits, and low-sodium milk.

Pregnancy/Nursing

Not recommended, especially during the second and third trimesters. Birth defects and fetal death may result. This drug passes into breast milk. Bottle-feed your baby if you must take this drug.

Seniors

Elderly patients may be more susceptible to side effects. Your doctor may prescribe a low dose, especially if kidney or liver function is impaired.

Warning

Many over-the-counter products contain potassium. Always read ingredient labels and do not take any nonprescription medications while on this drug. If you experience rapid or irregular heartbeats, sore throat, fever, severe vomiting or diarrhea, or excessive sweating, notify your doctor immediately.

Comments

ACE inhibitors are among the most commonly prescribed drugs for hypertension, which is referred to as the "silent killer" because there are often no symptoms. Untreated hypertension can lead to stroke, which affects more women than men—and the risk increases with each decade after age 35. Statistics indicate that African American women are at higher risk than are white women. A woman can decrease her risk of stroke and heart attack by making lifestyle changes—quit smoking, get sufficient aerobic exercise, start a low-fat diet, and take medications if necessary, including hormone-replacement therapy that may possibly protect the heart after menopause.

Brand Name
Veetids*

Generic Name
penicillin VK*

Type of Drug
Antibiotic (penicillin). This large class of drugs are among the most commonly prescribed. Your doctor will prescribe the correct antibiotic depending on the type of infection. Antibiotics are useless against viral infections such as colds and flu.

For
Various bacterial infections including those of the respiratory tract; "strep" throat; pneumonia; urinary-tract infections (UTIs).

Availability and Dosage
Tablets: 250 mg, 500 mg. Oral solution: 125 mg and 250 mg per 5 ml. Should be taken with a full glass of water on an empty stomach, 1 hour before or 2 hours after meals. It is essential to take the full course of treatment prescribed, even if your condition appears to be improving.

Side Effects
More common include nausea, upset stomach, diarrhea, and fungal infections. Others include white patches in the mouth, weakness, vaginal discharge and irritation, loss of appetite, itching, and rash.

Drug Interactions

Penicillin has the potential to interact with a wide variety of medications, including some oral contraceptives, diuretics, anticoagulants (blood thinners), nonsteroidal antiinflammatory drugs (NSAIDs), erythromycin, methotrexate, ACE inhibitors, and beta-blockers. Always inform your doctors of every medication you are taking, including nonprescription medicines, vitamins, herbal remedies, and dietary supplements. *Do not take any over-the-counter medications unless approved by your doctor.*

Food/Alcohol Interactions

Foods and beverages that have a high acid content may reduce the effectiveness of this drug. Your doctor or your pharmacist can provide you with a list of these. There are no special alcohol warnings.

Pregnancy/Nursing

No special warnings, although all drugs during pregnancy and breast-feeding should be avoided if possible. Before taking this drug, discuss with your doctor the benefits versus the potential risks.

Seniors

No special warnings. Take as prescribed and immediately inform your doctor of any persistent or troublesome side effects.

Warning

Penicillin antibiotics may interfere with the effectiveness of oral contraceptives containing estrogen. Unplanned pregnancies have resulted from this combination. You should use an additional method of birth control during your course of penicillin treatment. Penicillin allergies can be serious and sometimes fatal, although this occurs more frequently with the injectable form of the drug. Symptoms of penicillin allergy include difficulty in breathing, low blood pressure, skin blistering, swelling of the face or neck, and severe or watery diarrhea. *If you experience any of these, seek emergency medical treatment.*

Comments

Almost every office visit or prehospitalization examination includes the question, "Are you allergic to penicillin?" Penicillin allergies occur in up to 10% of people who take them. If you have a history of sensitivity to penicillin and/or cephalosporin antibiotics, asthma, hives, hay fever, or eczema, make sure this is noted in all of your medical records. You may wish to wear a medical identification tag and carry an ID card that lists this allergy along with all the medications you are currently taking.

venlafaxine

See Effexor*

Ventolin

See Proventil

verapamil SR

See Calan SR

Verelan

See Calan SR

Brand Name
Viagra*

Generic Name
sildenafil citrate

Type of Drug
Sexual stimulant.

For
Male erectile dysfunction (impotence). Viagra has not yet been approved for use by women, but some doctors are prescribing it at the request of their female patients. Some women are using their male partners' prescriptions. The side effects, drug interactions, and warning information in this profile pertains to men only, based on clinical trials and actual use.

Availability and Dosage
Tablets: 25 mg, 50 mg, 100 mg. Should be taken no more than once a day, 1 to 4 hours before sexual intercourse, depending on physician's instructions.

Side Effects
More common include headache, skin flushing, indigestion,

nasal congestion, urinary-tract infections (UTIs), diarrhea, and changes in vision including perceiving colors differently.

Drug Interactions

Sildenafil citrate may interact with erythromycin, antifungals such as itraconazole and ketaconazole, cimetidine, other medications for impotence, and nitroglycerin.

Food/Alcohol Interactions

No special warnings.

Pregnancy/Nursing

The effects of sildenafil citrate on fetal development are unknown. Do not use this drug if you are or plan to become pregnant or if you are breast-feeding.

Seniors

Older men may be more susceptible to side effects and are usually started at a low dose, which is increased as necessary by their doctors.

Warning

If your male partner is using Viagra, and you are in the same age bracket as 80% of the men who take it (50 and older), you may need a lubricant (e.g., Replens or Astroglide, both available over-the-counter) to minimize the effects of vaginal dryness and painful intercourse. The *New England Journal of Medicine* reported a significant increase in urinary-tract infections (UTIs) among the wives of Viagra users. The FDA has reports of at least 130 male deaths—most of them by heart attack—although a definitive link to Viagra has not been determined. This drug may be unsafe for use in patients who have a recent history of heart disease or stroke.

Comments

Viagra is on its way to becoming one of the most-prescribed new drugs. In the 6 months following its release in early 1998, 200,000 prescriptions were filled every week. Some women are not waiting for the drug to go through appropriate testing procedures to see if it improves common symptoms of female sexual dysfunction: decreased sex drive, vaginal dryness, and difficulty in achieving orgasm. Because the drug is FDA approved, doctors can prescribe it "off-label" for women, although some experts question its use in patients where safety and efficacy have not been established. Also, pharmacists may refuse to fill the prescriptions, and insurance companies are not likely to cover the $10-per-pill cost. Pilot studies are under way (including those by the American Foundation for Urological Diseases, Johns Hopkins University, and the pill's manufacturer, among others) to determine the effects of the drug in postmenopausal women. If you decide to use this drug, tell your doctor of any side effects you experience.

Vibramycin

See Doryx

Brand Name
Vicodin (also Vicodin-ES, Lorcet, Lortab, Norcet, Panacet, Zydone)

Generic Name

acetaminophen and hydrocodone bitartrate

Type of Drug

Narcotic/analgesic combination.

For

Relief of mild to moderate pain.

Availability and Dosage

These drugs come in varying strengths, including: Tablets: 500 mg acetaminophen with 2.5 mg, 5 mg, or 7.5 mg hydrocodone; 650 mg acetaminophen with 7.5 hydrocodone; 750 mg acetaminophen with 7.5 mg hydrocodone. Capsules: 500 mg acetaminophen with 5 mg hydrocodone. May be taken with or without food. Do not take more of this medicine than is prescribed.

Side Effects

More common include dizziness, nausea, vomiting, drowsiness, loss of appetite, and constipation. Others include weakness, headache, flushing, false sense of well-being, and stomach pain.

Drug Interactions

This drug may interact with central nervous system (CNS) depressants, some anticonvulsants, muscle relaxants, tranquilizers, benzodiazepines, tricyclic antidepressants, monoamine oxidase (MAO) inhibitor antidepressants, antihistamines, and anticoagulants (blood thinners). Do not take other medications containing acetaminophen, while you are on this drug. Always inform your doctors of every medication you are taking, including nonprescription medicines, vitamins, herbal remedies, and dietary supplements. *Do not take any over-the-counter medications unless approved by your doctor.*

Food/Alcohol Interactions

Avoid alcohol.

Pregnancy/Nursing

Not recommended.

Seniors

Elderly patients are at an increased risk for adverse side effects from the narcotic portion of this drug. Your doctor may start you on a low dose.

Warning

Do not take this drug within 14 days of taking a monoamine oxidase (MAO) inhibitor antidepressant (e.g., phenelzine, tranylcypromine) as serious interactions may result. Do not drive, operate machinery, or engage in any tasks requiring mental alertness until you know how this drug will affect you.

Comments

This combination drug is used for pain that does not respond to nonprescription pain relievers. Hydrocodone has a high risk of physical and psychological dependence. Make sure your doctor knows your complete medical history, including a history of alcohol or other substance abuse, head injury, or kidney or liver disease. Use caution when taking any over-the-counter products; they may contain acetaminophen, which could lead to an overdose when taken with this drug.

Brand Name
Vioxx

Generic Name

rofecoxib

Type of Drug

Nonsteroidal anti-inflammatory drug (NSAID). This drug differs from other NSAIDs in that scientists believe that it inhibits an enzyme called COX-2, which plays a role in pain and inflammation, while not inhibiting the COX-1 enzyme, which helps maintain normal stomach lining. Rofecoxib does not slow or halt the progress of arthritis.

For

Pain and inflammation of osteoarthritis; menstrual pain.

Availability and Dosage

Tablets: 12.5 mg, 25 mg. Oral suspension: 12.5 mg per 5 ml, 25 mg per 5 ml. To minimize stomach upset, take with food.

Side Effects

More common include diarrhea, headache, and heartburn. Others include sore throat, back pain, gas, and dizziness.

Drug Interactions

Rofecoxib can interact with angiotensin-converting-enzyme (ACE) inhibitors, anticoagulants (blood thinners), cyclosporine, fluconazole, other NSAIDs, diuretics, methotrexate, and lithium. Always inform your doctors of every medication you are taking, including nonprescription medicines, vitamins, herbal remedies, and dietary supplements. *Do not take any over-the-counter medications unless approved by your doctor.*

Food/Alcohol Interactions

Avoid or limit alcohol; it may aggravate stomach irritation.

Pregnancy/Nursing

Not recommended, especially during the last trimester. Discuss with your doctor the benefits versus the potential risks. It is not known whether rofecoxib passes into breast milk. Bottle-feed your baby if you must take this drug.

Seniors

Older patients may be more susceptible to side effects. Your doctor may prescribe a low dose.

Warning

Do not use rofecoxib if you have had an allergic reaction to aspirin or other NSAIDs. Although rofecoxib has a low potential for stomach ulcers, serious gastrointestinal ulcerations can occur without warning. Notify your doctor of any burning stomach pain, black or tarry stools, or vomiting.

Comments

Rofecoxib is one of the new class of "super-aspirins," designed to reduce pain and inflammation of osteoarthritis and other conditions. Almost 40 million Americans have some form of arthritis, 23 million of them women. Osteoarthritis is the breakdown of joint cartilage leading to pain and loss of movement; it affects nearly 12 million women which represent 74 percent of all cases. Ongoing research on this debilitating disease and other autoimmune disorders is focused on identifying genetic markers, with the hope of anticipating possible "triggers" that cause one person to develop the disease while leaving a similarly predisposed individual untouched.

warfarin

See Coumadin*

Brand Name
Wellbutrin (also Wellbutrin SR*)

Generic Name

bupropion hydrochloride

Type of drug

Antidepressant. This drug does not fall into the category of other antidepressants and is usually not prescribed until other types have failed to result in successful treatment.

For

Depression; smoking cessation.

Availability and Dosage

(Wellbutrin) Tablets: 75 mg, 100 mg. (Wellbutrin SR) Extended-release tablets: 50 mg, 100 mg, 150 mg. May be taken with or without food, but should probably not be taken at bedtime to reduce the risk of insomnia. Follow directions carefully when taking this medication, as the doses should be evenly spaced to reduce the risk of seizures. It may take up to 4 weeks before you see the effects of this medication.

Side Effects

More common include nausea, dry mouth, trembling, constipation, loss of appetite, diarrhea, fatigue, and dizziness. Others include difficulty in concentrating, vision changes, mood changes or hostile behavior, and drowsiness.

Drug Interactions

Bupropion has the potential to interact with many other medications, including some anticonvulsants, cimetidine, levodopa, tricyclic antidepressants, lithium, and some tranquilizers. Extra caution should be used with any monoamine oxidase (MAO) inhibitor antidepressant. Allow at least 14 days between stopping an MAO inhibitor and starting bupropion. Always inform your doctors of every medication you are taking, including nonprescription medicines, vitamins, herbal remedies, and dietary supplements. *Do not take any over-the-counter medications unless approved by your doctor.*

Food/Alcohol Interactions

Avoid alcohol. If you are a chronic drinker, you may need to gradually reduce your alcohol intake before starting this drug.

Pregnancy/Nursing

Not recommended. Bottle-feed your baby if you must take this drug.

Seniors

Older adults may have an increased risk of side effects, especially when rising abruptly from a sitting or reclining position. Your doctor may start you on a low dose.

Warning

Do not stop taking this drug without consulting your doctor. Abrupt withdrawal may result in serious side effects. If you experience movement disorders, rash, hallucinations, difficulty in breathing, or seizures, *seek emergency medical treatment immediately.*

Comments

Although initially developed and marketed as an antidepressant, bupropion is also marketed as a nonnicotine aid to smoking cessation (see Zyban). You will need to be regularly monitored by your doctor while on this drug.

Wymox

*See Amoxil**

Brand Name
Xalatan*

Generic Name
latanoprost

Type of Drug
Antiglaucoma; prostaglandin.

For
Glaucoma.

Availability and Dosage
Ophthalmic solution (eyedrops): 0.0005% strength. Usual dosage is 1 drop in each eye once daily. Not for internal use. Follow directions for applying the solution to your eyes. Wash your hands before use, and do not touch the dropper to your eye, finger, or any other surface. Remove contact lenses before applying, and wait at least 15 minutes before inserting contact lenses after treatment.

Side Effects
More common include burning and stinging of the eye, blurred vision, changes in eye color, dry eyes, and brown pigmentation of the iris. Others include increased tearing and eyelid pain. You may wish to wear dark glasses if this drug causes your eyes to become especially sensitive to light.

Drug Interactions
Latanoprost can interact with other eyedrops. Tell your ophthalmologist about any other solutions or ointments you are using in your eyes while on this medication, including over-the-counter eye products.

Food/Alcohol Interactions
No special warnings.

Pregnancy/Nursing
No special warnings, although all drugs during pregnancy and breast-feeding should be avoided if possible. Latanoprost may pass into breast milk. Before taking this drug, discuss with your doctor the benefits versus the potential risks.

Seniors

No special warnings. Take as prescribed and immediately inform your doctor of any persistent or troublesome side effects.

Warning

Serious side effects of this medication are rare, but any drug can cause an allergic reaction in people sensitive to it. If you have inflamed eyelids, eye discharge, skin rash or blistering, chest pain, or difficulty in breathing, contact your doctor immediately.

Comments

Glaucoma can come from a number of sources, including fluid pressure and poor blood flow to the eye. It causes progressive damage to the optic nerve. Latanoprost helps to reduce pressure in the eye. According to the World Health Organization, glaucoma is one of the leading causes of blindness in people over age 40. Other risk factors are family history and being of African descent. More than 7 million people worldwide are treated for glaucoma each year.

Brand Name
Xanax*

Generic Name

alprazolam*

Type of Drug

Benzodiazepine tranquilizer, antianxiety. Benzodiazepines are central nervous system (CNS) depressants and work on the part of the brain that controls emotion by slowing nervous-system transmissions. They are often the drug of choice to relieve the symptoms of anxiety but do not address the underlying cause.

For

Anxiety and anxiety disorders; tension; panic disorder; irritable bowel syndrome; depression; premenstrual syndrome (PMS).

Availability and Dosage

Tablets: 0.25 mg, 0.5 mg, 1 mg, 2 mg. May be taken with or without food. Do not take more of this drug than is prescribed. Alprazolam has a high potential for physical and psychological dependence. Do not abruptly stop taking this medicine without consulting your doctor. Your dose will need to be gradually reduced to avoid severe side effects.

Side Effects

More common include daytime drowsiness, weakness, dizziness, light-headedness, clumsiness, slurred speech, and headache. Others include strange dreams, fluid retention, fatigue, memory loss, changes in sex drive, constipation, and nausea. Notify your doctor immediately of any persistent or severe side effects while you are taking this drug.

Drug Interactions

Alprazolam has the potential to interact with a wide variety of medications, including antihistamines, anticonvulsants, cimetidine, erythromycin, levodopa, digoxin, oral contaceptives or other hormone drugs, other CNS depressants including diazepam, and any supplements that contain kava. Take antacids at least 1 hour before or after taking this drug. Always inform your doctors of every medication you are taking, including nonprescription medicines, vitamins, herbal remedies, and dietary supplements. *Do not take any over-the-counter medications unless approved by your doctor.*

Food/Alcohol Interactions

Avoid alcohol.

Pregnancy/Nursing

Not recommended. Increased risk of damage to the fetus, including respiratory problems and muscle weakness. Alprazolam passes into breast milk. Bottle-feeding your baby is recommended.

Seniors

Older adults have a higher risk of side effects, particularly drowsiness or dizziness. Your doctor may initially recommend a low dose.

Warning

Be sure to tell your doctor if you have a history of drug or alcohol dependence, depression or suicidal thoughts, asthma, narrow-angle glaucoma, sleep apnea, or kidney or liver disease. Use caution when driving, operating machinery, or performing tasks that require mental alertness until you know how this drug will affect you. Combining this drug with supplements that contain kava may result in intensified CNS-depressant effect.

Comments

You will need to be regularly monitored by your physician while on this medication, especially if you are taking it for a prolonged period of time. Women are often prescribed antianxiety agents while the underlying cause remains untreated. If you suspect that your symptoms are being prematurely ascribed to anxiety without a complete medical checkup, get a second opinion.

Brand Name
Xeloda

Generic Name

capecitabine

Type of Drug

Anticancer (antineoplastic).

For

Breast cancer. One of the newer anticancer drugs, this chemotherapy is usually prescribed when other therapies have not produced the desired results. Studies have shown that it can help shrink tumors significantly in some cases of advanced (metastatic) breast cancer.

Availability and Dosage

Tablets: 150 mg, 500 mg. Usually taken within 30 minutes after a meal. Follow your oncologist's instructions for dosage and timing.

Side Effects

More common include weakness, headache, constipation, indigestion, mild nausea, abdominal pain, dehydration, dry skin, drowsiness, fatigue, and general malaise. Report any side effects to your oncologist as soon as possible.

Drug Interactions

All drugs have the capacity to interact with other drugs. Capecitabine has few drug interactions but can be affected by anticoagulants (blood thinners) and aluminum hydroxide or magnesium hydroxide (e.g., Maalox). Always inform your doctors of every medication you are taking, including nonprescription medicines, vitamins, herbal remedies, and dietary supplements. *Do not take any over-the-counter medications unless approved by your doctor.*

Food/Alcohol Interactions

No special warnings.

Pregnancy/Nursing

Not recommended. Notify your doctor immediately if you think you have become pregnant while taking this drug. Capecitabine may pass into breast milk.

Seniors

Older adults may be more susceptible to gastrointestinal side effects, particularly those who are 80 and older.

Warning

A potentially serious side effect is a fever higher than 100.5. Stop taking this drug and notify your oncologist immediately. Other serious side effects include severe diarrhea, vomiting, pain, swelling in the mouth and throat, and "hand-foot syndrome," in which extremities become irritated, numb, and occasionally suffer extensive nerve damage.

Comments

Capecitabine usage needs to be closely monitored by your oncologist. Certain types of chemotherapy may cause premature menopause (technically defined as menopause occurring before age 40). You will need regular blood tests while taking this drug. Preliminary studies showed that capecitabine was generally much better tolerated and more successful in certain patients who had exhausted other options. It does not cure breast cancer but has been shown to slow the spread of this deadly disease, which claims the lives of more than 44,000 women each year.

Brand Name
Xenical

Generic Name

orlistat

Type of Drug

Lipase inhibitor (fat blocker).

For

Obesity management; weight loss. This drug is for people who are at least 30% overweight or have a body mass index (BMI) of

30 or above, to be used in conjunction with a mildly reduced-calorie, low-fat diet and appropriate exercise program.

Availability and Dosage

Capsules: 120 mg. Usual dose is 3 times a day during or after meals that contain no more than 30% fat. The drug attaches itself to the enzymes in your intestinal tract, called lipases, and keeps them from breaking down some of the fat you have eaten. The undigested fat cannot be absorbed and is eliminated.

Side Effects

More common include changes in bowel habits such as oily spotting, flatulence with discharge, oily or fatty stools, increased urgency and frequency, and fecal incontinence.

Drug Interactions

Orlistat can interact with other weight-loss medications and some cyclosporine antibiotics. Always inform your doctors of every medication you are taking, including nonprescription medicines, vitamins, herbal remedies, and dietary supplements. *Do not take any over-the-counter medications unless approved by your doctor.*

Food/Alcohol Interactions

No alcohol warnings. If you take orlistat with a meal that contains more than 30% fat, unpleasant side effects are more likely to occur. Orlistat can interfere with the absorption of some fat-soluble vitamins, including D, E, K, and beta-carotene. Take your vitamins at least 2 hours before or after taking orlistat.

Pregnancy/Nursing

Not recommended.

Seniors

No special warnings. Take as prescribed and immediately inform your doctor of any persistent or troublesome side effects.

Warning

This drug has the potential for abuse by people who have anorexia or bulimia. It should not be used by people who have gallbladder disease.

Comments

This drug was the subject of the largest study ever on an antiobesity agent—668 clinically overweight patients for 2 years. Following 1 year of treatment, orlistat (in combination with a proper diet) was shown to be more effective in reducing weight than diet alone. Patients lost an average of 13.4 pounds. Because this drug is relatively new (1999), its long-term effects are not known.

zafirlukast

See Accolate*

Brand Name
Zanaflex

Generic Name

tizanidine

Type of Drug

Muscle relaxant; antispasmodic. This drug alleviates spasticity and muscle cramping from certain medical conditions, including spinal injury.

For

Chronic muscle spasms associated with multiple sclerosis and cerebral palsy; uncontrolled muscle spasms.

Availability and Dosage

Tablets: 4 mg. Take this medication exactly as is prescribed. Your dosage may need to be adjusted during the first weeks of treatment. Do not change the amount or frequency of your dose on your own. Do not abruptly stop taking it without consulting your doctor. Your doctor will need to gradually reduce your dose.

Side Effects

More common include constipation, diarrhea, dizziness, light-headedness, back pain, drowsiness, dry mouth, and muscle weakness. Others include dry skin, mood changes, tremors, weight loss, loss of appetite, fever, nausea, and jaundice.

Drug Interactions

Tizanidine has the potential to interact with oral contraceptives, anticonvulsants, central nervous systems (CNS) depressants, antihistamines, narcotic painkillers, and antihypertensives. Always inform your doctors of every medication you are taking, including nonprescription medicines, vitamins, herbal remedies, and dietary supplements. *Do not take any over-the-counter medications unless approved by your doctor.*

Food/Alcohol Interactions

Avoid alcohol, as it will increase this drug's sedative effect.

Pregnancy/Nursing

Not recommended. Tizanidine may pass into breast milk. Although it has not been shown to cause ill effects, you may want to bottle-feed your baby if you must take this drug.

Seniors

Your doctor may prescribe a low dose to minimize the possibility of increased adverse effects.

Warning

You should wear a medical identification tag at all times and carry an ID card that lists all the medications you are currently taking. Make sure your doctor has your entire medical history, including a history of kidney or liver disease. You will need to be carefully monitored during the first weeks of drug therapy. If you vomit blood, pass black, tarry stools, have seizures, arrhythmias, hallucinations, or blurred vision, *seek emergency medical treatment*.

Comments

Tizanidine was the first new oral drug for spasticity when it was introduced in 1996. The drug does not cure multiple sclerosis, but in controlled tests of 450 patients who have MS and spinal injuries, 70% who took tizanidine showed various stages of improvement. Approximately 250,000 people in the United States have multiple sclerosis, two-thirds of them women. This inflammatory disease of the central nervous system—in which scarring of nerve fibers in the brain and spinal cord occurs—typically starts in young adults age 20 to 40. Symptoms vary, but include weakness, fatigue, vision problems, impaired coordination, slurred speech, short-term memory loss, depression, partial or complete paralysis, and bladder or bowel dysfunction. In the relapsing forms of the disease, symptoms may appear and disappear, and the disease can also go into spontaneous remission. The progressive form is marked by steady worsening of symptoms. Two interferon drugs are also used to treat multiple sclerosis (see Avonex).

Brand Name
Zantac*

Generic Name

ranitidine

Type of Drug

Histamine H_2 blocker; antiulcer. Histamine is a chemical that produces a variety of effects, including increased secretion of stomach acid. Antihistamines traditionally used for allergies do not block the effect of histamine on stomach acid.

For

Gastric ulcers; gastroesophageal reflux disease (GERD); prevention of stomach ulcers caused by nonsteroidal antiinflammatory drugs (NSAIDs).

Availability and Dosage

Tablets: 150 mg, 300 mg. Capsules: 150 mg, 300 mg. Effervescent tablets: 150 mg. Oral syrup: 15 mg per ml. May be taken with or without food.

Side Effects

More common include dizziness, headache, drowsiness, nausea, and abdominal pain. Others include anxiety, constipation, diarrhea, breast enlargement, hair loss (temporary), and insomnia.

Drug Interactions

Ranitidine may interact with ketoconazole, nifedipine, antidepressants, beta-blockers, glipizide, lidocaine, iron supplements, and anticoagulants (blood thinners). Aspirin and other nonsteroidal antiinflammatory drugs (NSAIDs) can cause or aggravate ulcers and gastric bleeding. Do not take antacids within 2 hours of taking ranitidine. Always inform your doctors of every medication you are taking, including nonprescription medicines, vitamins, herbal remedies, and dietary supplements. *Do not take any over-the-counter medications unless approved by your doctor.*

Food/Alcohol Interactions

Avoid alcohol. Avoid caffeinated foods and beverages. Acidic foods and beverages may irritate the stomach.

Pregnancy/Nursing

Not recommended. Ranitidine passes into breast milk, although there is no evidence of harm to the newborn. You may wish to bottle-feed your baby while you are taking this drug.

Seniors

There is an increased possibility of side effects, especially in people who have impaired kidney function. Your doctor may prescribe a low dose.

Warning

Make sure your doctor has your complete medical history, including a history of alcohol abuse or kidney or liver disease. If you vomit "coffee grounds" or pass black, tarry stools, *seek emergency medical treatment*. These could be symptoms of a bleeding ulcer.

Comments

Gastroesophageal reflux disease (GERD) occurs when stomach acid washes back up into the esophagus, resulting in heartburn. Nonprescription H_2 blockers are among most popular over-the-counter medications, but they do not cure GERD. The nonprescription form of ranitidine is Zantac 75 and is used for heartburn, indigestion, and upset stomach. Follow package directions carefully, do not take more often than needed, and consult your doctor if your symptoms worsen. Long-term use or high dosages of NSAIDs (aspirin, ibuprofen, ketoprofen, naproxen, flurbiprofen) can increase the possibility of developing an ulcer. Do not self-medicate using aspirin or other NSAIDs. The risk of ulcers increases if you are female, have a history of ulcers, are age 60 or over, use corticosteroids, smoke, or drink alcohol.

Brand Name
Zestoretic*

Generic Name

lisinopril and hydrochlorothiazide (HCTZ)

Type of Drug

Angiotensin-converting enzyme (ACE) inhibitor/diuretic combination. ACE inhibitors are antihypertensives used to treat high blood pressure (hypertension). They work by blocking an enzyme in the body that is required to produce a substance that causes blood vessels to tighten. When this enzyme is blocked, blood vessels are relaxed, blood pressure is lowered, the workload of the heart and arteries is reduced, and blood and oxygen supplies are increased. These drugs promote the loss of water and salt from the body, which results in the lowering of blood pressure.

For

High blood pressure (hypertension).

Availability and Dosage

Tablets: 2.5 mg, 5 mg, 10 mg, 20 mg, 30 mg, 40 mg. May be taken with or without food.

Side Effects

More common in women is a dry, hacking cough. Other side effects include headache, diarrhea, fatigue, dizziness, nausea, chest pain, and increased sun sensitivity.

Drug Interactions

This drug may interact with other heart medications and potassium-sparing diuretics, lithium, potassium supplements, antidiabetics, and nonsteroidal antiinflammatory drugs (NSAIDs). Do not take antacids within 2 hours of taking this drug. Always inform your doctors of every medication you are taking, including nonprescription medicines, vitamins, herbal remedies, and dietary supplements. *Do not take any over-the-counter medications unless approved by your doctor.*

Food/Alcohol Interactions

Avoid alcohol. Do not use salt substitutes or drink low-sodium milk.

Pregnancy/Nursing

Not recommended, especially during the second and third trimesters. Birth defects and fetal death may result. Bottle-feed your baby if you must take this drug.

Seniors

Increased side effects including dizziness may occur, especially if you have impaired kidney function. Your doctor may prescribe a low dose.

Warning

Women should use an effective method of birth control while taking this drug. If you become pregnant while on this drug, notify your doctor immediately. Make sure your doctor has your complete medical history, including a history of diabetes, lupus, gout, inflammation of the pancreas, or heart, liver, or kidney disease. Severe dizziness or light-headedness may be a symptom of hypotension (low blood pressure). Do not use sunlamps or tanning booths while you are taking this drug. Always use sunscreen with an SPF factor of at least 15, including on your lips.

Comments

The myth is that heart disease is the domain of men, but sobering statistics prove otherwise: Heart disease is the leading cause of death in American women over age 35. Hypertension—and its attendant risks of heart attack and stroke—is often called the "silent killer" because there are no warning signs or symptoms. It is more prevalent among heavy drinkers, the overweight or obese, and women who take oral contraceptives. It also disproportionately affects African Americans, Puerto Ricans, Cuban Americans, and Mexican Americans. You should have your blood pressure checked regularly and know where it falls under the following four stages: Stage 1 (mild hypertension) ranges from 140/90 to 159/99. Stage 2 (moderate hypertension) ranges from 160/100 to 179/109. Stage 3 (severe hypertension) ranges from 180/110 to 209/119. Stage 4 (very severe) is 210/120 and higher.

Brand Name
Zestril* (also Prinivil*)

Generic Name

lisinopril

Type of Drug

Angiotensin-converting enzyme (ACE) inhibitor. ACE inhibitors are antihypertensives used to treat high blood pressure (hypertension). They work by blocking an enzyme in the body that is required to produce a substance that causes blood vessels to tighten. When this enzyme is blocked, blood vessels are relaxed, blood pressure is lowered, the workload of the heart and arteries is reduced, and blood and oxygen supplies are increased.

For

High blood pressure (hypertension).

Availability and Dosage

Tablets: 5 mg, 10 mg, 20 mg, 40 mg. Usual dosage is once daily. May be taken with or without food.

Side Effects

More common in women is a dry, hacking cough. Others include headache, dizziness, tingling in the hands, feet, or around the mouth, muscle weakness, nausea, drowsiness, upset stomach, and rash.

Drug Interactions

This drug may interact with other heart medications and potassium-sparing diuretics, lithium, potassium supplements, antidiabetics, and nonsteroidal antiinflammatory drugs (NSAIDs). Do not take antacids within 2 hours of taking this drug. Always inform your doctors of every medication you are taking, including nonprescription medicines, vitamins, herbal remedies, and dietary supplements. *Do not take any over-the-counter medications unless approved by your doctor.*

Food/Alcohol Interactions

Limit or avoid alcohol, as it may precipitate an extreme drop in blood pressure.

Pregnancy/Nursing

Not recommended, especially during the second and third trimesters. Birth defects and fetal death may result. Bottle-feed your baby if you must take this drug.

Seniors

Increased side effects including dizziness may occur, especially if you have impaired kidney function. Your doctor may prescribe a low dose.

Warning

If you experience severe dizziness or light-headedness, this may be a symptom of hypotension (low blood pressure). This is more likely to occur during the first days of drug therapy. If you faint, tell your doctor. Make sure your doctor has your complete medical history, including a history of lupus, infections, or heart, liver, or kidney disease. If you experience chest pain, chills, fever, palpitations, shortness of breath, or swelling in face, hands, or feet, *seek emergency medical treatment.*

Comments

Heart disease is the leading cause of death in American women over age 35. There are several factors that contribute to heart disease: high cholesterol, smoking, obesity, and high blood pressure. For women overall, smoking is the greatest risk factor for heart attack and stroke. For women between age 65 and 74, hypertension is the greatest risk factor for heart attack, just slightly ahead of obesity. However, "central obesity"—having a waist larger than your hips—is a risk factor for women (to calculate this, divide your waist measurement by your hip measurement; it should be lower than 0.85). Also, see the above profile on lisinopril/HCTZ (Zestoretic).

Brand Name
Ziac*

Generic Name

bisoprolol and hydrochlorothiazide (HCTZ)

Type of Drug

Beta-blocker/thiazide diuretic combination. Beta-blockers block the response of the heart and blood vessels, lower the pulse rate, and reduce the force of the heartbeat, thereby reducing the workload of the heart. They are sometimes prescribed after a heart attack to prevent future attacks. Diuretics promote the loss of water and salt from the body, which results in the lowering of blood pressure.

For

High blood pressure (hypertension).

Availability and Dosage

Tablets: 2.5 mg, 5 mg, or 10 mg of bisoprolol combined with 6.25 mg of hydrochlorothiazide (HCTZ). May be taken with or without food. Do not abruptly stop taking this drug. Your doctor will need to gradually decrease your dose.

Side Effects

More common include drowsiness, dizziness, light-headedness, and decreased sex drive. Others include fatigue, anxiety, nervousness, insomnia, short-term memory loss, constipation, nausea, cramps, depression, nightmares, and sun sensitivity.

Drug Interactions

This drug may interact with a wide variety of medications, including other beta-blockers, antihypertensives, cimetidine, calcium channel blockers, thyroid drugs, lithium, insulin, nonsteroidal antiinflammatory drugs (NSAIDs) including aspirin, and drugs that contain aspirin, estrogens, and oral antidiabetics. Do not take monoamine oxidase (MAO) inhibitors within 2 weeks of taking bisoprolol/HCTZ. Always inform your doctors of every medication you are taking, including nonprescription medicines, vitamins, herbal remedies, and dietary supplements. *Do not take any over-the-counter medications unless approved by your doctor.*

Food/Alcohol Interactions

Avoid alcohol, as it can increase the sedative effect of this drug and cause an extreme drop in blood pressure. Avoid foods high in sodium.

Pregnancy/Nursing

Not recommended. Bottle-feed your baby if you must take this drug.

Seniors

Adverse reactions, especially dizziness and light-headedness, may be more pronounced in older patients.

Warning

If you are going to have surgery, make sure your doctor knows you are taking this drug. You must be carefully and regularly monitored while taking any antihypertensive drug. Make sure your doctor has your entire medical history, especially a history of bronchospasm, asthma, emphysema, diabetes, or heart, liver, or kidney disease.

Comments

Heart disease is the leading cause of death in American women over age 35. Stroke is the third-leading cause. (Cancer is the second-leading cause.) Death from cardiovascular disease accounts for half of all deaths among women and about six times more deaths than from breast cancer. Heart disease often goes undiagnosed in women under age 50, and yet women in that age group who have heart attacks are twice as likely to die as a result. Numerous studies have shown that women who visit emergency rooms for heart attack symptoms are less likely to receive medications or aggressive treatment. If you exhibit any of the warning signs of a heart attack—chest pains (pressure or heaviness in the chest or pain or pressure that radiates to the neck, shoulders, arms, or lower jaw), dizziness, or persistent heartburn or indigestion—and your doctor does not take your symptoms seriously, consult another physician or *seek emergency medical treatment.*

Brand Name
Ziagen

Generic Name
abacavir sulfate

Type of Drug
Antiviral; nucleoside reverse transcriptase inhibitor. This drug is proven to work only when used in combination with other antiretroviral drugs.

For
HIV.

Availability and Dosage
Tablets: 300 mg. Oral solution: 20 mg per ml. Drug management therapy for patients who have HIV infection or AIDS is a complex process involving a combination of drugs in what is now commonly referred to as an "AIDS cocktail." There is no one "cocktail"—these combinations, including protease inhibitors and nucleoside analogs, are providing increased life expectancy and dramatic improvement in symptoms for some patients. For example, zidovudine is used in one of the newer drugs (brand name Combivir) in combination with lamivudine in one tablet. Patients play a critical role in the management of their disease by taking medications for HIV and AIDS exactly as prescribed, in the proper dosages and at the proper times.

Side Effects
More common include nausea, weakness, headache, fatigue, loss of appetite, and diarrhea. Others include fever, vomiting, insomnia, overall swelling, and shortness of breath.

Drug Interactions
No significant drug interactions have been reported, but studies in this area continue. Always inform your doctors of every medication you are taking, including nonprescription medicines, vitamins, herbal remedies, and dietary supplements. *Do not take any over-the-counter medications unless approved by your doctor*.

Food/Alcohol Interactions
Avoid alcohol.

Pregnancy/Nursing

Not recommended. Women who have HIV should bottle-feed their babies to avoid transmission to the newborn.

Seniors

No special warnings. Take as prescribed and immediately inform your doctor of any persistent or troublesome side effects.

Warning

About 5% of HIV patients who take this drug suffer a hypersensitive reaction that is life-threatening. If you experience a severe allergic reaction at any time, you must stop taking this drug and contact your physician immediately. A severe reaction involves a skin rash plus two or more of the following symptoms: fever, nausea, vomiting, diarrhea, stomach pain, severe tiredness, achiness, and general ill feeling. If you are allergic to this drug you must never take it again, as more-severe symptoms could result in death. You should wear a medical identification tag at all times and carry an ID card that lists all the medications you are currently taking.

Comments

Although overall deaths from AIDS are on the decline, the disease is increasing faster among women than men and still affects minorities disproportionately. Women who have HIV often have difficulty accessing proper health care, and the prohibitive cost of the drugs involved ($16,000 or more a year) often excludes those who need them. Given the rise in heterosexually transmitted HIV, more prevention efforts—namely, insisting that partners use latex condoms—are being aimed at women. Although there is presently no cure for this disease, new drug trials and research continue. See the Women's Resource Directory at the back of this book for the names of organizations that have the latest information on treatments.

zidovudine (AZT)

See Retrovir

Brand Name
Zithromax*

Generic Name

azithromycin

Type of Drug

Antibiotic.

For

Various bacterial infections including those of the respiratory tract and the skin; sexually transmitted diseases (STD); urinary-tract infections (UTIs); infections of the cervix.

Availability and Dosage

Tablets: 250 mg, 600 mg. Capsules: 250 mg. Tablets may be taken with or without food. Capsules should be taken on an empty stomach, 1 hour before or 2 hours after meals. Take this drug for the full course of treatment prescribed.

Side Effects

More common include nausea, stomach pain, and diarrhea. Others include vomiting, dizziness, and headache.

Drug Interactions

Do not take this drug within 2 hours of taking antacids. This drug may also interact with anticoagulants (blood thinners), digoxin, triazolam, carbamazepine, and phenytoin. Always inform your doctors of every medication you are taking, including nonprescription medicines, vitamins, herbal remedies, and dietary supplements.

Food/Alcohol Interactions

Avoid or limit alcohol.

Pregnancy/Nursing

No special warnings, although all drugs during pregnancy and breast-feeding should be avoided if possible. Before taking this drug, discuss with your doctor the benefits versus the potential risks.

Seniors

No special warnings. Take as prescribed and immediately inform your doctor of any persistent or troublesome side effects.

Warning

If you have an allergy to azithromycin, erythromycin, or any macrolide antibiotic, you should not take this drug. Make sure your doctor knows if you have a history of liver disease.

Comments

This large class of drugs are among the most commonly prescribed, resulting in such widespread use that the bacteria they were developed to kill have become resistant to them. These "resistant" forms are then passed from person to person, further causing the spread of infections that become even more difficult to treat. Some antibiotics work against a limited number of microorganisms. Broad-spectrum antibiotics are effective against a variety of bacteria. Your doctor will prescribe the correct antibiotic depending on the type of infection. Antibiotics are useless against viral infections such as colds and flu.

Brand Name
Zocor*

Generic Name

simvastatin

Type of Drug

Cholesterol-lowering. When diet, exercise, and weight loss fail to reduce total and LDL (low-density lipoprotein, or "bad") cholesterol, this drug may be prescribed as part of a total cholesterol-management program to reduce the risk of stroke and heart attack.

For

High cholesterol.

Availability and Dosage

Tablets: 5 mg, 10 mg, 20 mg, 40 mg, 80 mg. May be taken with or without food, usually in the evening.

Side Effects

More common include constipation, diarrhea, muscle aches and pains, dizziness, and headache. Others include heartburn, weakness, insomnia, and nausea.

Drug Interactions

Simvastatin can interact with erythromycin, immune system suppressants, digoxin, anticoagulants (blood thinners), ketoconazole, spironolactone, and cimetidine. Do not take niacin while taking this drug. Always inform your doctors of every medication you are taking, including nonprescription medicines, vitamins, herbal remedies, and dietary supplements. *Do not take any over-the-counter medications unless approved by your doctor.*

Food/Alcohol Interactions

Avoid alcohol. This drug is designed to be used in conjunction with a healthy diet and appropriate exercise program to lower cholesterol.

Pregnancy/Nursing

A woman must never become pregnant while on this drug. Women of childbearing age should not take simvastatin unless the possibility of pregnancy has been ruled out. Use a reliable form of birth control while taking this medication. If you become pregnant while on this drug, contact your doctor immediately. Bottle-feed your baby if you must take this drug.

Seniors

No special warnings. Take as prescribed and immediately inform your doctor of any persistent or troublesome side effects.

Warning

You must be regularly monitored while on this drug. Liver-function tests will be needed. Make sure your doctor has your complete medical history, including a history of diabetes, low blood pressure, seizures, muscle disease or weakness, recent surgery, or liver disease. This drug should be used with caution by people who consume large amounts of alcohol.

Comments

In 1999, simvastatin (Zocor) became the first cholesterol drug to receive FDA clearance for use in raising levels of "good" cholesterol (high-density, or HDL). Low levels of "good" cholesterol and high levels of "bad" cholesterol (low-density, or LDL, and triglycerides) are associated with an increased risk of heart disease, the number-one killer of women in the United States. Some research indicates that a high triglyceride level may present a greater risk for women than it does for men. Your total cholesterol level should be 200 or less, slightly higher if you're over age 65. Between 200 and 240 may be responsive to diet and exercise alone; if not, drug therapy may help. Artery-clogging LDL cholesterol should be between 100 to 130. The total cholesterol-to-HDL ratio should not be higher than 4.5 to 1 The optimum ratio is 3.5 to 1. The ratio is determined by dividing the HDL cholesterol level into the total cholesterol level. For example, a total cholesterol of 200 mg and an HDL of 50 mg would be interpreted as 4 to 1. Risk factors—smoking, hypertension, diabetes, and obesity—are also important in determining whether a cholesterol-lowering drug may be necessary.

zolmitriptan

See Zomig

Brand Name
Zoloft*

Generic Name

sertraline

Type of Drug

Selective serotonin reuptake inhibitor (SSRI) antidepressant. This drug is in a newer class of antidepressants that work by raising the brain's level of serotonin, a chemical associated with mood and mental alertness. It can also help to relieve the repetitive rituals and anxiety associated with obsessive-compulsive disorder.

For

Depression; obsessive-compulsive disorder (OCD).

Availability and Dosage

Tablets: 50 mg, 100 mg. Food may affect the blood levels of this drug. Take on an empty stomach 1 hour before or 2 hours after meals.

Side Effects

More often include headache, tremor, and nausea. Others include dry mouth, drowsiness, sleep disturbances, indigestion, changes in appetite, and sexual dysfunction (decreased sexual desire or difficulty in achieving orgasm).

Drug Interactions

Any SSRI drug has the potential to interact with many other drugs, including lithium, diazepam, cimetidine, other antidepressants, sumatriptan, anticoagulants (blood thinners), tramadol, and venlafaxine. Do not take a monoamine oxidase (MAO) inhibitor antidepressant within 14 days of taking this drug. Interactions can also occur with nonprescription medications for allergies, coughs, and colds that contain dextromethorpan. Always inform your doctors of every medication you are taking, including nonprescription medicines, vitamins, herbal remedies, and dietary supplements. *Do not take any over-the-counter medications unless approved by your doctor.*

Food/Alcohol Interactions

Avoid alcohol. Avoid or limit caffeine, as it may increase the central nervous system (CNS) stimulant effects of the drug.

Pregnancy/Nursing

No special warnings, although all drugs during pregnancy and breast-feeding should be avoided if possible. Before taking this drug, discuss with your doctor the benefits versus the potential risks. This drug passes into breast milk, but without any known effects. You may wish to bottle-feed your baby if you must take this drug.

Seniors

No special warnings. Take as prescribed and immediately inform your doctor of any persistent or troublesome side effects. Your doctor may prescribe a low dose.

Warning

A rare but potentially serious condition known as "serotonin syndrome" may result from the combination of venlafaxine (Effexor) and sertraline. If you experience shivering, agitation, confusion, loss of coordination, or twitching, *seek emergency medical treatment*. The use of any antidepressant requires careful and regular monitoring by a physician, including blood tests. Sertraline may also cause a marked decrease in sexual drive and an increase in sexual dysfunction. Discuss such problems with your doctor or a therapist.

Comments

With the development of this newer class of antidepressants (SSRIs), some doctors have all but abandoned the "older" classes, such as tricyclic antidepressants, citing that newer drugs are more effective and have fewer side effects. Women, for example, were shown to respond more favorably to sertraline (Zoloft) than to a tricyclic in some of the drug studies. But a 1999 report by the Agency for Health Care Policy and Research of Health and Human Services indicates that it is more important to treat the type of depression using the appropriate drug rather than to insist that the new drugs have rendered the old ones obsolete. This issue is especially important to women, who reportedly outnumber men 2 to 1 in treatment for major depression. For nonmajor depression (including dysthymia, a chronic, low-grade form of the disorder), the ratio jumps to 10 to 1. There is some controversy over whether women actually experience depression more often than men do, or whether they are more likely to seek treatment and therefore are more statistically visible. Before taking any antidepressant make sure that your doctor has conducted a thorough evaluation and determined a course of treatment that includes behavioral therapy. If you suspect that you are being given an antidepressant as a "quick fix" without proper physical and psychological examinations, get a second opinion.

zolpidem

*See Ambien**

Brand Name
Zomig

Generic Name
zolmitriptan

Type of Drug
Antimigraine. This drug is used to treat migraine headache attacks. Migraines are the most common neurological disease, with an estimated 28 million sufferers in the United States, 18 million of them women. About half of all women's migraine headaches are believed to be linked to estrogen; in these cases, migraines can disappear entirely after menopause. Doctors often prescribe calcium channel blockers, beta-blockers, and tricyclic antidepressants to prevent frequent migraines.

For
Migraine headache. Not to be used for tension or other types of headaches.

Availability and Dosage
Tablets: 2.5 mg, 5 mg. This drug should be taken at the first signs of a migraine attack, with or without aura (the warning sign that often precedes an attack). Do not take this medicine more often than is prescribed, and do not exceed 10 mg in 24 hours. This drug is for treatment of migraine attack only; it should never be used as a pain reliever for any other condition.

Side Effects
More common include dizziness, drowsiness, fatigue, muscle weakness, and dry mouth. Others include indigestion, anxiety, itching, feelings of cold, and skin tingling.

Drug Interactions

Zolmitriptan should not be taken within 24 hours of the following drugs: monoamine oxidase (MAO) inhibitor antidepressants, dihydroergotamine or other ergot medication. Always inform your doctors of every medication you are taking, including nonprescription medicines, vitamins, herbal remedies, and dietary supplements. *Do not take any over-the-counter medications unless approved by your doctor.*

Food/Alcohol Interactions

Avoid alcohol and caffeine. Do not skip meals or fast. Your doctor should provide you with a list of foods, drinks, and additives that may trigger a migraine.

Pregnancy/Nursing

Not recommended. If you wish to breast-feed your baby while on this drug, first discuss it with your doctor.

Seniors

No special warnings. Take as prescribed and immediately inform your doctor of any persistent or troublesome side effects.

Warning

Do not smoke while on this drug, as it can increase adverse side effects related to the heart. Make sure that your doctor knows of any history of heart disease, angina, arrhythmia, rapid heartbeat, stroke, hypertension, or kidney or liver disease.

Comments

Migraine is a complex, debilitating disease and not just another name for headache. Migraine "triggers" are different in each case but generally include certain foods, bright lights, excessive noise, stress, lack of sleep, changes in temperature, and many more. The migraine is often preceded by an "aura" of flashing lights following by intense pain, vision disturbances, nausea, and vomiting. Over-the-counter medications specifically formulated for migraine are now available, but always check with your doctor or your pharmacist before self-medicating. There is no cure, and many people are finding nondrug therapeutic relief in biofeedback, massage, and acupuncture.

Brand Name
Zostrix

Generic Name

capsaicin

Type of Drug

Topical analgesic.

For

Temporary relief of neuralgia (nerve pain); herpes zoster (shingles); herpes simplex type 1 (cold sores, fever blisters), herpes simplex type 2 (genital herpes), psoriasis, rheumatoid arthritis, osteoarthritis; itching; irritations of the vulva; postsurgical pain.

Availability and Dosage

Topical cream. Follow instructions for application and do not apply to inflamed or broken skin. When using this medication for arthritis or other joint pain, wait 30 minutes after application before washing your hands.

Side Effects

More common include burning or stinging at the application site. Others include skin warmth or redness.

Drug Interactions

No special warnings, although all drugs have the ability to interact with other drugs. Report any problems to your doctor or your pharmacist. Always inform your doctors of every medication you are taking, including nonprescription medicines, vitamins, herbal remedies, and dietary supplements.

Food/Alcohol Interactions

No special warnings.

Pregnancy/Nursing

No special warnings, although all drugs during pregnancy and breast-feeding should be avoided if possible. Before taking this drug, discuss with your doctor the benefits versus the potential risks.

Seniors

No special warnings. Take as prescribed and immediately inform your doctor of any persistent or troublesome side effects.

Warning

Tell your doctor if you have a history of allergies to hot peppers, as capsaicin is derived from them. Keep away from the eyes and mucous membranes. If you wear contact lenses, insert them before using this cream.

Comments

Capsaicin is available over-the-counter. The information above applies to OTC medications that contain capsaicin. Follow package directions carefully, and consult your doctor or your pharmacist if you have any questions.

Zovia

See Oral Contraceptives

Brand Name

Zovirax

Generic Name

acyclovir

Type of Drug

Antiviral.

For

Treatment of herpes simplex (genitals, mucous membranes, central nervous system); herpes zoster (shingles); varicella (chicken pox).

Availability and Dosage

Tablets: 400 mg, 800 mg. Capsules: 200 mg. Topical ointment: 5%. Oral suspension: 200 mg per 5 ml. Dosages and forms will vary depending on the condition being treated. The oral form may be taken with or without food. Do not apply the topical form intravaginally.

Side Effects

Oral forms: headache, nausea, vomiting, and dizziness. Topical ointment: irritation, burning (more common in women), itching, and vaginal inflammation.

Drug Interactions

The topical ointment form may interact with other topical medications. The oral form may interact with zidovudine (AZT), lithium, methotrexate, and gold compounds. It may also interact with prescription and nonprescription pain relievers that contain acetaminophen or aspirin. Always inform your doctors of every medication you are taking, including nonprescription medicines, vitamins, herbal remedies, and dietary supplements.

Food/Alcohol Interactions

No special warnings.

Pregnancy/Nursing

Not recommended. Acyclovir passes into breast milk, but without any known effects. You may wish to bottle-feed your baby if you must take this drug.

Seniors

No special warnings. Take as prescribed and immediately inform your doctor of any persistent or troublesome side effects. Your doctor may prescribe a low dose of the oral form.

Warning

Acyclovir does not cure herpes, nor does it prevent the spread of infection, but it can slow the growth rate of the virus. Genital herpes is spread by sexual contact, especially when there are sores or blisters on the vulva, the vaginal or anal area, or when a pelvic exam has discovered sores on the cervix. But herpes can also be transmitted even when there are no sores visible. Viral particles may be shedding on the skin that may not be easily detected. The use of condoms by your male partner is recommended at all times. Genital herpes can be transmitted to a newborn and increase his or her risk of brain damage and blindness. If you know or suspect you have herpes, make sure that you tell your ob/gyn. Evidence suggests that women who have genital herpes may be more likely to develop cervical cancer. It is essential that you get an annual Pap smear.

Comments

There is no known cure for genital herpes, although patients now have better treatment options for this viral disease. Acyclovir has been proven to be a safe and effective treatment to help patients who have recurrent outbreaks. Clinical trials are now under way to develop a herpes vaccine, which some researchers predict will be available by 2003. The FDA is also expected to approve

POCkit, a herpes blood test that can be taken anytime and show results in six minutes instead of the traditional "swab tests" that can be done only when sores are present and take several days to provide results.

Brand Name
Zyban*

Generic Name
bupropion HCL

Type of Drug
Nonnicotine smoking-cessation aid. This drug may double your chances of success in quitting smoking, especially when combined with a smoking-cessation program that includes therapy.

For
Reducing nicotine withdrawal symptoms when quitting smoking.

Availability and Dosage
Extended-release tablets: 150 mg. May be taken with or without food. The usual length of treatment is 7 to 12 weeks. Do not take more of this medicine than is prescribed.

Side Effects
More common include dry mouth and difficulty in sleeping. Others include skin rash and shakiness.

Drug Interactions
This drug may interact with tricyclic antidepressants, fluoxetine, lithium, levadopa, carbamazepine, and phenytoin. Do not take this drug within 14 days of taking a monoamine oxidase (MAO) inhibitor antidepressant. Always inform your doctors of every medication you are taking, including nonprescription medicines, vitamins, herbal remedies, and dietary supplements. *Do not take any over-the-counter medications unless approved by your doctor.*

Food/Alcohol Interactions
Avoid alcohol, as it may increase the risk of seizures. If you are a chronic drinker, you may need to gradually reduce your alcohol intake before starting this drug.

Pregnancy/Nursing

Not recommended. Bottle-feed your baby if you must take this drug.

Seniors

If you have reduced kidney or liver function, your doctor may prescribe a low dose.

Warning

Make sure your doctor has your complete medical history, including a history of seizures, alcohol or substance abuse, anorexia, bulimia, suicidal thoughts, manic depression, or liver or kidney disease. Approximately 1 in 1,000 people will have a seizure while taking bupropion. If you experience seizure, palpitations, hallucinations, or difficulty in breathing, *seek emergency medical treatment.*

Comments

This drug was originally developed and marketed as an antidepressant (see Wellbutrin), but it is chemically unrelated to tricyclic, tetracyclic, selective serotonin reuptake inhibitors (SSRIs), or other known antidepressant agents. If you plan to use a nonprescription nicotine patch or gum while taking this drug, consult your doctor before starting that therapy. The combination may result in high blood pressure. In 1999, the Internal Revenue Service concluded that because nicotine is addictive—and therefore no different from alcohol or substance-abuse treatment—prescription drugs and programs for smoking cessation are tax deductible.

Zydone

See Vicodin

Brand Name
Zyloprim

Generic Name
allopurinol*

Type of Drug
Antigout.

For

Gout; prevention of high levels of uric acid in the blood, including those associated with radiation or chemotherapy for cancer.

Availability and Dosage

Tablets: 100 mg, 300 mg. Should be taken with food.

Side Effects

More common include skin rash, itching, and hives. Others include nausea, drowsiness, headache, stomach pain, and diarrhea.

Drug Interactions

Allopurinol may interact with cyclophosphamide, anticoagulants (blood thinners), some antidiabetics, some penicillin antibiotics, and diuretics. Do not take vitamin C or iron supplements while taking this drug. Always inform your doctors of every medication you are taking, including nonprescription medicines, vitamins, herbal remedies, and dietary supplements. *Do not take any over-the-counter medications unless approved by your doctor.*

Food/Alcohol Interactions

Avoid alcohol. Drink a minimum of 10 glasses of water a day to minimize formation of kidney crystals or stones.

Pregnancy/Nursing

Not recommended. Allopurinol passes into breast milk. Bottle-feed your baby if you must take this drug.

Seniors

No special warnings. Take as prescribed and immediately inform your doctors of any persistent or troublesome side effects.

Warning

If you develop a skin rash or itching, scaly skin, fever, chills, or sore throat, contact your doctor immediately. Any of these could be a sign of serious allergic reaction to this drug. Do not drive or operate machinery until you know how this medication will affect you.

Comments

This drug is useful only in helping to prevent gout attacks by decreasing uric acid in the body; it will not affect an attack already in progress. An excess of uric acid can cause kidney stones. Uric acid rises slightly in women around the time of menopause, but not all elevations in uric acid need to be treated, as there are various stages of gout. Allopurinol is also used for other medical conditions that result from excess uric acid, including gouty arthritis (crystal arthritis), in which joint fluid forms crystals. These crystals are more commonly seen around the big toe, the knee, the ankle, and the foot instep.

Brand Name
Zyrtec*

Generic Name
cetirizine HCL

Type of Drug
Antihistamine. This drug counteracts the effects of histamine, a chemical released in the body that can cause itching and swelling.

For
Relief of symptoms caused by seasonal allergies.

Availability and Dosage
Tablets: 5 mg, 10 mg. Oral syrup: 5 mg per ml. Usual tablet dose is 10 mg once a day. May be taken with or without food.

Side Effects
More common include dry mouth, fatigue, and drowsiness.

Drug Interactions
No special warnings, although all drugs have the ability to interact with other drugs. Report any problems to your doctor or your pharmacist. Always inform your doctors of every medication you are taking, including nonprescription medicines, vitamins, herbal remedies, and dietary supplements.

Food/Alcohol Interactions
No special warnings, although you should avoid alcohol if you experience drowsiness as a side effect of this drug. Drink plenty of water while taking any antihistamine.

Pregnancy/Nursing
Not recommended. Cetirizine passes into breast milk. Bottle-feed your baby if you must take this drug.

Seniors

If you have impaired kidney or liver function, your doctor may prescribe a low dose.

Warning

Although this drug is usually well tolerated and does not cause as much sedation as other types of antihistamines, drowsiness is the most common side effect. Use caution when taking this drug with any other drug known to cause drowsiness, including some antianxiety or antidepressant medications, painkillers, and drugs for insomnia.

Comments

There are dozens of over-the-counter antihistamines available, and many people self-medicate, using them for everything from hay fever to hives. You should not take any OTC antihistamine if you are pregnant. Antihistamines have the potential to interact with many different drugs, including those taken for heart disease, diabetes, and other conditions. Follow package directions carefully, and always check with your doctor or your pharmacist before taking an OTC antihistamine if you are on any prescription drug.

You and Your Pharmacist

Twenty-three seconds. That's how much time elapses between the beginning of an office visit with your doctor and the first time he or she interrupts you, according to a 1998 University of Rochester study. As a female patient, you may not even get that far. As we have said before, women should strive for the ideal—open, relaxed, informative, and honest communication with their doctors. But once again, reality intervenes: In our time-crunched world of managed care and jam-packed waiting rooms, you are as likely to be examined by one of the "new" health profession-als—a nurse practitioner (NP) or a physician's assistant (PA). Qualified and skilled, yes. And we're for any system that gets us out of that crammed waiting room that much faster. But when it comes to getting detailed information about your drug therapy, there's no guarantee that an NP or a PA can spend any more time with you than your doctor can.

It's long past time for every woman to develop an additional health care partnership—one with her pharmacist. As the baby boomers age and many of our seniors are thriving well into their eighties, nineties, and beyond, pharmacists are now one of our most valuable health resources—and often our most overlooked. Some of us might have grown up with the traditional picture of an inaccessible white-coated person dispensing pills from behind an inexplicably high counter, but in many ways the new role of today's pharmacist goes back further, to the days when pharma-cists knew their customers individually, knew what medicines they were taking and how they were supposed to work, com-municated closely with their family doctors, and regularly coun-seled their customers.

New Pharmacists, New Pharmacies

Like all professionals, pharmacists have reacted to changing mar-ket conditions in order to remain up-to-date and competitive. The shift from pill dispenser to consultant is growing as the pharmacy profession continues to reinvent itself to keep pace with the un-precedented amount of health care information coming at us from every angle. With drug companies spending close to $2 bil-lion a year on prescription drug advertising in print and televi-sion—much of it aimed at women—it's beneficial to have someone to help translate all of those friendly, upbeat, warm and fuzzy ads into straightforward medical information.

The American Pharmaceutical Association, for example, refers to the new pharmacists as "pharmaceutical care managers," to illustrate their move from behind the counter to play an upfront, pivotal role in health care. The new pharmacy consists of personalized consulting booths; "brown bag reviews" (where customers bring in all of their medications to discuss drug interactions, side effects, and how the medications work together); case management for high-risk customers (people who have asthma, hypertension, diabetes, and other chronic disorders); pharmacist house calls; specialized compounding services that provide customized dosage forms; and wellness programs that offer basic blood pressure, blood glucose, and cholesterol testing, as well as information on drug and nondrug therapies, diet, and exercise in a total health-care management environment.

Many Doctors—One Pharmacy

We now know that women see more doctors, get more prescriptions, and buy more over-the-counter products than men do. New studies show that they may process and respond differently to some medications, as they go through the hormonal stages of life—menstruation, pregnancy, nursing, perimenopause, and postmenopause. Seeing several doctors may be unavoidable, but try to get all your prescriptions filled at one pharmacy, preferably one that is computerized. Today's comprehensive drug databases keep track of minor and major side effects, drug interactions, overdose warnings, what to do when you miss a dose, and other essential information. By having all of your prescriptions at one pharmacy, your pharmacist can see your complete prescription medication picture at a glance. This could prove lifesaving in the event of interacting drugs prescribed by different doctors.

This is not to say that pharmacists don't make mistakes. They do, some of them serious, even fatal. No matter how high-tech health care becomes, the possibility for human error always exists. Examine your medication carefully before taking it: Is the brand name and/or generic name on the label correct? Some drug names look and sound almost exactly alike and have led to serious illness or death when confused by the dispensing pharmacist. Is the dosage correct? Did you receive a full refill or a partial one? If you have the least suspicion that you received the wrong medication, dosage, number of pills, or notice any other discrepancy, take your prescription back to the pharmacy immediately and ask your pharmacist to verify the information. Laws now require that when a patient receives a prescription drug they haven't taken before, the pharmacist must personally provide information to that customer.

What Should You Ask Your Pharmacist?

According to the American Pharmaceutical Association, thousands of people fail to get better, spend more than they have to, and end up in the hospital simply because they did not take their medication properly. Improper use of medicines also costs the U.S. economy an estimated $15 billion each year. The FDA states that about one-half of all women take their medications improperly. The biggest mistakes are 1) taking less medicine than is prescribed, 2) taking more medicine than is prescribed, 3) stopping too soon, and 4) failing to refill prescriptions.

Before taking any new medication, ask your pharmacist the following:

What is the name of the medication?

This sounds simple, but the thousands of generic and brand names can be mind-boggling. A doctor may tell you the name of one drug during your examination, and when you pick up the prescription it has a completely different name. It may be the generic substitute, but never assume anything. Always verify with your pharmacist that it is the correct medication.

When and how do I take it?

The pharmacy instruction sheet that comes with your drug should give basic information, but don't hesitate to double-check with your pharmacist. Do I take this medicine with food? Should I take it at the same time every day? When should I refill, if necessary? Should I avoid alcohol, certain foods, or activities? What should I do if I miss a dose?

Does this medicine contain anything that can cause an allergic reaction?

This is where using the same pharmacy is especially useful. They can note in their computer records any allergic reactions you have had to any ingredients in both prescription and nonprescription drugs.

Should I expect any side effects?

The subject of side effects can be a tricky one: You want to feel better, you know you need the medication, and yet there is a list of unpleasant things that can happen to you if you take it. There is an intriguing phenomenon in medical school known as Munchausen's syndrome, in which some medical students are convinced that they have whatever disease they are studying at the time. I know women who seem to approach drug information using a variation on that theme—if they don't read about side effects, they can't get them. Others simply dismiss such information as unimportant or irrelevant. The key here is balance—staying informed about possible problems without the accompanying apprehension, plus an understanding of which side effects are likely to be serious and which are merely annoying. Your pharmacist may help you understand the difference and offer advice. Of course, you should always consult your physician or other health care provider if serious reactions occur.

Is it safe to become pregnant or breast-feed while taking this medication?

This information is often sketchy, due to the understandable absence of pregnant women from drug trials. The best course is to avoid all medications, but that's not always possible. Although we know that most drugs have never been proven harmful, this is not sufficient evidence of their absolute safety, either. Certain drugs, however, are known to cause birth defects and other fetal conditions and should never be taken during pregnancy or nursing. Your pharmacist should know what these are. If not, check with your doctor before taking any prescription or nonprescription drugs.

How should I store my medications?

Despite its name, the bathroom medicine cabinet is not the best place to keep your medications. Regular exposure to moisture and warmth can break down ingredients in some drugs. Storage instructions are usually indicated on the label or drug insert sheet.

About Generic Drugs

Seventeen years after a drug is patented by a pharmaceutical company, its formula becomes public property. Once a patent expires, other pharmaceutical companies are free to manufacture and sell their own version of the drug. This is where generic drugs come in: Because duplicating a formula using the original developer's recipe takes less research and development, and the manufacturer passes those savings on to the consumer, generics can be 40 to 50 percent less expensive than their brand-name equivalents. These are manufactured under FDA guidelines for generic drugs, and most generics are as safe and effective as their brand-name counterparts.

In the past ten years, patents on many popular drugs have expired, and generics have become big business. The topic is not without controversy—some pharmaceutical companies caution that a generic drug may be up to 20 percent less effective than the brand-name one. Some manufacturers of generics counter those claims by stating that 1984 FDA standards not only protect consumers but have helped to control rising health-care costs by alleviating the skyrocketing price of many prescription drugs.

Both sides are accurate, to a point: FDA standards do require generic drugs to have the same active ingredients, strengths, and forms as their brand-name counterparts. However, the burden of proof on the manufacturer applies only to *bioequivalency*—that the drug is absorbed and utilized in the body the same way—which is not the same as *identical*. The law allows a 10 to 20 percent variation in this area, even though most generic drugs usually do not deviate by more than 5 or 6 percent.

Another misconception is that brand-name drugs are sold by large, well-known companies and generics are sold by smaller, questionable firms. In fact, a pharmaceutical company that markets a brand-name drug may sell the same active ingredient to a dozen other companies, so the main ingredient in a generic you purchase may come from the company that makes the brand-name drug.

As a consumer, you will have to do what you do for any other major purchase—ask questions and comparison shop. Despite the overall safety of generics, there are differences among certain drugs that call for caution, including drugs for heart disease and neurological and psychiatric disorders. In some cases, the speed and accuracy with which a drug enters the bloodstream needs to be exacting. For women, this can be of special importance as more information comes to light about how drugs may be metabolized and cleared differently in women's bodies.

When getting your prescriptions filled, always ask your pharmacist if the generic equivalent is acceptable. If it is, tell your doctor to specifically prescribe the generic name on your prescription. Many pharmacies are now dispensing prescriptions only "as written," meaning that you could end up spending much more for a brand name when a less expensive generic drug would have been just as effective. Keep in mind, however, that not all drugs have generic equivalents available for sale. These are the newer drugs whose patents may be years away from expiring, and there are simply no alternatives.

Safe Drug Use

Most of us don't even think of drugs until we need them, and then we are in the position of trying to find out everything about a medication while under the additional stress of being ill. Much of safe drug use is common sense and good judgment, whether it's something as simple as never taking your medicine in the dark or keeping all medications away from children and pets. Following are selected tips on safe drug use from the Council on Family Health.

When your medicine is prescribed

Inform your physician about any other prescription and nonprescription medicines you are currently taking. Tell your physician or your pharmacist about any allergies or personal medical conditions you have, particularly pregnancy, high blood pressure, glaucoma, or diabetes. Be sure you fully understand all instructions before leaving your doctor's office or your pharmacy.

Protect yourself against tampering

Read the label to determine what seals and other protective features are used on the product. Inspect the packaging for signs of tampering. Examine the medicine itself to check for capsules or tablets that differ from the others. Do not use medicine from packages that have cuts, tears, or other imperfections. If in doubt, return questionable products to your pharmacy.

Read the labels on both prescription and nonprescription drugs to learn

The medicine's active ingredients.
What symptoms the medicine will relieve.
How much to take, when to take it, and when not to take it.
When to stop using the medicine.
Warnings.
If and when to consult a doctor.
Side effects and drug interactions.

When taking prescription medicines

Never take any medicine that has been prescribed for a friend or relative, and never allow a friend or relative to use yours. Never take more medicine than is prescribed. Two pills are not better than one; they may at best be ineffective or at worst dangerous.

When taking all medicines

Check the expiration date on the label. After that date, the medicine may lose its potency and in some cases may be harmful. Discard them immediately.

Safely dispose of all out-of-date medicines by flushing them down the toilet or putting them in the garbage disposal rather than in a trash can, where a child or pet may find them.

Keep all medicines in their original containers with the labels, including nonprescription medicines.

Always replace child-resistant caps carefully. If there are no young children in your household, you may request prescription drugs without child-resistant caps.

If you are pregnant or nursing a baby
It is especially important to consult your physician or your pharmacist before taking any prescription or nonprescription medicine.

If you are elderly
As you get older, changes in your body may make you more susceptible to side effects or drug interactions. Always tell your doctor exactly what medicines you are taking, including nonprescription ones.

(Source: Council on Family Health, Washington, D.C. Adapted with permission.)

Keeping Track

Women have no shortage of lists, files, and other paperwork in our lives, but the following may prove life-saving. They will certainly help you keep an organized account of your drug therapy and can give you, your doctor, and your pharmacist an overall look at your total drug-management program.

- Keep a medication journal or diary. It doesn't have to be complicated or sophisticated. Choose a method that fits your schedule and lifestyle, which can mean simply jotting down the names of the medications you took that day, to a detailed account of drugs, dosages, times taken, and side effects.
- If you take multiple medications, or are on them for an extended period of time, keeping a record can prove indispensable. Every time you take a medication, write down the name, the dosage, and the time. This is especially important when taking more than one drug day after day, as it's easy to become confused. Note any side effects or symptoms whether you think they're drug related or not. Over time, you may see a pattern emerge that can prove useful in adjusting medications or dosages.
- Drug recordkeeping is essential for elderly women, women with chronic illnesses, and women seeing numerous doctors, all of whom run an increased risk of overmedication, oversedation, and even "doubling up" (taking both the generic *and* the brand-name forms of a drug). If a doctor, pharmacist, or other health care professional sees a patient's "grocery list" of drugs, they may be alerted to the possibility of overmedication.

- Keep at least three copies of a list with the following information: prescription drugs and the name of the prescribing health care professional; all nonprescription medications; and vitamins, herbal remedies, and dietary supplements. Keep one copy at home, carry one copy with you (with a medical ID tag if you have a chronic condition or are using a drug that has potentially serious interactions), and give one copy to a trusted family member. Update it regularly and give each of your health care providers a copy. Never assume that all of your doctors know what you are taking. They don't—unless you tell them.

- Save the package insert that comes with each drug, even if you think you'll never wade through all of that frustrating, flea-size type. Thankfully, some print ads now feature patient information in a convenient question-and-answer format, but it may not have the complete prescribing information that is on the package insert. Store your package inserts and pharmacy instruction sheets in a large envelope or file folder.

Drugs in Cyberspace

Many prescription drugs now have their own Web sites on the Internet. You can enter the drug's brand or generic name as a keyword to see a list of "hits" containing that drug. Many of them use www., then the name of the drug, then .com. Pharmaceutical companies also have their own Web sites with information on many of their products. Keep in mind that a drug's manufacturer may choose to put a more positive spin on product summaries and advertising copy. However, most of them also offer full package-insert information (usually titled "Prescribing Information") that comes complete with cautions and warnings.

Ordering prescription drugs on-line is relatively uncharted and unaccredited territory, but it will no doubt become a booming industry if and when more people become accustomed to and comfortable with the process. There are more than 400 on-line pharmacies, some requiring your doctor's examination report and prescription, and others offering "quickie" on-line evaluations resulting in a ready-to-fill prescription. The National Association of Boards of Pharmacy is pioneering a certification process to meet the association's licensure and compliance requirements. To qualify, on-line pharmacies must meet a 17-point pharmacy practice criteria including verification of prescriber and patient identity, patient confidentiality, and patient education about the drugs they are using.

In the meantime, use caution when ordering drugs on-line.

The FDA acknowledges that many on-line sites are lawful enterprises that genuinely offer privacy, convenience, and traditional safeguards. Buying on-line offers greater availability of drugs, and access to comparison shopping. However, there are "rogue sites" using the Internet as an outlet for illegal products and practices. The FDA offers the following tips:

- Check the National Association of Boards of Pharmacy Web site at *www.nabp.net* to determine if the site is licensed.
- Make sure that the site provides access to a registered pharmacist to answer your questions.
- Avoid sites that do not properly identify themselves or their location, or do not have a U.S. address and phone number to contact if there is a problem, particularly if they specialize in selling Viagra or weight-loss drugs such as Xenical (orlistat).
- Do not buy drugs from sites that provide prescription drugs for first-time use without a physical exam.

Over-the-Counter Medications

There are thousands of them, we see dozens of advertisements for them every day, they are certainly accessible, and millions of Americans use them safely and regularly with little or no ill effects. But nonprescription, or over-the-counter (OTC), medications can contain the same or similar ingredients as those used in prescription drugs and so can cause side effects and, in some cases, significant interactions with one another or with prescription drugs. A general rule of thumb for OTCs is to follow package directions carefully, do not increase the dosage or take for longer than is recommended, and notify your doctor if your symptoms do not improve or if they get worse. Your pharmacist can be your first and best source of information about the following OTC medications.

Oral analgesics

Pain is usually a symptom of an underlying condition, can be acute or chronic, mild or severe, temporary or long-lasting. Nonprescription pain relievers include aspirin, acetaminophen, and other nonsteroidal antiinflammatory drugs (NSAIDs), and are used for everything from headaches to menstrual cramps to arthritis. Such pain relievers can interact with many prescription drugs (including blood-thinners) and, in the case of NSAIDs (including aspirin), carry the risk of stomach irritation and gastric bleeding. The combination of acetaminophen and regular alcohol use has been implicated in liver problems. Pain relievers for migraine headaches often contain caffeine—a substance that can interact with certain drugs and cause caffeine withdrawal when stopped.

Appetite suppressants

Many of these drugs contain phenylpropanolamine (PPA), a decongestant found in many cough, cold, and sinus medications. PPA is a stimulant and can cause nervousness, palpitations, and insomnia. Package warnings state that people who have heart disease, hypertension, diabetes, or thyroid disease should not take these drugs without a doctor's supervision. Combining them with caffeine or caffeine-containing products can cause overstimulation. PPA should never be taken with any monoamine oxidase (MAO) inhibitor antidepressant. OTC appetite suppressants are indicated for short-term use only; their effectiveness decreases with prolonged use.

Sleep aids

The main ingredients in these preparations are antihistamines, which are generally used to control symptoms of colds, allergies, and sinus problems. If you've ever taken an OTC antihistamine, you have probably experienced drowsiness as a side effect. A subgroup of antihistamines includes the ingredients diphenhydramine and doxylamine, the main components in most OTC sleep aids. Common side effects are dry mouth, dizziness, fatigue, and lethargy. Antihistamines can interact with many prescription drugs, including benzodiazepines and any central nervous system (CNS) depressant. Sleep aids are intended for short-term use only. Chronic insomnia may be a sign of an underlying condition such as depression.

Antacids and histamine H_2 blockers

There are four histamine H_2 blockers on the Top 200 Prescriptions of 1998—cimetidine, famotidine, nizatadine, and ranitidine—and all four have OTC versions that are used for heartburn and acid indigestion. These acid reducers are among the most popular and best-selling nonprescription medications, as are regular antacids, which are usually quicker acting. Antacids and acid reducers can interfere with the absorption of many prescription medications, including heart drugs, antidepressants, some asthma medications, and benzodiazepines. In some cases, doses of antacids and other drugs need to be separated by at least 2 hours. Long-term use can mask the symptoms of an ulcer or gastroesophageal reflux disease (GERD).

Vaginal yeast infection antifungals

The introduction of OTC antifungal medications to treat vaginal yeast infections means that women no longer have to run to their doctors every time these irritating and often persistent episodes occur. They come in vaginal suppository, cream, and tablet form and are designed for a limited course of treatment. If you have been previously diagnosed and treated, and familiar symptoms recur, these products can be convenient and appropriate. Unfortunately, they are sometimes used in place of proper medical diagnosis. Do not self-medicate with OTC antifungals. If your symptoms do not improve or if they worsen, you may have a bacterial vaginal infection that may require antibiotic treatment.

Women's Resource Directory

The organizations and resources listed below are arranged according to condition, disease, disorder, or topic. The names, addresses, phone numbers, and Web sites were accurate to the best of our knowledge at the time of publication. Toll-free telephone numbers (those with 800, 877, or 888 prefixes) are included whenever possible.

If you choose to write for information, a postcard request is sufficient. Be sure to indicate a specific topic, as some of these organizations have numerous brochures available on a wide range of subjects. There may be a local branch of the organization you seek, so consult your local telephone book first. You can also do an on-line search using a keyword (osteoporosis, arthritis, breast cancer, etc.), as the Web contains thousands of women's health sites on individual topics as well as links to other sites.

If there is a fee for any information from the following organizations, they will send you a list of materials available for sale (books or videocassettes, for example). In almost all cases, however, the pamphlets and brochures they provide are free.

AIDS

CDC National AIDS Hotline
P.O. Box 13827
Research Triangle Park, NC 27709
800–342–AIDS 24 hours a day
800–344–7432 (Spanish) 8 A.M.–2 P.M. every day
800–243–7889 (TTY service for the hearing impaired) 10 A.M.–10 P.M. Monday–Friday. Trained information specialists offer anonymous, confidential information about HIV and AIDS and provide referrals to appropriate services.

AIDS Treatment Information Service (ATIS)
www.hivatis.org
Provides information about federally approved treatment guidelines including the HIV Treatment Guidelines for Adults and Adolescents, which can be downloaded from their Web site.

The AIDS Clinical Trials Information Service (ACTIS)
800–874–2572
Provides the latest information on clinical trials of experimental drugs and other therapies for people at all stages of HIV infection.
www.actis.org

Aging

The National Center on Women and Aging
Heller Graduate School MS 035
Brandeis University
Waltham, MA 02454–9110
www.brandeis.edu/heller/national/ind.html

National Institute on Aging
Building 31, Room 5C27
31 Center Drive, MSC 2292
Bethesda, MD 20892
www.nih.gov/nia

Alcoholism

Alcoholics Anonymous (AA)
475 Riverside Drive, 11th Floor
New York, NY 10015
(Also consult local telephone book listings)
www.alcoholics-anonymous.org

National Council on Alcoholism and Drug Dependence
12 W. 21st St.
New York, NY 10010
800-NCA-CALL
(Refers callers to local NCADD affiliates)
www.ncadd.org

Allergy and Asthma

American Academy of Allergy, Asthma and Immunology
611 East Wells St.
Milwaukee, WI 53202
800–822–ASMA (hotline)
www.aaaai.org

National Jewish Medical and Research Center
1400 Jackson St.
Denver, CO 80206
800–222–5864
www.njc.org

Alzheimer's Disease

Alzheimer's Association
919 N. Michigan Ave., Suite 1100
Chicago, IL 60611–1676
800–272–3900
(Also consult local telephone book listings)
www.alz.org

Anorexia (see Eating Disorders)

Anxiety

Anxiety Disorders Association of America
11900 Parklawn Dr., Suite 100
Rockville, MD 20852
301–231–9350
www.adaa.org

American Psychiatric Association
Division of Public Affairs, Code P-H
1400 K Street NW
Washington, DC 20005
202–682–6220
www.psych.org

National Institute of Mental Health (NIMH)
Public Inquiries
6001 Executive Blvd. RM. 8184 MSC 9663
Bethesda, MD 20892-9663
301–443–4513
www.nimh.nih.gov
(Note: NIMH has hundreds of brochures on numerous topics; be
sure to specifically request information on anxiety.)

Arthritis

Arthritis Foundation
1330 W. Peachtree St.
Atlanta, GA 30309
800–283–7800
(Also consult local telephone book listings)
www.arthritis.org

National Institute of Arthritis and Musculoskeletal and Skin
Diseases
Building 31, Room 4C05
Bethesda, MD 20892-2350
301–496–8188
877–226–4267
www.nih.gov/niams

Attention Deficit Hyperactivity Disorder (ADHD)

ADD Warehouse
800–233–9273
www.addwarehouse.com

Children and Adults with Attention Deficit Disorders
800–233–4050
www.chadd.org

Bulimia (see Eating Disorders)

Cancer

American Cancer Society
National Office
1599 Clifton Road, N.E.
Atlanta, GA 30329
800–ACS–2345
(Also consult local telephone book listings)
www.cancer.org

College of American Pathologists
325 Waukegan Road
Northfield, IL 60093
800–323–4040
www.papsmear.org
Register on the Web site to get email reminders to make an appointment.

National Cancer Institute
Office of Cancer Communications
Building 31, Room 10A03, MSC 2580
Bethesda, MD 20892-2580
800–4CANCER
www.nci.nih.gov

Women's Cancer Network
c/o Gynecologic Cancer Foundation
401 N. Michigan Avenue
Chicago, IL 60611
312–644–6610
800–444–4441

Cancer, Breast

Y-Me National Organization for Breast Cancer Information and Support
212 W. Van Buren St.
Chicago, IL 60607-3908
800–221–2141 (hotline)
www.Y-me.org

The Susan G. Komen Breast Cancer Foundation
5005 LBJ Freeway, Suite 250
Dallas, TX 75244
800–462–9273 (Breast Care Helpline)
www.breastcancerinfo.com

Cancer, Ovarian

Ovarian Cancer National Alliance
910 17th St NW Suite 413
Washington, DC 20006
202–331–1332
www.ovariancancer.org

Cancer, Skin

Skin Cancer Foundation
P.O. Box 561
New York, NY 10156
800–SKIN490
www.skincancer.org

Chronic Fatigue Syndrome

The CFIDS Association of America, Inc.
P.O. Box 220398
Charlotte, NC 28222–0398
800–442–3437
www.cfids.org

Contraception

Plan B (Emergency contraceptive)
Women's Capital Corporation
P.O. Box 5026
Bellevue, WA 98009–5026
888–NOT–2–LATE (Emergency Contraception Hotline)
www.go2planb.com

Planned Parenthood Federation of America, Inc.
800–230–PLAN
(Also consult local telephone book listings)
www.plannedparenthood.org

Cystitis (see Urinary Tract Infections)

Depression

National Institute of Mental Health (NIMH)
Information Resources and Inquiries Branch

Office of Scientific Information, Room 15C
5900 Fishers Lane, Room 15–105
Rockville, MD 20857
301–443–4513
www.nimh.nih.gov
(Note: NIMH has hundreds of brochures on various topics; be sure to specifically request information on depression.)

American Psychiatric Association
Division of Public Affairs, Code P–H
1400 K Street NW
Washington, DC 20005
202–682–6220
www.psych.org

Diabetes

American Diabetes Association
National Center
1701 N. Beauregard St.
Alexandria, VA 22311
800–232–3472
(Also consult local telephone book listings)
www.diabetes.org

Eating Disorders

National Association of Anorexia Nervosa and Associated Disorders
P.O. Box 7
Highland Park, IL 60035
847–831–3438
www.anad.org

Overeaters Anonymous, Inc.
World Service Office
6075 Zenith Court, NE
Rio Rancho, NM 87124
505–891–2664
www.overeatersanonymous.org
(Consult local telephone book listings)

Endometriosis

The Endometriosis Association
8585 N. 76th Place
Milwaukee, WI 53223
800–992–3636
www.endometriosisassn.org

Epilepsy

The Epilepsy Foundation
4351 Garden City Drive
Landover, MD 20785
800–EFA–1000
www.efa.org

Glaucoma

The Glaucoma Foundation
116 John St. Suite 1605
New York, NY 10038
800–452–8266·(hotline)
www.glaucoma-foundation.org

Headache (including Migraine)

American Council for Headache Education
19 Mantua Road
Mt. Royal, NJ 08061
800–255–ACHE
www.achenet.org

National Headache Foundation
428 W. St. James Place, 2nd Floor
Chicago, IL 60614–2750
888–NHF–5552
www.headaches.org

Heart Disease

American Heart Association
7272 Greenville Ave.
Dallas, TX 75231
800–AHA–USA1 (800–242–8721)
www.americanheart.org
(Also consult local telephone book listings)

AHA National Women's Heart Disease and Stroke Campaign
888–MY-HEART (888–69–43278)

National Heart, Lung, and Blood Institute
Information Center
P.O. Box 30105
Bethesda, MD 20824–0105
800–575–WELL (800–575–9355)
www.nhlbi.nih.gov

Herpes

American Social Health Association
P.O. Box 13827
Research Triangle Park, NC 27709
800–227–8922 (CDC Sexually Transmitted Diseases Hotline)
www.ashastd.org

High Blood Pressure (Hypertension)

American Heart Association
7272 Greenville Ave.
Dallas, TX 75231
800-AHA-USA1 (800–242–8721)
www.americanheart.org

National Heart, Lung, and Blood Institute
Information Center
P.O. Box 30105
Bethesda, MD 20824–0105
800–575-WELL (800–575–9355)
www.nhlbi.nih.gov

Hysterectomy

Hysterectomy Educational Resources and Services Foundation
(HERS)
422 Bryn Mawr Ave.
Bala Cynwyd, PA 19004
610–667–7757
www.ccon.com/hers

Infectious Diseases

Centers for Disease Control (CDC)
1600 Clifton Road
Atlanta, GA 30333
404–639–7230 (Women's Health)
800–311–3435
www.cdc.gov

Infertility

RESOLVE, Inc.
1310 Broadway
Somerville, MA 02144–1731
617–623–0744
617–623–1156
www.resolve.org

Kidney Disease

National Kidney Foundation
30 E. 33rd Street
New York, NY 10016
800–622–9010
(Also consult local telephone book listings)
www.kidney.org

American Kidney Fund
6110 Executive Bld., Suite 1010
Rockville, MD 20852
800–638–8299
www.kidneyfund.org

Lupus

Lupus Foundation of America, Inc.
1300 Piccard Drive., Suite 200
Rockville, MD 20850–4303
800–558–0121
www.lupus.org

Medications (see also Pharmaceuticals)

DES Information
DES (diethylstilbestrol) is a synthetic hormone that was widely
prescribed to pregnant women between 1938 and 1971 to prevent miscarriage. Women and children who were exposed to
this drug may experience serious health problems. The National
Cancer Institute has produced a series of free booklets designed
to answer questions and provide resources. For a list of titles,
call DES Action, 800–337–9288.
www.desaction.org

Food and Drug Administration (FDA)
HFE88
5600 Fishers Lane
Rockville, MD 20857
888-463-6332
(Also consult local telephone book government listings)
www.fda.gov/womens
Sponsors "Take Time to Care" program concerning women and
medications.

Free and Low-Cost Prescription Drugs
Cost Containment Research Institute
611 Pennsylvania Avenue, SE, Suite 1010

Washington, DC 20003–4303
202–637–0038
202–637–0001
www.institute-dc.org
Information for certain qualified individuals to receive drugs at little or no cost.

MedWatch
U.S. Food and Drug Administration Medical Products Reporting System
888-INFO-FDA
If you have had a serious adverse reaction to a drug, you can request forms to report your experience. The information you supply, including your identity, is confidential and legally protected. This valuable program has been instrumental in the withdrawal of potentially dangerous drugs from the market.
www.fda.gov/medwatch

Menopause

North American Menopause Society
P.O. Box 94527
Cleveland, OH 44101–4527
800–774–5342
www.menopause.org

Mitral Valve Prolapse (MVP)

Mitral Valve Prolapse Center of Alabama
800 Montclair Road, Suite 370
Birmingham, AL 35213
800–541–8602
www.mvprolapse.com

Multiple Sclerosis

Multiple Sclerosis Association of America
706 Haddonfield Road
Cherry Hill, NJ 08002
800–LEARN–MS
(Also consult local telephone book listings)
www.msaa.com

Osteoporosis

National Osteoporosis Foundation
1232 22nd Street NW
Washington, DC 20037–1292
877–868–4520
www.nof.org

Obesity

Weight-control Information Network
1 Win Way
Bethesda, MD 20892–3665
877–946–4627
www.niddk.nih.gov

Pain

American Chronic Pain Association
P.O. Box 850
Rocklin, CA 95677
916–632–0922
(Also consult local telephone book listings)
www.theacpa.org

Parkinson's Disease

American Parkinson's Disease Association
250 Hylan Bld., Suite 4B
Staten Island, NY 10305–1946
800–223–2732
(Also consult local telephone book listings)
www.apdaparkinson.com

Pharmacists

American Association of Colleges of Pharmacy
1426 Prince St.
Alexandria, VA 22314
703–739–2330
www.aacp.org

American Society of Health-System Pharmacists
7272 Wisconsin Avenue
Bethesda, MD 20814
301–657–3000
www.ashp.org

National Association of Chain Drug Stores
413 North Lee St.
P.O. Box 1417-D49
Alexandria, VA 22313–1480
703–549–3001
www.nacds.org

Pharmaceuticals

American Pharmaceutical Association
2215 Constitution Ave. NW
Washington, DC 20037-2985
800-237-AphA
www.aphanet.org

Consumer Healthcare Products Association
1150 Connecticut Ave. NW
Washington, DC 20036
202-429-9260
www.chpa-info.org

Pharmaceutical Research and Manufacturers of America
1100 15th Street NW
Washington, DC 20005
www.phrma.org

Pregnancy

American College of Obstetricians and Gynecologists Resource
Center
409 12th Street SW
Washington, DC 20024-2188
202-638-5577
www.acog.org

Premenstrual Syndrome (PMS)

PMS Access
P.O. Box 9326
Madison, WI 53715
800-222-4767

Rheumatoid Arthritis (see Arthritis)

Rosacea

National Rosacea Society
800 S. Northwest Highway, #200
Barrington, IL 60010
888-NO-BLUSH
www.rosacea.org

Sexually Transmitted Diseases

American Social Health Association
P.O. Box 13827
Research Triangle Park, NC 27709
800-227-8922 (CDC National STD Hotline)
www.ashastd.org

Stroke

National Stroke Association
96 Inverness Dr. E, Suite I
Englewood, CO 80112-5112
800–787–6537
www.stroke.org

Ulcers

Centers for Disease Control (CDC)
1600 Clifton Road
Atlanta, GA 30333
404–639–7230
800–311–3435
www.cdc.gov

Urinary Tract Infections (UTIs)

Interstitial Cystitis Association of America, Inc.
51 Monroe St., Suite 1402
Rockville, MD 20850
800–435–7422
www.ichelp.org

Women's Health

Agency for Healthcare Research and Quality (AHRQ)
Women's Health Program
U.S. Department of Health and Human Services
200 Independence Avenue, SW
Washington, DC 20201
877–696–6775
www.ahcpr.gov

The American Medical Women's Association
801 N. Fairfax St., Suite 400
Alexandria, VA 22314
703–838–0500
www.amwa-doc.org

Council on Family Health
1155 Connecticut Ave. NW, Suite 400
Washington, DC 20036
202–429–6600
www.cfhinfo.org

Health Gate Data Corp
25 Corporate Drive
Burlington, MA 01803
800–434–GATE (4283)
www.healthgate.com

National Caucus and Center on Black Aged, Inc.
1424 K Street, NW, Suite 500
Washington, DC 20005
202–637–8400
www.ncba-blackaged.org

National Latina Health Organization (NLHO)
P.O. Box 7587
Oakland, CA 94801
510–534–1362
E-mail: *latinahlth@aol.com*

Office of Minority Health
P.O. Box 37337
Washington, DC 20013–7337
800–444–6472
www.omhrc.gov

Partnership for Women's Health at Columbia
The Journal of Gender-Specific Medicine
CPMC, PH 8-105
622 W. 168th St.
New York, NY 10032
212–305–9514
www.mmhc.com
The first publication to explore gender-related differences in
health care, current research, and news in gender-specific medicine.

Women's Health America
429 Gammon Place
P.O. Box 259690
Madison, WI 53725
800–222–4767 (National Women's Health Hotline)
www.womenshealth.com

Women's Health Initiative
Women between the ages of 50 and 79 are needed for studies conducted on cancer, heart disease, and osteoporosis at forty nationwide centers. The WHI provides certain medical exams at no cost to the participant for up to twelve years. There are no experimental drugs, no medical trainees involved, and no monetary compensation to join the study. For more information, call 800–97-WOMEN.

Appendix 1: Medical Conditions

Below is a list of medical conditions followed by selected brand-name and generic prescription drugs that may be used to treat either the condition or the symptoms of the condition. This cross-reference includes *only* the brand-name and generic drugs mentioned in this book. Consult your physician if you have questions about these or any other drugs prescribed for your particular condition. For more information on each of these drugs, see part 1—Prescription Drug Profiles.

Acne
Accutane
A/T/S
E.E.S.
E-Mycin
Erycette
Ery-Tab
erythromycin
erythromycin, topical
isotretinoin
Retin-A
tretinoin
T-Stat

Acquired Immune Deficiency Syndrome (AIDS), see HIV

Allergies
Allegra
beclomethasone
Beconase AQ
cetirizine
Claritin
Claritin-D 12 HR
Claritin-D 24 HR
cromolyn sodium
cyproheptadine
fexofenadine hydrochloride
Flonase
Flovent
fluticasone propionate
Intal
loratadine 12 Hr
loratadine 24 Hr
loratadine/pseudoephedrine
mometasone furoate
Nasalcrom
Nasonex
Periactin
Vancenase AQ
Vancenase AQ DS
Vanceril Inhaler
Zyrtec

Alzheimer's disease
Aricept
Cognex
donepezil
tacrine hydrochloride

Angina
amlodipine
Calan SR
Cardizem
Cardizem CD
Cardizem SR
Dilacor SR
diltiazem hydrochloride
Lopressor
metoprolol tartrate
nifedipine
Norvasc
Procardia XL

Toprol XL
verapamil SR

Anxiety
alprazolam
Alzapam
atenolol
Ativan
BuSpar
buspirone
Centrax
clorazepate dipotassium
diazepam
Librium
Lopressor
lorazepam
metoprolol tartrate
Nardil
phenelzine sulfate
prazepam
Tenormin
Toprol XL
Tranxene
Valium
Xanax

Arthritis (see also Osteoarthritis; Rheumatoid Arthritis)
Advil
Arava
Cytotec
ibuprofen
Indocin
indomethacin
leflunomide
Medipren
Motrin
misoprostol
Nuprin

Asthma
Accolate
albuterol
Azmacort Aerosol
Deltasone

Liquid Pred
Medrol
methylprednisolone
Meticorten
Nasacort Aerosol
nifedipine
Orasone
prednisone
Procardia XL
Proventil
salmeterol xinafoate
Serevent
triamcinolone acetonide
Ventolin
zafirlukast

Attention Deficit Hyperactivity Disorder (ADHD)
Adderall
amphetamine

Bulimia
amitriptyline
Elavil
Endep
fluoxetine
Prozac

Cancer, breast
cyclophosphamide
Cytoxan
Evista
fluoxymesterone
Halotestin
methotrexate
Nolvadex
raloxifene
Rheumatrex
tamoxifen citrate

Cancer, ovarian
Climara
cyclophosphamide
Cytoxan
Estrace
Estraderm

estradiol
Estraguard

Cancer, other
cyclophosphamide
Cytoxan
methotrexate
Rheumatrex

Candidiasis
Diflucan
fluconazole
Terazol 3
Terazol 7
terconazole

Cholesterol-lowering
atorvastatin calcium
fluvastatin
gemfibrozil
Lescol
Lipitor
Lopid
lovastatin
Mevacor
Pravachol
pravastatin

Contraceptive, injection
Depo-Provera

Contraceptive, oral
Alesse-21
Alesse-28
Brevicon
Demulen 1/35
Demulen 1/50
Desogen
desogestrel and ethinyl
    estradiol
Estrostep
Estrostep Fe
ethynodial diacetate and
    ethinyl estradiol
Genora 0.5/35
Genora 1/35
Genora 1/50

Intercon 0.5/35
Intercon 1/35
Intercon 1/50
Jenest-28
Levlen
Levlite
levonorgestrel and ethinyl
    estradiol
Levora 0.15/30
Loestrin 1.5/30
Loestrin 1/20
Loestrin Fe 1.5/30
Loestrin Fe 1/20
Lo-Ovral
Mircette
Modicon
N.E.E. 1/35
N.E.E. 1/50
Necon 0.5/35
Necon 1/35
Necon 1/50
Necon 10/11
Nelova 1/35
Nelova 1/50M
Nelova 10/11
Nordette
Norethin 1/35
Norethin 1/50M
norethindrone acetate and
    ethinyl estradiol
norethindrone and ethinyl
    estradiol
norethindrone and
    mestranol
norgestimate and ethinyl
    estradiol
norgestrel and ethinyl
    estradiol
Norinyl 1+35
Norinyl 1+50
Ortho Tri-Cyclen
Ortho-Cept
Ortho-Cyclen
Ortho-Novum 1/35
Ortho-Novum 1/50

Ortho-Novum 10/11 28
Ortho-Novum 7–7–7 28
Ovcon-35
Ovcon-50
Ovral
Tri-Levlen
Tri-Norinyl 28
Triphasil
Trivora
Zovia 1/35E
Zovia 1/50E

Depression
alprazolam
amitriptyline
bupropion hydrochloride
clorazepate dipotassium
Depakote
Desyrel
divalproex
Effexor
Elavil
Endep
fluoxetine
fluvoxamine
gabapentin
imipramine hydrochloride
Luvox
Nardil
nefazodone
Neurontoin
paroxetine
Paxil
phenelzine sulfate
Prozac
sertraline
Serzone
Tofranil
Tranxene
trazodone
venlafaxine
Wellbutrin
Wellbutrin SR
Zoloft

Diabetes, Type I (Insulin Dependent)
Humalin 70/30
Humalin N
Humalin R
insulin

Diabetes, Type II (Non-insulin-Dependent)
Actos
Amaryl
Avandia
glimepiride
glipizide
Glucophage
Glucotrol
Glucotrol XL
metformin hydrochloride
pioglitazone
rosiglitazone

Edema
Aldactone
Diaqua
Esidrix
hydrochlorothiazide (HCTZ)
HydroDIURAL
spironolactone

Endometriosis
Cycrin
medroxyprogesterone acetate
nafarelin acetate
Provera
Synarel

Epileptic seizures, see Seizures

Fluid Retention, see Edema

Gallstones
Actigall
ursodiol USP

Gastroesophageal reflux disease (GERD)
cimetidine
famotidine
omeprazole
Pepcid
Prilosec
Propulsid
ranitidine
Tagamet
Zantac

Genital Warts
Aldara
Condylox
imiquimod
podofilox

Glaucoma
timolol
Timoptic XE

Gout
allopurinol
Zyloprim

HIV
Combiver
Crixivan
indinavir sulfate
Norvir
Retrovir
ritonavir
zidovudine (AZT)

Headaches, migraine
Amerge
amitriptyline
Ansaid
Betapace
carbamazepine
Elavil
Endep
flurbiprofen
Imitrex
Isoptin
Lopressor

Maxalt
metoprolol tartrate
naratriptan hydrochloride
nifedipine
Procardia XL
rizatriptan benzoate
sotalol
sumatriptan
Tegretol
Toprol XL
verapamil
zolmitriptan
Zomig

Headaches, other
Advil
ibuprofen
ketoprofen
Medipren
Motrin
Nuprin
Orudis
Rufen

Heart Arrhythmia
Betapace
Calan SR
Isoptin
Isoptin SR
sotalol
verapamil
Verelan

Heart Conditions
Altace
amlodipine
atenolol
Calan SR
Capoten
captopril
Cardizem
Cardizem CD
Cardizem SR
Diaqua
Dilacor SR
diltiazem hydrochloride

enalapril maleate
Esidrix
furosemide
hydrochlorothiazide
(HCTZ)
HydroDIURAL
Inderal
Isoptin
Lasix
Lopressor (also Toprol XL)
metoprolol tartrate
nifedipine
nitroglycerin
Nitrostat
Norvasc
Procardia XL
propranolol
ramipril
Tenormin
Vasotec
verapamil SR
Verelan

Herpes
acyclovir
famciclovir
Famvir
valacyclovir
Valtrex
Zovirax

**High Blood Pressure
(Hypertension)**
Accupril
Aldactone
Altace
amlodipine
atenolol
benazepril
Calan SR
Capoten
captopril
Cardura
Cozaar
Diaqua
doxazosin

Dyazide
enalapril maleate
Esidrix
felodipine
fosinopril
furosemide
hydrochlorothiazide
(HCTZ)
HydroDIURAL
Hytrin
Hyzaar
Inderal
Kato
K-Dur 10
K-Dur 20
Klor-Con
Lasix
lisinopril
Lopressor
losartan potassium
losartan/hydrochlorothia-
zide (HCTZ)
Lotensin
metoprolol tartrate
Micro-K Extencaps
Monopril
nifedipine
Norvasc
Plendil
potassium chloride
Prinivil
Procardia XL
propranolol
quinapril
ramipril
spironolactone
Tenormin
terazosin
Toprol XL
triamterene
Vasotec
verapamil SR
Zestril

Infections, bacterial
  amoxicillin and potassium
    clavulanate
  Augmentin
  Bactroban
  cefprozil
  Ceftin
  cefuroxime axetil
  Cefzil
  cephalexin
  Floxin
  Keflet
  Keflex
  Lorabid
  loracarbef
  MetroGel
  metronidazole
  mupirocin
  ofloxacin
  penicillin VK
  Sumycin
  tetracycline HCL
  Veetids
  Zithromax

Infections, fungal
  betamethasone and
    clotrimazole
  Diflucan
  fluconazole
  itraconazole
  ketoconazole
  Lotrisone
  Nizoral
  Sporanox

Infections, respiratory tract
  amoxicillin
  Amoxil
  azithromycin
  Biaxin
  Biomox
  cephalexin
  clarithromycin
  E.E.S.

E-Mycin
Ery-Tab
Erythrocin
erythromycin
Keflet
Keflex
Lorabid
loracarbef
Polymox
Trimox
Wymox
Zithromax

Infections, skin
  amoxicillin
  Amoxil
  azithromycin
  Bactroban
  Biomox
  cephalexin
  Cipro
  ciprofloxacin
  Deltasone
  Keflet
  Keflex
  Liquid Pred
  Lorabid
  loracarbef
  Meticorten
  mupirocin
  Orasone
  Polymox
  prednisone
  Trimox
  Wymox
  Zithromax

**Infections, urinary tract
(UTIs)**
  amoxicillin
  Amoxil
  azithromycin
  Bactrim
  Biomox
  cephalexin

Cipro
ciprofloxacin
Cotrim
Cotrim DS
E.E.S.
E-Mycin
Ery-Tab
Erythrocin
erythromycin (oral)
Flagyl
flavoxate hydrochloride
Floxin
Gantrisin
Keflet
Keflex
Levaquin
levofloxacin
Lorabid
loracarbef
Macrobid
nitrofurantoin
ofloxacin
Polymox
Protostat
Septra
Septra DS
sulfisoxazole
trimethoprim and
    sulfamethoxazole
Trimox
Urispas
Wymox
Zithromax

Infertility
Clomid
clomiphene

Insomnia
Alzapam
Ambien
Ativan
diazepam
Halcion
Restoril

temazepam
triazolam
Valium
zolpidem

Irritable Bowel Syndrome (IBS)
alprazolam
Alzapam
Ativan
Bentyl
Centrax
clorazepate dipotassium
dicyclomine hydrochloride
lorazepam
prazepam
Tranxene
Xanax

Lupus
Deltasone
Liquid Pred
Meticorten
Orasone
prednisone

Menopause
conjugated estrogens
conjugated estrogens and
    medroxyprogesterone
estropipate
Evista
Ogen
Premarin
Premphase
Prempro
raloxifene HCl

Menstrual Pain
Ansaid
flurbiprofen
ibuprofen
Motrin
Naprelan
Naprosyn
naproxen sodium

rofecoxib
Vioxx

Motion Sickness

Antivert
meclizine
Phenergan suppository
promethazine

Multiple Sclerosis

amantadine
Avonex
Betaseron
Deltasone
interferon beta 1-a
interferon beta 1-b
Liquid Pred
Meticorten
Orasone
prednisone
Symmetrel

Obesity

Adipex-P
Daspex
Fastin
Ionamin
Mazanor
mazindol
Meridia
orlistat
phentermine
sibutramine hydrochloride
monohydrate
Xenical

Obsessive-Compulsive Disorder (OCD)

fluoxetine
fluvoxamine
Luvox
Prozac
sertraline
Zoloft

Osteoarthritis (also see Arthritis)

Ansaid
capsaicin
Celebrex
celecoxib
Daypro
diclofenac sodium
flurbiprofen
ibuprofen
ketoprofen
Motrin
nabumetone
Naprelan
Naprosyn
naproxen
naproxen sodium
Orudis
Orudis SR
oxaprozin
Relafen
rofecoxib
Vioxx
Zostrix

Osteoporosis

alendorate sodium
calcitonin salmon
Fosamax
Miacalcin

Pain

acetaminophen and
codeine phosphate
acetaminophen and
hydrocodone bitartrate
acetaminophen and
oxycodone
hydrochloride
carisoprodol
cyclobenzaprine
Darvocet-N 100
Endocet
Flexeril
ibuprofen
ketoprofen

Lorcet
Lortab
Motrin
~~Naprelan~~
naproxen
naproxen sodium
Naprosyn
Norcet
Orudis
Orudis SR
Panacet
Percocet
phenazopyridine
   hydrochloride
Propacet 100
propoxyphene napsylate
   and acetaminophen
Pyridium
rofecoxib
Roxicet
Roxilox
Soma
tramadol
Tylox
Tylenol with Codeine
Ultram
Vicodin
Vicodin-ES
Vioxx
Zydone

Panic Disorder
alprazolam
Alzapam
Ativan
Centrax
clonazepam
clorazepate dipotassium
diazepam
Klonopin
lorazepam
paroxetine
Paxil
prazepam
Tranxene

Valium
Xanax

Parkinson's Disease
amantadine
carbidopa and levodopa
Eldepryl
Mirapex
pramipexole
selegiline
Sinemet
Sinemet CR
Symmetrel

**Premenstrual Syndrome
(PMS)**
alprazolam
BuSpar
buspirone
Cycrin
medroxyprogesterone
Provera
Xanax

Psoriasis
calcipotriene
cyclosporine
Dovonex
methotrexate
Neoral
Rheumatrex
Sandimmune
SangCya

**Rheumatoid Arthritis (also
see Arthritis)**
Advil
Ansaid
Arava
auranofin
capsaicin
Celebrex
celecoxib
cyclosporine
Daypro
Deltasone
Enbrel

etanercept
flurbiprofen
ibuprofen
ketoprofen
leflunomide
Liquid Pred
Medipren
Medrol
methotrexate
methylprednisolone
Meticorten
Motrin
nabumetone
Naprelan
Naprosyn
naproxen
naproxen sodium
Neoral
Nuprin
Orasone
Orudis
Orudis SR
oxaprozin
prednisone
Relafen
Rheumatrex
Ridaura
Sandimmune
Sang Eya
Zostrix

Rosacea
MetroGel
metronidazole

Seizures
carbamazepine
clonazepam
Depakote
Dilantin
divalproex
Klonopin
phenytoin
Tegretol

Sexually Transmitted Diseases (STDs)
acyclovir
Aldara
amoxicillin
amoxil
azithromycin
Biomox
Condylox
E.E.S.
E-Mycin
E-Mycin
Erythrocin
erythromycin
Floxin
imiquimod
ofloxacin
podofilox
Polymox
Trimox
valacyclovir
Valtrex
Wymox
Zithromax
Zovirax

Shingles
acyclovir
capsaicin
famciclovir
Famvir
valacyclovir
Valtrex
Zostrix
Zovirax

Thyroid
Levothroid
levothyroxine
Levoxine
Levoxyl
Synthroid
Synthrox

Ulcers
Axid
cimetidine
Cytotec
famotidine
misoprostol
nizatidine
Pepcid
ranitidine
Tagamet
Zantac

Vaginal Infections
Flagyl
MetroGel
metronidazole
Protostat
Terazol 3
Terazol 7
terconazole

Appendix 2: Top 200 Prescriptions—United States 1998

Based on the number of prescriptions dispensed in the United States

Brand Name	Generic	Manufacturer
Premarin	conjugated estrogens	Wyeth-Ayerst
Synthroid	levothyroxine	Knoll
Trimox	amoxicillin	Apothecon
Hydrocodone w/APAP	hydrocodone w/APAP	Watson
Prozac	fluoxetine	Lilly
Prilosec	omeprazole	Astra
Zithromax	azithromycin	Pfizer
Lipitor	atorvastatin	Parke-Davis
Norvasc	amlodipine	Pfizer
Claritin	loratadine	Schering
Lanoxin	digoxin	Glaxo Wellcome
Zoloft	sertraline	Pfizer
Albuterol Aerosol	albuterol	Warrick
Paxil	paroxetine	SmithKline Beecham
amoxicillin	amoxicillin	Teva Pharmaceuticals
Prempro	conjugated estrogens/ medroxyprogesterone	Wyeth-Ayerst
Zestril	lisinopril	Zeneca
Vasotec	enalapril	Merck
Augmentin	amoxicillin/clavulanate	SmithKline Beecham
cephalexin	cephalexin	Teva Pharmaceuticals
Zocor	simvastatin	Merck
Glucophage	metformin	Bristol-Myers Squibb
Coumadin	warfarin	Dupont
acetaminophen/ codeine	acetaminophen/codeine	Teva Pharmaceuticals
ibuprofen	ibuprofen	Greenstone

Brand Name	Generic	Manufacturer
furosemide	furosemide	Mylan
Cipro	ciprofloxacin	Bayer
trimethoprim/ sulfamethoxazole	trimethoprim/ sulfamethoxazole	Teva Pharmaceuticals
Cardizem CD	diltiazem	Hoechst Marion Roussel
Pravachol	pravastatin	Bristol-Myers Squibb
Biaxin	clarithromycin	Abbott
propoxyphene napsylate/APAP	propoxyphene napsylate/ APAP	Mylan
Levoxyl	levothyroxine	Jones
Procardia XL	nifedipine	Pfizer
prednisone	prednisone	Schein
Prevacid	lansoprazole	Tap Pharmaceuticals
Ultram	tramadol	McNeil
alprazolam	alprazolam	Greenstone
Ambien	zolpidem	Searle
Amoxil	amoxicillin	SmithKline Beecham
Accupril	quinapril	Parke-Davis
K-Dur 20	potassium chloride	Schering
Glucotrol XL	glipizide	Pfizer
hydrocodone/APAP	hydrocodone/APAP	Mallinckrodt
Triamterene/HCTZ	triamterene/HCTZ	Geneva
Ortho Tri-Cyclen	norgestimate/ethinyl estradiol	Ortho Pharmaceuticals
Lotensin	benazepril	Novartis
Prinivil	lisinopril	Merck
Hytrin	terazosin	Abbott
Veetids	penicillin VK	Apothecon
propoxyphene napsylate/APAP	propoxyphene napsylate/APAP	Teva Pharmaceuticals
Relafen	nabumetone	SmithKline Beecham
Zyrtec	cetirizine	Pfizer
Cardura	doxazosin	Pfizer

Brand Name	Generic	Manufacturer
Claritin-D 12 HR	loratadine/ pseudoephedrine	Schering
Allegra	fexofenadine	Hoechst Marion Roussel
Pepcid	famotidine	Merck
Triphasil	L-norgestrel/ethinyl estradiol	Wyeth-Ayerst
Humalin N	human insulin—NPH	Lilly
Dilantin	phenytoin	Parke-Davis
Ortho-Novum 7/7/7	norethindrone/ethinyl estradiol	Ortho Pharmaceuticals
atenolol	atenolol	Geneva
Toprol-XL	metoprolol	Astra
Flonase	fluticasone	Glaxo Wellcome
lorazepam	lorazepam	Mylan
amitriptyline	amitriptyline	Mylan
Cefzil	cefprozil	Bristol-Myers Squibb
Depakote	divalproex	Abbott
Imdur	isosorbide mononitrate S.A.	Schering
Viagra	sildenafil citrate	Pfizer
Diflucan	fluconazole	Pfizer
Propulsid	cisapride	Janssen
alprazolam	alprazolam	Geneva
triamterene/HCTZ	triamterene/HCTZ	Mylan
atenolol	atenolol	Mylan
Fosamax	alendronate	Merck
Adalat CC	nifedipine	Bayer
Cozaar	losartan	Merck
atenolol	atenolol	ESI Lederle
Lescol	fluvastatin	Novartis
hydrocodone/APAP	hydrocodone/APAP	Qualitest
albuterol Nebulizer Solution	albuterol	Warrick

Brand Name	Generic	Manufacturer
glyburide	glyburide	Copley
Wellbutrin SR	bupropion HCL	Glaxo Wellcome
Vancenase AQ DS	beclomethasone	Schering
Zithromax Suspension	azithromycin	Pfizer
clonazepam	clonazepam	Teva Pharmaceuticals
naproxen	naproxen	Teva Pharmaceuticals
carisoprodol	carisoprodol	Schein
Daypro	oxaprozin	Searle
Monopril	fosinopril	Bristol-Myers Squibb
Ceftin	cefuroxime	Glaxo Wellcome
Claritin-D 24 HR	loratadine/pseudoephedrine	Schering
hydrochlorothiazide	hydrochlorothiazide	Purepac
acetaminophen/ codeine	acetaminophen/codeine	Purepac
Nitrostat	nitroglycerin	Parke-Davis
Atrovent Inhalation	ipratropium	Boehr Ingel
Humulin 70/30	human insulin 70/30	Lilly
Rezulin	troglitazone	Parke-Davis
Lotrisone	clotrimoxazole/ betamethasone	Schering
Serevent	salmeterol	Glaxo Wellcome
Ziac	bisoprolol/HCTZ	Wyeth-Ayerst
hydrochlorothiazide	hydrochlorothiazide	ESI Lederle
Cycrin	medroxyprogesterone	ESI Lederle
ibuprofen	ibuprofen	Par
Lo/Ovral 28	norgestrel/ethinyl estradiol	Wyeth-Ayerst
diazepam	diazepam	Mylan
Xalatan	latanoprost	Pharmacia & Upjohn
Imitrex	sumatriptan	Glaxo Wellcome
Roxicet	oxycodone/APAP	Roxane
metoprolol tartrate	metoprolol	Mylan
verapamil SR	verapamil	Zenith
furosemide oral	furosemide	Watson Pharmaceuticals

Brand Name	Generic	Manufacturer
medroxyprogesterone	medroxyprogesterone	Greenstone
Desogen	desogestrel/ethinyl estradiol	Organon
Ery-Tab	erythromycin	Abbott
Mevacor	lovastatin	Merck
Ortho-Cyclen	norgestimate/ethinyl estradiol	Ortho Pharmaceuticals
Azmacort	triamcinolone aerosol	Rhone-Poulenc Rorer
Klor-Con	potassium chloride	Upsher-Smith
Cyclobenzaprine	cyclobenzaprine	Schein
Neurontin	gabapentin	Parke-Davis
ranitidine	ranitidine	Novopharm
penicillin VK	penicillin VK	Teva Pharmaceuticals
lorazepam	lorazepam	Purepac
Axid	nizatidine	Lilly
Risperdal	risperidone	Janssen
Bactroban	mupirocin	SmithKline Beecham
hydrochlorothiazide	hydrochlorothiazide	Zenith
cyclobenzaprine	cyclobenzaprine	Mylan
Zantac	ranitidine	Glaxo Wellcome
Macrobid	nitrofurantoin	Procter & Gamble
Serzone	nefazodone	Bristol-Myers Squibb
temazepam	temazepam	Mylan
clonidine	clonidine	Mylan
cephalexin	cephalexin	Apothecan
verapamil SR	verapamil	Mylan
guaifenesin/ phenylpropanolamine	guaifenesin/ phenylpropanolamine	Duramed
Flovent	fluticasone propionate	Glaxo Wellcome
glyburide	glyburide	Greenstone
naproxen	naproxen	Mylan
BuSpar	buspirone	Bristol-Myers Squibb
furosemide	furosemide	Zenith
Levaquin	levofloxacin	Ortho Pharmaceutical
Tri-Levlen	L-norgestrel/ethinyl estradiol	Berlex

Brand Name	Generic	Manufacturer
Zestoretic	lisinopril/ hydrochlorothiazide	Zeneca
Hyzaar	losartan/ hydrochlorothiazide	Merck
neomycin/polymyxin/HC	neomycin/polymyxin/HC	Schein
estradiol	estradiol	Watson
Loestrin-FE 1.5/30	norethindrone/ethinyl estradiol	Parke-Davis
methylprednisolone	methylprednisolone	Duramed
Provera	medroxyprogesterone	Pharmacia & Upjohn
Ortho-Cept	desogestrel/ethinyl estradiol	Ortho Pharmaceutical
ranitidine	ranitidine	Mylan
alprazolam	alprazolam	Purepac
Tobradex	tobramycin/ dexamethasone	Alcon Laboratories
Phenergan Suppository	promethazine	Wyeth-Ayerst
Estraderm	estradiol	Novartis
Estrace	estradiol	Bristol-Myers Squibb
allopurinol	allopurinol	Mylan
potassium chloride	potassium chloride	ETHEX
propranolol LA	propranolol LA	ESI Lederle
Loestrin-Fe 1/20	norethindrone/ethinyl estradiol	Parke-Davis
Humulin R	human insulin regular	Lilly
Elocon	mometasone	Schering
tamoxifen	tamoxifen	Barr
gemfibrozil	gemfibrozil	Teva Pharmaceuticals
Lasix	furosemide	Hoechst Marion Roussel
ranitidine	ranitidine	Geneva
Endocet	oxycodone/APAP	Endo
Altace	ramipril	Hoechst Marion Roussel
Effexor	venlafaxine	Wyeth-Ayerst
Timoptic XE	timolol	Merck

Brand Name	Generic	Manufacturer
Diovan	valsartan	Novartis
Rhinocort	budesonide	Astra
Xanax	alprazolam	Pharmacia & Upjohn
Deltasone	prednisone	Pharmacia & Upjohn
warfarin	warfarin	Barr
Lotrel	amlodipine/benazepril	Novartis
Climara	estradiol	Berlex
Plendil	felodipine SR	Astra
cimetidine	cimetidine	Mylan
glipizide	glipizide	Mylan
Alesse 28	levonorgestrel/ethinyl estradiol	Wyeth-Ayerst
albuterol aerosol	albuterol	Zenith
trazodone	trazodone	Sidmak
Miacalcin Nasal	calcitonin salmon	Novartis
Necon 1/35	norethindrone/ethinyl estradiol	Watson Pharmaceuticals
Amaryl	glimepiride	Hoechst Marion Roussel
Propacet 100	propoxyphene napsylate/ APAP	Teva Pharmaceuticals
metoprolol tartrate	metoprolol	Geneva
Lorabid	loracarbef	Lilly
Accolate	zafirlukast	Zeneca
Sumycin	tetracycline HCL	Apothecon
Zyban	bupropion HCL SR	Glaxo Wellcome
promethazine tabs	promethazine	ESI Lederle
Dyazide	hydrochlorothiazide/ triamterene	SmithKline Beecham
Adderall	amphetamine mixed salts	Shire Richwood
amitriptyline	amitriptyline	Sidmark
Retin-A	tretinoin	Ortho Derm

Reprinted by permission from *American Druggist,* February 1999 issue.

Appendix 3: Quick Reference Guide to Drug Profiles

Brand Name	Generic	For	Type of Drug
Asterisk* indicates that the drug is on the Top 200 Prescriptions for 1998			
abacavir sulfate, see Ziagen			
Accolate*	zafirlukast	Prevention and treatment of chronic (not acute) asthma	Antileukotriene
Accupril*	quinapril	High blood pressure; congestive heart failure	ACE inhibitor
Accutane	isotretinoin	Acne	Antiacne
acetaminophen and codeine phosphate*, see Tylenol with Codeine			
acetaminophen and hydrocodone bitartrate, see Vicodin			
acetaminophen and oxycodone hydrochloride, see Percocet			
Actigall	ursodiol USP	Prevention of gallstone formation in obese patients experiencing rapid weight loss	Bile acid
Actos	pioglitazone	Type II non-insulin-dependent diabetes mellitus (NIDDM)	Antidiabetic
acyclovir, see Zovirax			
Adalat CC*, see Procardia XL*			
Adipex-P, see Fastin			
Adderall*	amphetamine mixed salts	Attention deficit hyperactivity disorder (ADHD)	Amphetamine
Advil, see Motrin			

Brand Name	Generic	For	Type of Drug
Alatone, see Aldactone			
albuterol*, see Proventil			
Aldactone	spironolactone	High blood pressure, edema	Diuretic; antihypertensive
Aldara	imiquimod	External genital and perianal warts	Antimitotic, antiinflammatory; chemical remover
alendorate sodium, see Fosamax*			
Alesse 21 and Alesse 28*, see Oral Contraceptives			
Allegra*	fexofenadine hydrochloride	Relief of symptoms of seasonal allergies and allergic rhinitis	Antihistamine
allopurinol*, see Zyloprim			
alprazolam*, see Xanax*			
Altace*	ramipril	High blood pressure, congestive heart failure	ACE inhibitor
Alzapam, see Ativan*			
amantadine, see Symmetrel			
Amaryl*	glimepiride	Type II non-insulin–dependent diabetes mellitus (NIDDM)	Antidiabetic
Ambien*	zolpidem	Insomnia, including difficulty staying asleep or awakening too early	Sedative; CNS depressant
Amerge	naratriptan hydrochloride	Short-term relief for acute migraine	Antimigraine
amitriptyline*, see Elavil*			
amlodipine, see Norvasc*			
amlodipine/benazepril, see Lotrel*			
amoxicillin*, see Amoxil*			
amoxicillin and clavulanic acid, see Augmentin*			

Brand Name	Generic	For	Type of Drug
Amoxil* (also Biomox, Polymox, Trimox*, Wymox)	amoxicillin*	Various infections, including urinary tract, respiratory tract; skin infections, gonorrhea	Antibiotic
amphetamine mixed salts, see Adderall*			
anastrozole, see Arimidex			
Ansaid	flurbiprofen	Relief of symptoms of rheumatoid arthritis & osteoarthritis, inc. joint pain, inflammation, stiffness, swelling; menstrual pain; migraine	NSAID
Antivert	meclizine	Motion sickness; prevent vomiting and nausea; vertigo or dizziness	Antiemetic; antihistamine
Arava	leflunomide	Slows damage to joints and reduces symptoms of rheumatoid arthritis	Antirheumatic
Aricept	donepezil	Alzheimer's disease	Acetylcholinesterase inhibitor (chemical nerve-muscle coordinator)
Arimidex	anastrozole	Breast cancer	Anticancer (antineoplastic)
aspirin, see Easprin			
atenolol, see Tenormin			
Ativan (also Alzapam)	lorazepam*	Anxiety, agitation; panic attacks, irritable bowel syndrome (IBS); insomnia	Benzodiazepine tranquilizer
Atorvastatin calcium, see Lipitor			
Atrovent*	ipratropium	Bronchial spasms associated with bronchitis and emphysema	Anticholinergic; bronchodilator
A/T/S, see Ery-Tab*			
Augmentin*	amoxicillin and potassium clavulanate	Bacterial infections	Antibiotic

Brand Name	Generic	For	Type of Drug
auranofin, see Ridaura			
Avandia	rosiglitazone	Type II non-insulin-dependent diabetes mellitus (NIDDM)	Antidiabetic
Avonex	interferon beta 1-a	Multiple sclerosis	Interferon
Axid*	nizatidine	Stomach and duodenal ulcers, heartburn, GERD	Histamine H2 blocker; antiulcer
azithromycin, see Zithromax*			
Azmacort Aerosol* (also Nasacort Aerosol)	triamcinolone acetonide	Chronic asthma. (Nasacort is used to relieve hay fever symptoms and allergic rhinitis)	Corticosteroid inhaler
Bactrim (also Septra, Septra DS, Cotrim, Cotrim DS)	trimethoprim and sulfamethoxazole	Urinary-tract infections (UTIs), bronchitis	Antiinfective; sulfa
Bactroban*	mupirocin	Impetigo, minor bacterial skin infections	Topical antibiotic
beclomethasone, see Vancenase AQ			
Beconase AQ, see Vancenase AQ			
benazepril, see Lotensin*			
Bentyl	dicyclomine hydrochloride	Irritable bowel syndrome (IBS); spastic colon	Antispasmodic
betamethasone and clotrimazole, see Lotrisone*			
Betapace	sotalol hydrochloride	High blood pressure; arrhythmias;migraines	Beta-blocker
Betaseron, see Avonex			
Biaxin*	clarithromycin	Sinus and respiratory-tract infections; strep throat; pneumonia	Antibiotic
Biomox, see Amoxil*			

Brand Name	Generic	For	Type of Drug
bisoprolol HCTZ, see Ziac*			
Brevicon, see Oral Contraceptives			
budesonide, see Rhinocort*			
bupropion, see Wellbutrin			
bupropion HCl, see Zyban*			
BuSpar*	buspirone	Anxiety, symptoms of PMS including aches, cramps, fatigue	Antianxiety; tranquilizer
buspirone, see BuSpar*			
Calan SR (also Calan, Isoptin, Isoptin SR, Verelan)	verapamil SR*	Angina pectoris, irregular heartbeat, high bp. Calan SR is used only to treat high blood pressure	Calcium channel blocker
calcipotriene, see Dovonex			
calcitonin salmon, see Miacalcin Nasal*			
capecitabine, see Xeloda			
Capoten	captopril	High blood pressure; congestive heart failure	ACE inhibitor
capsaicin, see Zostrix			
captopril, see Capoten			
carbamazepine, see Tegretol			
carbidopa and levodopa, see Sinemet			
Cardizem CD* (also Cardizem, Cardizem SR, Dilacor SR)	diltiazem hydrochloride	Angina pectoris	Calcium channel blocker
Cardura*	doxazosin	High blood pressure	Antihypertensive
carisoprodol*, see Soma			
cefprozil*, see Cefzil*			

Brand Name	Generic	For	Type of Drug
Ceftin*	cefuroxime axetil	Bacterial infections	Antibiotic
cefuroxime axetil, see Ceftin*			
Cefzil*	cefprozil	Bacterial infections, including those of the middle ear, skin, upper and lower respiratory tract	Antibiotic
Celebrex	celecoxib	Relief of symptoms of osteoarthritis and rheumatoid arthritis	NSAID
celecoxib, see Celebrex			
Celexa	citalopram hydrobromide	Depression	Antidepressant
Cenestin	synthetic conjugated estrogens	Relief of menopausal symptoms	Estrogen (synthetic)
Centrax	prazepam	Anxiety; agitation; irritable bowel syndrome (IBS); tension, panic attacks, fatigue	Benzodiazepine
cephalexin*, see Keflex			
cephradine, see Velosef			
cetirizine HCl, see Zyrtec*			
chlordiazepoxide, see Librium			
cimetidine* see Tagamet			
Cipro*	ciprofloxacin	Urinary-tract infections (UTIs); skin and bone infections; bronchitis; pneumonia	Antibiotic
ciprofloxacin, see Cipro*			
citalopram hydrobromide, see Celexa			
clarithromycin, see Biaxin*			

Brand Name	Generic	For	Type of Drug
Claritin* (also **Claritin-D 12 Hour***, **Claritin-D 24 Hour***)	loratadine (12 Hr and 24 Hr are loratadine pseudoephedrine sulfate)	Symptoms of seasonal and other allergies	Antihistamine
Claritin D 12 hr and 24 hr, see Claritin*			
Climara* , see Estrace*			
Clomid	clomiphene	Infertility	Fertility
clomiphene, see Clomid			
clonazepam, see Klonopin			
clorazepate dipotassium, see Tranxene			
Cognex	tacrine hydrochloride	Alzheimer's disease	Cholinesterase Inhibitor (chemical nerve-muscle coordinator)
CombiPatch	estradiol/ norethindrone acetate	Relief of menopausal symptoms	Estrogen
Combivir, see Retrovir			
Condylox	podofilox	External genital warts	Antimitotic; chemical remover
conjugated estrogens, see Premarin*			
conjugated estrogens, synthetic, see Cenestin			

Brand Name	Generic	For	Type of Drug
Cotrim, see Bactrim			
Coumadin*	warfarin	Reduce the risk of blood clots	Anticoagulant
Cozaar*	losartan potassium	High blood pressure	Antihypertensive
Crixivan	indinavir sulfate	Advanced HIV infection, usually used in conjunction with other drugs	Antiviral
cromolyn sodium, see Intal			
cyclobenzaprine*, see Flexeril			
cyclophosphamide, see Cytoxan			
Cycrin*, see Provera*			
cyproheptadine, see Periactin			
Cytotec	misoprostol	Preventing stomach ulcers, especially associated with taking NSAIDs for arthritis; duodenal ulcers	Antiulcer
Cytoxan	cyclophosphamide	Cancer (breast, ovarian, other types)	Anticancer (antineoplastic)
Darvocet-N 100 (also Propacet 100)	propoxyphene napsylate and acetaminophen	Pain relief	Narcotic analgesic
Daspex, see Fastin			
Daypro*	oxaprozin	Relief of symptoms associated with rheumatoid arthritis and osteoarthritis; joint pain, inflammation, stiffness, swelling	NSAID
Deltasone* (also Orasone, Liquid Pred, Meticorten)	prednisone*	Relief of inflammation and symptoms associated with rheumatoid arthritis; lupus; multiple sclerosis; severe asthma; skin diseases	Corticosteroid
Demulen, see Oral Contraceptives			
Depakote*	divalproex sodium	Seizure disorders, including epilepsy; manic-depression (bipolar disorder); migraine	Anticonvulsant

Brand Name	Generic	For	Type of Drug
Depo-Provera	medroxyprog-esterone acetate	Birth control (injection by a health practitioner)	Contraceptive (injection); progestin
Desogen*, see Oral Contraceptives			
desogestrel/ethinyl estradiol, see Oral contraceptives			
Desyrel	trazodone*	Depression; panic disorder	Antidepressant
Detrol	tolterodine tartrate	Overactive bladder	Anticholinergic; bladder sedative
diazepam*, see Valium			
dicyclomine hydrochloride, see Bentyl			
diethylpropion, see Tenuate			
Diflucan*	fluconazole	Candidiasis fungal infections including vaginal yeast infections; thrush (infections of mouth or throat); infections of the central nervous system	Antifungal
digoxin, see Lanoxin*			
dihydroergotamine mesylate, see Migranal			
Dilacor SR, see Cardizem CD*			
Dilantin*	phenytoin	Certain types of epileptic seizures	Anticonvulsant
diltiazem hydrochloride, see Cardizem CD*			

Brand Name	Generic	For	Type of Drug
Diovan (also Diovan HCT)	valsartan (valsartan/ hydrochloroth- iazide HCT)	High blood pressure	Antihypertensive; angiotensin-receptor blocker
divalproex sodium, see Depakote*			
donepezil, see Aricept			
Doryx (also Vibramycin)	doxycycline hyclate	Various bacterial infections; UTIs; chlamydia; fevers caused by ticks and lice including Lyme disease and Rocky Mountain spotted fever	Antibiotic
Dovonex	calcipotriene	Plaque psoriasis	Antipsoriatic
doxazosin, see Cardura*			
doxycycline hyclate, see Doryx			
Dyazide*	triamterene and hydrochloroth- iazide (HCTZ)	High blood pressure; edema	Diuretic
E-Mycin, see Ery-Tab*			
E.E.S., see Ery-Tab*			
Easprin (also ZORprin)	aspirin	Relief of pain and inflammation, including symptoms of arthritis; fever reducer; prevent blood clot formation	NSAID; analgesic; blood thinner
Effexor*	venlafaxine	Depression	Antidepressant
Elavil (also Endep)	amitriptyline*	Depression; bulimia; chronic pain; migraine	Tricyclic antidepressant
Eldepryl	selegiline	Parkinson's disease	Antiparkinsonian; selective MAO inhibitor
Elocon*	mometasone furoate	Relief of swelling, redness, itching, and discomfort of many skin problems	Topical corticosteroid

Brand Name	Generic	For	Type of Drug
enalapril maleate, see Vasotec*			
Enbrel	etanercept	Relief of symptoms of rheumatoid arthritis	Antirheumatic
Endep, see Elavil			
Endocet*, see Percocet			
Entex	guaifenesin/ phenyl- propanolamine*	Relief of allergy symptoms; symptoms of the common cold or other respiratory ailments	Nasal decongestant/ expectorant combination
Ery-Tab* (also E-Mycin, E.E.S.)	erythromycin (E.E.S.)— erythromycin ethylsuccinate)	Various infections, including urinary tract infections (UTIs); acne; chlamydia; gonorrhea: bacterial endocarditis; pelvic inflammatory disease (PID); respiratory-tract infections	Antibiotic
Erycette, see Ery-Tab*			
erythromycin, see Ery-Tab*			
Esidrix (also HydroDIURAL,	hydrochloroth- iazide (HCTZ)*	High blood pressure; congestive heart failure; edema	Diuretic antihypertensive
Eskalith (also Lithobid, Lithonate)	lithium	Treatment of the manic phase of manic-depression (bipolar disorder)	Antimanic
Estrace* (also Climara*, Estraderm*, FemPatch)	estradiol*	Relief of menopausal symptoms; postmenopausal osteoporosis; ovarian failure; breast cancer	Estrogen
Estraderm,* see Estrace*			
estradiol,* see Estrace*			
estradiol/norethindrone acetate, see CombiPatch			
estropipate, see Ogen			

Brand Name	Generic	For	Type of Drug
Estrostep, see Oral Contraceptives			
etanercept, see Enbrel			
ethynodial diacetate and ethinyl estradiol, see Oral Contraceptives			
Evista	raloxifene HCl	Osteoporosis in postmenopausal women; breast cancer	Selective estrogen receptor motivator (SERM)
famciclovir, see Famvir			
famotidine, see Pepcid*			
Famvir	famciclovir	Herpes zoster (shingles); genital herpes (herpes simplex)	Antiviral
Fastin (also Adipex-P, Ionamin)	phentermine	Obesity and short-term appetite suppression; Duchenne's muscular dystrophy	Appetite suppressant
felodipine, see Plendil*			
FemPatch, see Estrace*			
fexofenadine hydrochloride, see Allegra*			
Flagyl (also Protostat)	metronidazole	Vaginal yeast infections; UTIs; abdominal infections; lower respiratory-tract infections	Antibiotic; antiparasitic
flavoxate hydrochloride, see Urispas			
Flexeril	cyclobenzaprine*	Muscle spasms, stiffness, pain	Muscle relaxant
Flonase* (also Flovent*)	fluticasone propionate	Relief of seasonal or chronic allergies; allergic rhinitis; asthma	Corticosteroid

Brand Name	Generic	For	Type of Drug
Flovent, see Flonase*			
Floxin	ofloxacin	STDs including chlamydia; chronic bronchitis and pneumonia; UTIs; various bacterial infections	Antibiotic
fluconazole, see Diflucan*			
fluoxetine, see Prozac*			
fluoxymesterone, see Halotestin			
flurbiprofen, see Ansaid			
fluticasone propionate, see Flonase*			
fluvastatin, see Lescol*			
fluvoxamine, see Luvox			
Fosamax*	alendorate sodium	Osteoporosis	Aminobiphosphonate (bone resorption inhibitor)
fosinopril, see Monopril*			
fosfomycin tromethamine, see Monurol			
furosemide, see Lasix*			
gabapentin, see Neurontin*			
Gantrisin	sulfisoxazole	UTIs, kidney infections, cystitis	Antiinfective; sulfa
gemfibrozil*, see Lopid			
Genora, see Oral Contraceptives			
glimepiride, see Amaryl*			
glipizide, see Glucotrol			

Brand Name	Generic	For	Type of Drug
Glucophage*	metformin hydrochloride	Type II (non-insulin–dependent) diabetes mellitus (NIDDM)	Antidiabetic
Glucotrol (also Glucotrol XL*)	glipizide	Type II (non-insulin–dependent) diabetes mellitus (NIDDM)	Antidiabetic
guaifenesin/phenylpropanolamine*, see Entex			
Halcion	triazolam	Insomnia; frequent nighttime awakening	Benzodiazepine sedative; CNS depressant
Halotestin	fluoxymesterone	Certain types of advanced breast cancer or for women who have breast tumors promoted by female hormones	Androgen (male hormone)
Humalin 70/30* (also Humalin N*, Humalin R*)	insulin	Type I insulin-dependent diabetes	Antidiabetic
hydrochlorothiazide (HCTZ)*, see Esidrix			
hydrochlorothiazide (HCTZ) and triamterene, see Dyazide*			
HydroDIURAL, see Esidrix			
hydroxychloroquine, see Plaquenil			
Hytrin*	terazosin HCl	Mild to moderate high blood pressure	Antihypertensive
Hyzaar*	losartan potassium/ hydrochlorothiazide (HCTZ)	High blood pressure	Antihypertensive
ibuprofen*, see Motrin			

Brand Name	Generic	For	Type of Drug
imipramine hydrochloride, see Tofranil			
imiquimod, see Aldara			
Imdur*	isosorbide mononitrate	Recurrent angina	Antianginal
Imitrex*	sumatriptan	Migraine headaches	Antimigraine
Inderal	propranolol	High blood pressure; angina; irregular heartbeats	Beta-blocker
Indinavir sulfate, see Crixivan			
Indocin	indomethacin	Arthritis inflammation	NSAID
indomethacin, see Indocin			
Intal	cromolyn sodium	Allergic rhinitis; chronic asthma	Antiallergy; antiasthmatic
Intercon, see Oral Contraceptives			
Interferon beta-1a, see Avonex			
Ionamin, see Fastin			
ipratropium, see Atrovent*			
Isoptin, see Calan SR			
isosorbide mononitrate S.A., see Imdur*			
isotretinoin, see Accutane			
itraconazole, see Sporanox			
Jenest-28, see Oral Contraceptives			
K-Dur 20* (also K-Dur 10, Micro-K Extencaps, Klor-Con, Kato)	potassium chloride*	Mild hypertension; replaces depleted potassium levels in the blood	Potassium supplement

Brand Name	Generic	For	Type of Drug
Kato, see K-Dur 20*			
Keflet, see Keflex			
Keflex (also Keflet)	cephalexin*	UTIs; respiratory tract infections; various bacterial infections; skin and bone infections	Cephalosporin antibiotic
ketoconazole, see Nizoral			
ketoprofen, see Orudis			
Klonopin	clonazepam	Epilepsy; convulsive disorders; panic attacks, petit mal seizures; schizophrenia	Anticonvulsant; benzodiazepine
Klor-Con, see K-Dur 20*			
Lamisil	terbinafine HCl	Nail infections; skin infections	Antifungal
Lanoxicaps, see Lanoxin*			
lansoprazole, see Prevacid			
Lanoxin* (also Lanoxicaps)	digoxin	Congestive heart failure	Digitalis
Lasix*	furosemide	High blood pressure; congestive heart failure; kidney dysfunction; accumulation of fluid in the lungs	Diuretic; antihypertensive
latanoprost, see Xalatan*			
leflunomide, see Arava			
Lescol*	fluvastatin	High cholesterol	Cholesterol-lowering
Levaquin*	levofloxacin	Respiratory-tract infections; UTIs	Antibiotic
Levlen, see Oral Contraceptives			
Levlite, see			
Oral Contraceptives			
levofloxacin, see Levaquin*			
levonorgestrel, see Plan B			

Brand Name	Generic	For	Type of Drug
levonorgestrel/ethinyl estradiol, see Oral Contraceptives			
levonorgestrel/ethinyl estradiol, see Preven			
Levora, see Oral Contraceptives			
Levothroid, see Synthroid*			
levothyroxine, see Synthroid*			
Levoxine, see Synthroid*			
Levoxyl*, see Synthroid*			
Librium	chlordiazepoxide	Anxiety disorders	Benzodiazepine
Lipitor*	atorvastatin calcium	High cholesterol	Cholesterol-lowering
Liquid Pred, see Deltasone*			
lisinopril, see Zestril*			
lisinopril/HCTZ, see Zestoretic*			
lithium, see Eskalith			
Lithobid, see Eskalith			
Lithonate, see Eskalith			
Lo-Ovral 28*, see Oral Contraceptives			
Loestrin, see Oral Contraceptives			
Lopid	gemfibrozil*	Very high levels of blood triglycerides	Cholesterol-lowering
Lopressor (also Toprol XL*)	metoprolol tartrate	Angina pectoris, high blood pressure; heart attack; migraine headache; anxiety	Beta-blocker
Lorabid*	loracarbef	Bacterial infections, including middle ear, upper and lower respiratory tract, skin, and UTIs	Cephalosporin antibiotic

Brand Name	Generic	For	Type of Drug
loracarbef, see Lorabid*			
loratadine, see Claritin*			
loratadine/pseudoephedrine, see Claritin-D*			
lorazepam*, see Ativan			
Lorcet, see Vicodin			
Lortab, see Vicodin			
losartan potassium/HCTZ, see Hyzaar*			
losartan potassium, see Cozaar*			
Lotensin*	benazepril	High blood pressure	ACE inhibitor
Lotrel*	amlodipine/ benazepril	High blood pressure	Calcium channel blocker/ACE inhibitor
Lotrisone*	betamethasone and clotrimazole	Fungal infection or rash	Topical corticosteroid; antifungal
lovastatin, see Mevacor*			
Luvox	fluvoxamine	Obsessive-compulsive disorder (OCD); depression	SSRI antidepressant
Macrobid* (also Macrodantin)	nitrofurantoin	Urinary-tract infections (UTIs)	Antiinfective
Macrodantin, see Macrobid*			
Maxalt	rizatriptan benzoate	Short-term treatment of migraine headaches	Antimigraine
Mazanor (also Sanorex)	mazindol	Appetite suppression; short-term treatment of obesity	Appetite suppressant
mazinol, see Mazanor			
meclizine, see Antivert			

Brand Name	Generic	For	Type of Drug
Medipren, see Motrin			
Medrol	methylprednisolone*	Reduce inflammation of rheumatoid arthritis and severe asthma	Corticosteroid
medroxyprogesterone*, see Provera*			
medroxyprogesterone acetate, see Depo-Provera			
Meridia	sibutramine hydrochloride monohydrate	Obesity	Appetite suppressant
metformin hydrochloride, see Glucophage*			
methotrexate, see Rheumatrex			
methylprednisolone*, see Medrol			
Meticorten, see Deltasone*			
metoprolol tartrate*, see Lopressor			
MetroGel	metronidazole	Rosacea, various bacterial infections; sexually transmitted diseases (STDs). The intravaginal gel form is for bacterial vaginosis	Oral and topical antibiotic; antiparasitic
metronidazole, see Flagyl and MetroGel			
Mevacor*	lovastatin	High cholesterol	Cholesterol-lowering
Miacalcin Nasal*	calcitonin salmon	Osteoporosis	Nasal spray for osteoporosis (bone resorption inhibitor)

Brand Name	Generic	For	Type of Drug
Micro-K Extencaps, see K-Dur 20*			
Migranal	dihydroergota-mine mesylate	Active migraine. Not a migraine preventive.	Antimigraine
Mirapex	pramipexole	Parkinson's disease	Antiparkinsonian
Mircette, see Oral Contraceptives			
misoprostol, see Cytotec			
Modicon, see Oral Contraceptives			
mometasone, see Elocon*			
Monopril*	fosinopril	High blood pressure	ACE inhibitor
Monurol	fosfomycin tromethamine	Bladder infections; urinary-tract infections (UTIs)	Antibiotic
Motrin (also Advil, Nuprin, Medipren, Rufen)	ibuprofen*	Pain and inflammation; menstrual pain; headache; severe inflammation of arthritis, rheumatoid arthritis, and osteoarthritis	NSAID
mupirocin, see Bactroban			
N.E.E., see Oral Contraceptives			
nabumetone, see Relafen*			
nafarelin acetate, see Synarel			
Naprosyn (also Naprelan)	naproxen*	Pain and inflammation of rheumatoid arthritis and osteoarthritis	NSAID
naproxen*, see Naprosyn			
naratriptan hydrochloride, see Amerge			
Nardil	phenelzine sulfate	Depression; anxiety; phobias	MAO inhibitor
Nasacort Aerosol, see Azmacort Aerosol*			

Brand Name	Generic	For	Type of Drug
Nasalcrom, see Intal			
Nasonex	mometasone furoate monohydrate	Prevention of symptoms of seasonal allergies; allergic rhinitis	Corticosteroid nasal spray
Necon, see Oral Contraceptives			
nefazodone, see Serzone*			
Nelova, see Oral Contraceptives			
Neoral, see Sandimmune			
Neurontin*	gabapentin	Treatment of epileptic seizures in adults; depression	Anticonvulsant
nifedipine, see Procardia XL			
Nitro-Dur, see Nitrostat			
nitrofurantoin, see Macrobid*			
nitroglycerin, see Nitrostat*			
Nitrostat (also **Nitro-Dur**)	nitroglycerin	Acute sudden-onset anginal pain; coronary artery disease	Antianginal
nizatidine, see Axid*			
Nizoral	ketoconazole	Various fungal infections; thrush, candidiasis; ringworm; athlete's foot; seborrheic dermatitis	Antifungal
Nolvadex	tamoxifen citrate	Postmastectomy, to suppress recurring breast cancer, to reduce the risk of breast cancer in high-risk women	Antiestrogen; anticancer (antineoplastic)
Norcet, see Vicodin			
Nordette, see Oral Contraceptives			
Norethin, see Oral Contraceptives			
norethindrone and ethinyl estradiol, see Oral Contraceptives			
norethindrone and mestranol, see Oral Contraceptives			

Brand Name	Generic	For	Type of Drug
norethindrone acetate and ethinyl acetate, see Oral Contraceptives			
norgestimate and ethinyl estradiol, see Oral Contraceptives			
norgestrel and ethinyl estradiol, see Oral Contraceptives			
Norinyl, see Oral Contraceptives			
Norvasc*	amlodipine	High blood pressure; angina pectoris	Calcium channel blocker
Norvir	ritonavir	HIV infection	Antiviral; protease inhibitor
Nuprin, see Motrin			
ofloxacin, see Floxin			
Ogen	estropipate	Estrogen replacement	Estrogen
omeprazole, see Prilosec*			
Oral Contraceptives (group listing in part 1)			
Orasone, see Deltasone*			
orlistat, see Xenical			
Ortho-Cept*, see Oral Contraceptives			
Ortho-Novum, see Oral Contraceptives			
Ortho-Cyclen*, see Oral Contraceptives			
Ortho Tri-Cyclen*, see Oral Contraceptives			

Brand Name	Generic	For	Type of Drug
Orudis (also Oruvail)	ketoprofen	Pain relief; relief of symptoms of rheumatoid arthritis and osteoarthritis	NSAID
Oruvail, see Orudis			
Ovcon, see Oral Contraceptives			
Ovral, see Oral Contraceptives			
oxaprozin, see Daypro*			
Panacet, see Vicodin			
Parnate	tranylcypromine sulfate	Depression	MAO inhibitor
paroxetine, see Paxil*			
Paxil*	paroxetine	Depression; panic disorders	SSRI antidepressant
penicillin VK*, see Veetids*			
Pepcid*	famotidine	Decreasing stomach acid; stomach and duodenal ulcers; gastroesophageal reflux disease (GERD)	Histamine H_2 blocker
Percocet (also Endocet*, Roxicet*, Roxilox*, Tylox)	acetaminophen and oxycodone hydrochloride	Pain relief	Narcotic analgesic
Periactin	cyproheptadine	Relief of symptoms of seasonal allergies; skin rash; itching; or hives caused by allergies; anorexia	Antihistamine; antiemetic
phenazopyridine hydrochloride, see Pyridium			
phenelzine sulfate, see Nardil			
Phenergan Suppository*	promethazine	Motion sickness, nausea, vomiting	Antihistamine; antiemetic
phentermine, see Fastin			

Brand Name	Generic	For	Type of Drug
phenytoin*, see Dilantin*			
pioglitazone, see Actos			
Plan B	levonorgestrel	Emergency contraception (the "morning after" pill)	Progestin; postcoital contraceptive
Plaquenil*	hydroxychloro-quine	Symptoms of rheumatoid arthritis: swelling, joint pain, stiffness; symptoms of lupus; treatment of malaria	Antimalarial; antiinflammatory
Plendil*	felodipine	Mild to moderate hypertension	Calcium channel blocker
podofilox, see Condylox			
Polymox, see Amoxil*			
potassium chloride*, see K-Dur 20*			
pramipexole, see Mirapex			
Pravachol*	pravastatin	High blood cholesterol	Cholesterol-lowering
pravastatin, see Pravachol*			
prazepam, see Centrax			
prednisone*, see Deltasone*			
Premarin*	conjugated estrogens	Menopausal symptoms; prevention of osteoporosis	Estrogen
Premphase, see Prempro*			
Prempro* (also Premphase)	conjugated estrogens and medroxyprogesterone	Menopausal symptoms	Estrogen
Prevacid*	lansoprazole	Duodenal ulcers; gastroesophageal reflux disease (GERD)	Antiulcer
Preven	levonorgestrel and ethinyl estradiol	Emergency contraception (the "morning after" pill)	Progestin/estrogen; post-coital contraceptive kit

Brand Name	Generic	For	Type of Drug
Prilosec*	omeprazole	Short-term treatment of active duodenal ulcers; gastric ulcers; GERD	Antiulcer
Prinivil*, see Zestril*			
Procardia XL* (also **Adalat CC***)	nifedipine	Angina; high blood pressure including pregnancy-related related high blood pressure; migraine headache	Calcium channel blocker
promethazine, see Phenergan			
Propacet 100, see Darvocet-N 100			
propoxyphene napsylate and acetaminophen, see Darvocet-N 100			
propranolol, see Inderal			
Protostat, see Flagyl			
Proventil (also **Ventolin**)	albuterol*	Asthma; bronchial spasms	Bronchodilator
Provera* (also **Cycrin***)	medroxyprog-esterone acetate	Irregular menstrual periods or to correct a hormone imbalance that may cause abnormal uterine bleeding; endometriosis; premenstrual syndrome (PMS)	Progestin
Prozac*	fluoxetine	Depression; bulimia; OCD	SSRI antidepressant
Pyridium	phenazopyridine hydrochloride	Urinary-tract infection (UTI) pain relief	Urinary-tract analgesic
quinapril, see Accupril*			
raloxifene, see Evista			
ramipril, see Altace*			
ranitidine, see Zantac*			

Brand Name	Generic	For	Type of Drug
Relafen*	nabumetone	Rheumatoid arthritis, osteoarthritis	NSAID
Restoril	temazepam	Short-term treatment of insomnia;	Benzodiazepine
Retin-A*	tretinoin	Acne	Topical antiacne
Retrovir	zidovudine (AZT)	HIV	Antiviral
Rheumatrex	methotrexate	Certain types of cancer and leukemia; rheumatoid arthritis; psoriasis	Anticancer, antipsoriatic; antirheumatic
Rhinocort*	budesonide	Relief of symptoms of hay fever, allergic rhinitis; prevention of nasal polyp regrowth after surgery	Corticosteroid
Ridaura	auranofin	Rheumatoid arthritis: to reduce joint pain, swelling, tenderness	Antiinflammatory; antiarthritic; gold compound
Risperdal*	risperidone	Symptoms of psychosis	Antipsychotic
risperidone, see Risperdal*			
ritonavir, see Norvir			
rizatriptan beazoate, see Maxalt			
rofecoxib, see Vioxx			
rosiglitazone, see Avandia			
Roxicet*, see Percocet			
Roxilox, see Percocet			
Rufen, see Motrin			
salmeterol xinafoate, see Serevent*			
Sandimmune (also Neoral, SangCya)	cyclosporine	Prevention of organ rejection after heart, kidney, or liver transplant	Immunosuppressive agent
SangCya, see Sandimmune			
Sanorex, see Mazanor			

Brand Name	Generic	For	Type of Drug
seleginine, see Eldepryl			
Septra, see Bactrim			
Septra DS, see Bactrim			
Serevent*	salmeterol xinafoate	Relief of symptoms of chronic (not acute) asthma	Bronchodilator
Serophene, see Clomid			
sertraline, see Zoloft*			
Serzone*	nefazodone	Depression	Antidepressant
sibutramine hydrochloride monohydrate, see Meridia			
sildenafil citrate, see Viagra*			
simvastatin, see Zocor*			
Sinemet (also Sinemet CR)	carbidopa and levodopa	Parkinson's disease	Antiparkinsonian
Soma	carisoprodol*	Painful muscle conditions	Muscle relaxant
sotalol HCl, see Betapace			
spironolactone, see Aldactone			
Sporanox	itraconazole	Fungal infections	Antifungal
sulfisoxazole, see Gantrisin			
sumatriptan, see Imitrex*			
Sumycin*	tetracycline hydrochloride	Various bacterial infections	Antibiotic
Symmetrel	amantadine	Parkinson's disease; fatigue associated with multiple sclerosis	Antiparkinsonian
Synarel	nafarelin acetate	Endometriosis, menstrual cramps; abnormal menstrual bleeding	Gonadotropin-releasing hormone nasal spray

Brand Name	Generic	For	Type of Drug
Synthroid* (also Levoxyl*, Levoxine, Levothroid, Synthrox)	levothyroxine	Thyroid disorders	Thyroid hormone
Synthrox, see Synthroid*			
T-Stat, see Ery-Tab*			
tacrine hydrochloride, see Cognex			
Tagamet	cimetidine*	Stomach ulcers; duodenal ulcers; gastroesophageal reflux disease (GERD)	Histamine H_2 blocker
tamoxifen citrate, see Nolvadex			
Tasmar	tolcapone	Parkinson's disease	Antiparkinsonian
Tegretol	carbamazepine	Seizure disorders; certain emotional disorders including manic-depression; severe jaw pain; migraine	Anticonvulsant
temazepam* , see Restoril			
Tenormin	atenolol	High blood pressure; angina pectoris, irregular heartbeat; anxiety	Beta-blocker
Tenuate	diethylpropion	Short-term weight reduction	Nonamphetamine appetite suppressant
Terazol 3 (also Terazol 7)	terconazole	Candidiases, specifically vaginal yeast infections	Antifungal
terazosin, see Hytrin*			
terbinafine HCl, see Lamisil			
terconazole, see Terazol 3			
tetracycline, see Sumycin			
theophylline, see Theo-Dur			
timolol, see Timoptic XE*			

Brand Name	Generic	For	Type of Drug
Timoptic XE*	timolol	Reduction of internal eye pressure in certain types of glaucoma	Beta-blocker (ophthalmic)
tizanidine, see Zanaflex			
Tobradex*	tobramycin/ dexamethasone	Prevention or treatment of eye infections; to suppress inflammation	Antibiotic/corticosteroid combination
tobramycin/dexamethasone, see Tobradex*			
Tofranil	imipramine hydrochloride	Depression	Tricyclic antidepressant
tolcapone, see Tasmar			
tolterodine tartrate, see Detrol			
Toprol XL* , see Lopressor			
tramadol HCl, see Ultram*			
tranylcypromine sulfate, see Parnate			
Tranxene	clorazepate dipotassium	Anxiety; anxiety-related insomnia; irritable bowel syndrome (IBS)	Benzodiazepine
trazodone, see Desyrel			
tretinoin, see Retin-A*			
Tri-Levlen, see Oral Contraceptives			
Tri-Norinyl, see Oral Contraceptives			
triamcinolone acetonide, see Azmacort Aerosol*			
triamterene and hydrochlorothiazide, see Dyazide*			

Brand Name	Generic	For	Type of Drug
triazolam, see Halcion			
trimethoprim and sulfamethoxazole, see Bactrim			
Trimox, see Amoxil*			
TriPhasil*, see Oral Contraceptives			
Trivora, see Oral Contraceptives			
Tylenol with Codeine	acetaminophen and codeine phosphate*	Moderate to severe pain relief	Narcotic/analgesic combination
Tylox, see Percocet			
Ultracef, see Duricef			
Ultram*	tramadol HCl	Relief of mild to moderate pain	Analgesic
Urispas	flavoxate hydrochloride	Urinary tract spasms; relief of painful and frequent urination; pubic area pain	Antispasmodic
ursodiol USP, see Actigall			
valacyclovir HCl, see Valtrex			
Valium	diazepam*	Anxiety disorders; panic attacks; muscle spasms; tremors; insomnia	Benzodiazepine tranquilizer; CNS depressant
valsartan, see Diovan*			
Valtrex	valacyclovir HCl	Recurrent genital herpes; herpes zoster (shingles)	Antiviral
Vancenase AQ (also Vancenase AQ DS*, Beconase AQ, Vanceril Inhaler)	beclomethasone	Nasal inflammation; relief of hay fever symptoms; prevention of nasal polyps after surgical removal	Corticosteroid aerosol

Brand Name	Generic	For	Type of Drug
Vanceril Inhaler, see Vancenase AQ			
Vasotec*	enalapril maleate	High blood pressure; congestive heart failure; diabetic kidney disease	ACE inhibitor
Veetids*	penicillin VK*	Bacterial infections	Antibiotic
venlafaxine, see Effexor*			
Ventolin, see Proventil			
verapamil SR*, see Calan SR			
Verelan, see Calan SR			
Viagra*	sidenafil citrate	Male erectile dysfunction. Viagra has not yet been approved for use by women, but some doctors are prescribing it to their female patients and some women are using their partners' prescriptions. Studies on determining the drug's effect on women should be completed in 2002.	Sexual stimulant
Vibramycin, see Doryx			
Vicodin (also Vicodin-ES, Lorcet, Lortab, Norcet, Panacet, Zydone)	acetaminophen and hydrocodone bitartrate	Mild to moderate pain	Narcotic/analgesic combination
Vioxx	rofecoxib	Pain and inflammation of osteoarthritis; menstrual pain	NSAID
warfarin, see Coumadin*			
Wellbutrin (also Wellbutrin SR*)	bupropion hydrochloride	Depression	Antidepressant
Wymox, see Amoxil*			
Xalatan*	latanoprost	Glaucoma	Antiglaucoma; prostaglandin

Brand Name	Generic	For	Type of Drug
Xanax*	alprazolam*	Anxiety and anxiety disorders; tension; panic disorder; irritable bowel syndrome (IBS); depression; PMS	Benzodiazepine tranquilizer; antianxiety
Xeloda	capecitabine	Breast cancer	Anticancer (antineoplastic)
Xenical	orlistat	Obesity management	Lipase inhibitor (fat blocker)
zafirlukast, see Accolate*			
Zanaflex	tizanidine	Chronic muscle stiffness associated with multiple sclerosis and cerebral palsy; uncontrolled muscle spasms	Muscle relaxant
Zantac*	ranitidine	Gastric ulcers; GERD; to prevent stomach ulcers caused by NSAIDs	Histamine H_2 blocker; antiulcer
Zestoretic*	lisinopril and hydrochlorothiazide (HCTZ)	High blood pressure	ACE inhibitor
Zestril* (also Prinivil*)	lisinopril	High blood pressure	ACE inhibitor
Ziac*	bisoprolol/ hydrochlorothiazide (HCTZ)	High blood pressure	Beta-blocker and thiazide diuretic combination
Ziagen	abacavir sulfate	HIV. Used in combination with other drugs	Antiretroviral
zidovudine (AZT), see Retrovir			
Zithromax*	azithromycin	Various bacterial infections, including respiratory tract, STDs, skin infections, UTIs and infections of the cervix	Antibiotic
Zocor*	simvastatin	High blood cholesterol	Cholesterol-lowering
zolmitriptan, see Zomig			
Zoloft*	sertraline	Depression; obsessive-compulsive disorder (OCD)	SSRI antidepressant
zolpidem, see Ambien*			

Brand Name	Generic	For	Type of Drug
Zomig	zolmitriptan	Migraine headache	Antimigraine
ZORprin, see Easprin			
Zostrix	capsaicin	Temporary relief from neuralgia (nerve pain); pain associated with herpes zoster (shingles), psoriasis, rheumatoid arthritis, osteoarthritis; itching; irritations of the vulva; herpes simplex type 1 (cold sores, fever blisters); herpes simplex type 2 (genital herpes); postsurgical pain	Topical analgesic
Zovia, see Oral Contraceptives			
Zovirax	acyclovir	Treatment of herpes simplex (genitals, mucous membranes, central nervous system); herpes zoster (shingles); varicella (chicken pox)	Antiviral
Zyban*	bupropion HCL	Reduction of withdrawal symptoms of smoking cessation	Nonnicotine smoking-cessation aid; antidepressant
Zydone, see Vicodin			
Zyloprim	allopurinol*	Gout; prevention of high levels of uric acid in the blood, including those associated with radiation or chemotherapy for cancer	Antigout
Zyrtec*	cetirizine HCL	Relief of symptoms of seasonal and year-round allergies	Antihistamine

About the Authors

Julie Catalano is an award-winning writer whose articles on women's health and fitness have appeared in national publications for twenty years. A member of the American Society of Journalists and Authors, she lives in San Antonio, Texas.

Robert L. Rowan, M.D., is a clinical professor teaching at New York University School of Medicine.